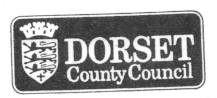

Body Treatments and Dietetics for the Beauty Therapist

by

Ann Gallant

F.S.H.B.Th. Int.B.Th.Dip. DRE.(Tutor),
Teacher's Certificate in Further Education

Formerly Lecturer Responsible
for Beauty Therapy at
Chichester College of Higher Technology and
Gloucestershire College of Arts and
Technology

Stanley Thornes (Publishers) Ltd

First published in 1978 by

Stanley Thornes (Publishers) Ltd.,
Old Station Drive, Leckhampton
CHELTENHAM GL53 0DN

Reprinted 1981
Reprinted 1982
Reprinted 1983 with minor corrections
Reprinted 1985 with minor corrections
Reprinted 1987
Reprinted 1988
Reprinted 1989
Reprinted 1990

ISBN 0 85950 400 X Library edition
     0 85950 401 8 Student edition

Printed and bound in Great Britain at The Bath Press, Avon

Preface

This new book, *BODY TREATMENTS AND DIETETICS FOR THE BEAUTY THERAPIST*, is designed to cover all aspects of Body Therapy important to the trainee Beauty Therapist or practitioner, and should prove an invaluable guide to practice and procedures in Beauty Therapy.

Encompassing figure assessment, exercise, diet and nutrition, as well as clinic procedures for established and advanced practical Body Therapy, the book deals in depth with the related anatomical and science information necessary to ensure safe and efficient clinic applications.

Written in response to a need for sound information on Body Therapy, this book in combination with the earlier *PRINCIPLES AND TECHNIQUES FOR THE BEAUTY SPECIALIST*, forms a complete guide to professional Beauty Therapy practice. It also fulfills the course requirements for all the major examination boards, including City and Guilds Beauty Therapy Certificate 761, International Health and Beauty Therapist's Diploma (NHBC), and CIDESCO examinations.

I would like to acknowledge all the valuable assistance I have received from students and staff at Gloucester College, particularly those involved in acting as models for illustrations. My particular thanks go to John Rounce for checking the science content, and to Leo Palladino for his continuing encouragement and advice throughout. Special thanks go to Julie Moret for all her help and to John Hudson for the superb photography upon which the line illustrations were based; also to Angela Lumley for her excellent final illustrations and sympathetic approach to the Beauty Therapy artistry.

Ann Gallant   July 1978

Contents

Chapter 1

The Total Approach to Body Treatment

Body treatments are a very challenging and rewarding part of the beauty therapist's work, requiring skill and judgement in order to achieve success. For *results* are what are required; mainly in slimming and figure improvement, through salon treatments and home diet and exercise plans. Growing awareness of the link between obesity and disease has established the need to be the right weight, if personal health is to be maintained. So it is natural that beauty therapists will find a large proportion of their work is biased towards *reduction*, either generally or specifically in one area of the body. This increases the need for knowledge of body function and makes an understanding of nutrition an essential element for success in modern therapy practice.

The work itself is very varied and provides opportunities for close personal contact with clients, treating and guiding them towards desired results. Whether for figure improvement, relaxation, or toning purposes, caring for the individual remains constant and makes the therapist's work very rewarding. Renewed interest in personal health and beauty in recent years has increased the range of possible salon treatments, and has produced new apparatus in response to this growing figure-awareness in both men and women. Many minor figure faults can be corrected with treatment and home guidance; with electrical therapy playing an important part in the improvement. So a sound knowledge of the electrical systems available and their effects on the body becomes necessary, to ensure safe and effective treatment.

The improved standards of treatment, and expertise, in body work has brought recognition of the more preventative role beauty therapy can play in maintaining physical health, and creating a feeling of well being. Exercise routines, diet guidance, and relaxation treatment can all act naturally to keep the individual in peak form, free from the stress and strain of modern life. Recognition of these natural benefits from treatment is reflected in the growth of leisure centres, sports complexes and clinics all offering different forms of acti
Apart from the obvious benefits of a fit body

an attractive figure, the value of avoiding minor aches and pains associated with muscular fatigue or being overweight, is gradually gaining public acceptance.

This wider range of treatment, and change in emphasis to include health maintenance, has increased both the therapist's responsibility in treatment and the need for more information on background factors that will affect the progress and results possible.

THE TOTAL APPROACH

Success in body therapy relies on adopting a *total approach* to treatment, combining diet, exercise and salon applications to achieve results. To decide the combination of treatment which will prove the most successful, the therapist will need to have good verbal ability to discover the cause and history of the figure problem, by putting the client at her ease and gaining her confidence. The total approach also relies heavily on the therapist's skill in *figure analysis*, to know when a routine can be successful, or whether the problem is beyond the help of the therapist and needs medical scrutiny. Knowing when, and when not, to treat, is an important area of decision for the therapist, and is one often taken in isolation. Frequently the decision is made solely on knowledge of body structure and function, and all personal resources are needed to plan effective and safe routines.

The therapist's work is slowly changing to include many treatments that are undertaken in medical agreement to improve or maintain health, or as a preventative measure. Obesity control, stress treatments, post-natal guidance, and post-cardiac routines are all areas of work becoming increasingly important to the fully competent and knowledgeable body therapist. This provides great scope and opportunity for use of personal initiative in treatment choice and planning, and brings an entirely new facet of work into the therapist's field of reference. Being accepted as part of a team associated with health maintenance brings new dimensions to the work of the therapist; ones she must be prepared to meet. To work as part of a dedicated team, and accept the medical requirements presented, requires a truly professional attitude to both therapy and clients.

There is also a need to give willingly of personal time and interest to help clients achieve their goals. Stamina and fitness are necessary to ensure that the actual treatment can be completed without undue fatigue or muscular strain. The work is demanding, both physically and mentally, and the therapist needs resilience to cope with her busy days. The results and achievements, however, make it all worthwhile, for, by being able to help in a caring way to guide the client to a better understanding of her body's needs, it also helps her towards a more attractive and healthy figure.

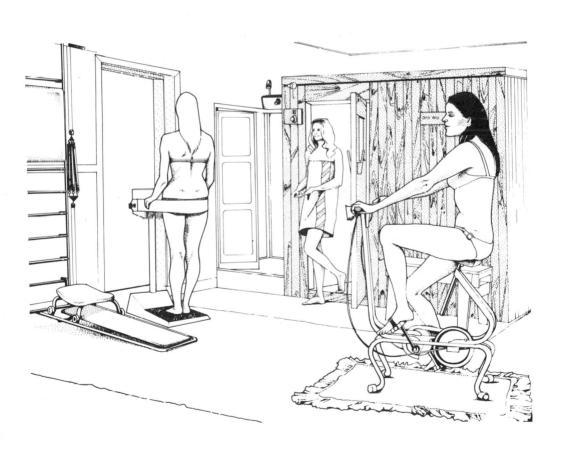

CONSULTATION TECHNIQUES

A consultation prior to or linked with the initial treatment, provides an opportunity for the therapist to meet the client and obtain certain information from her, which will help to determine the treatment plan. By adopting a sympathetic but professional attitude to the client, a rapport can develop which increases the client's confidence and co-operation. Having created an atmosphere in which the client's problems can be discussed freely, without embarrassment, the real purpose of the treatment will become more readily apparent.

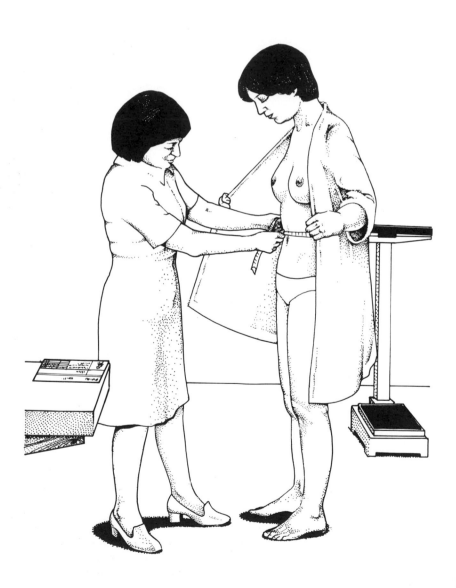

Tact has to be employed in consultation techniques, particularly with the older client, who may, initially, feel too embarrassed to discuss the full extent of her figure worries, especially if confronted with a very young and slim therapist. It is often not possible to gain all the information required by conversation alone, and it may be preferable to combine a manual treatment so as to gain a better understanding of the existing condition. Through personal contact with the client, her anxiety can be dispelled, and a good working relationship formed. The manual massage relaxes the client and extends the therapist's knowledge of the body. In quiet conversation background factors can be discussed, including diet, exercise, and the possible form the treatment should take.

Analysis of the figure is a skilled task, and will only be totally successful if the approach to the client is correct. To assess the figure and its potential improvement it is necessary to record the actual statistics and also gain a general background history to the figure problem. Discussion regarding the figure faults, gynaecological and medical history, and the social pattern of life followed, will provide valuable information on which to base the treatment plan. It will also provide guidance as to the extent of client co-operation and involvement with the treatment that is likely. Clients that need a lot of support, and those that can help themselves, both rely on the therapist's skill and judgement in consultation to devise the correct plan for their needs.

Client Handling

Taking accurate measurements can be an embarrassing time for both the therapist and client if not approached professionally and with some regard for the client's feelings. Extremely overweight individuals may only require initially that their *weight* is recorded, unless they wish to record for posterity their actual measurements prior to reduction. Therapists who are in tune with their client's feelings will let their modesty dictate the way in which the measurements are taken. Older women may prefer to retain their bra and pants, and as long as these do not present a false picture, it is permissible initially to record the measurements, noting this fact. Ideally all measurements should be taken without restricting or uplifting underwear, with the client naked, but it is unnecessary to cause embarrassment over this point, with the risk of losing a client. As the client's well being and happiness is the main aim, it is not sensible to cause distress by dictating the manner in which the figure knowledge should be obtained.

Extremely shy or highly strung individuals do not always have to be measured on their first visit, although a general form of treatment can proceed, whilst they become familiar with the routine, and so relax. It is often more beneficial to have them overcome their tension through a pleasant treatment and skilful client handling, before embarking on the figure record and analysis. It is wise to remember that therapy clients have a choice about where, and from whom, they receive their treatment, and as they pay for a caring and effective service, that is what they should receive.

Measurements should be taken around the fullest part of an area, and for general reduction, the bust, waist, hips and thighs are adequate for most purposes. Improvement, or reduction in a specific area will require more detailed measurements to be taken, and periodically a general set of body measurements, to ensure the figure is not becoming out of proportion.

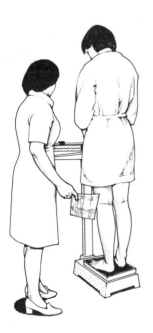

Weighing the client may be undertaken at suitable intervals, depending on the purpose of the treatment. If reducing, the weight checks should be close enough together to encourage the client, but not be so close as to dishearten when a weight loss is not evident. For general reduction an overall downward trend is the aim, and this must be discussed with the client, so that static periods, with no weight loss or even slight weight gains, are understood.

The weight checks must be accurate and, like the measurements, be recorded on the client's personal record card. A salon gown may be worn for modesty if preferred, and it will then need to be worn on every occasion to avoid discrepancies. Clients wishing to appear their lightest may prefer to be weighed naked: either method is satisfactory as long as it is constant. By recording the client's progress and weight changes systematically, much encouragement can be given during static periods to show the overall improvement achieved, which should spur the client to further efforts.

Encouragement and a fairly firm but honest approach are the most effective means of achieving the results the client desires. The purpose of consultation is to ensure that the aim of the treatment is realized, safely and successfully, through a total approach devised at a professional therapy level.

CLIENTS' RECORD CARDS

In body therapy the initial treatment is linked with a consultation to establish the client's figure diagnosis, and the possible pattern of future treatment. At this first treatment information is gathered which helps the therapist to establish the client's background, and provides guidance as to the form the treatment should take.

A client's personal record card should be completed as a reference, which then acts as a blueprint for all the following salon routines, and background guidance for the client. The information taken will indicate the best way results can be achieved effectively without harm to the client. The card is kept in the therapy clinic, in the reference file, under the relevant section, according to the client's name, and initial, to avoid confusion. These files of clients' records are important, and show the total business completed within the salon.

Record card information needed includes:

(*a*) The client's name, initial, and address.
(*b*) A telephone number where she can be reached if an appointment has to be changed.
(*c*) Client's age, and the number and ages of her children.
(*d*) Medical history
    – major operations and physical conditions which would affect treatment.
    – serious illnesses she has had.
    – any medication she is on.
    – gynaecological history.
(*e*) Doctor's name and address.
(*f*) Weight, height, and initial measurements.
(*g*) Figure diagnosis.
(*h*) Record of treatments completed.

The card records fully the salon applications completed, and any effects experienced after treatment which might require altering the routine. The card also has space to record periodic checks on weight and measurements if the client is on a reduction and figure improvement programme. Keeping an accurate personal and treatment record helps the therapist in several ways to achieve results. It helps to ensure no unsuitable or harmful treatment is given, as the physical details obtained can be checked against the contra-indication lists for specific treatment routines. The *contra-indications*, or reasons why the treatment cannot be given, differ with different systems of therapy, all of which must be known. However, certain physical conditions – such as high blood pressure – exclude the client from most forms of treatment involving general vascular stimulation.

Health and Beauty Clinic

NAME	ADDRESS	Telephone
Mrs Smith	24 Blackburn Ave. Hamilton. Essex	Ham. 2343

MEDICAL HISTORY, and approval for Treatment	Name of Physician
Age 26 yrs. Recent childbirth. Child six weeks - 15·11·77 No other children. Post-natal examination Medical approval given.	Dr. Taylor

	Date	Treatment Completed	Height 5·6	Measurements				Weight
	24·9·77	Figure diagnosis. Manual massage.		A 39	B 40½	C 34	D 38	69 kg
	1·10·77	Vacuum massage. Midriff and hips.		E 23	F 17			
	15·10·77	Muscle contraction. Hip-Abdominal + Thighs						68 kg
	22·10·77	" " "		A 37	B 36	C 33	D 37	
	5·11·77	Vacuum and muscle contraction		E 22	F 16½			67 kg
	26·11·77	" " "						66 kg

Client's Record Card

The general medical history is necessary for the same reasons, particularly with obese, menopausal and post-natal clients. Here medical approval for the treatment should be obtained by the client prior to its commencement. The medical history, and number and ages of children, will help to build a picture of the client's life style and circumstances. This will give guidance as to the type of diet, and amount of exercise that can be incorporated into the figure improvement plan. It may also give insight into the time and financial commitment that the client is able to give to her salon applications: how much will have to be achieved from personal home effort will then be evident. *Time* proves more of a restriction than money for many clients, due either to work or family responsibilities. The treatment organization will rest heavily on this information, to make best use of the time available.

The figure diagnosis gives an analysis of the figure, its body type, postural faults, fat distribution, and figure faults. On this information, with height, weight and measurements, rests the choice of treatment and its ideal pattern of application. The figure diagnosis is the pivot point of most successful figure improvement and reduction plans, and is dealt with fully in Chapter 2.

The record of treatments completed, with the measurements and weight loss progress, can indicate where a change of treatment is necessary. If results are not being achieved or a period of static performance is apparent from the record card details, then the combination or bias of the treatment can be altered to improve matters. Weight records over a period will indicate where more stringency or attention to the diet is needed. The reasons for the lack of weight loss can then be discussed frankly, and remedies suggested, before the client becomes depressed with the results. The need for client co-operation is very evident on the diet aspects, to achieve the full results possible in the improvement plans.

The *long term* results of clients on reduction plans can be used to encourage them through difficult or static patches. With skilful client handling and conversation they can be reminded of their achievements, and the overall pattern of reduction and figure improvement accomplished to date. This may promote further interest in their total plan, if enthusiasm is flagging after months of diet, exercise and salon applications.

The client's card is also important in instances of staff changes or illness, and makes it possible for a new therapist to take over in a fully professional and competent manner, and so maintain client satisfaction. In this way valuable clients are not lost to a business because of the inevitable movement of qualified staff. If a high standard of work and a responsible attitude to the clients' well being and progress is maintained within the beauty business, clients will accept changes without any loss of confidence.

Clients' record cards are one example of this more professional approach in action. They safeguard the client, assure her of an effective and suitable routine, and form a history of her condition and progress in treatment.

PURPOSE AND ORGANIZATION OF TREATMENT

It is important to establish initially the purpose of the treatment in order to plan the most effective and enjoyable routine. A different attitude is necessary for *relaxation therapy* to that of *reduction programmes*, and the therapist must adjust her client handling and general approach accordingly.

The organization, or form, of the planned treatment will depend on its purpose, and will enable the therapist to guide her client as regards the time and cost likely to be expended. Treatments for relaxation or sports massage can be given on an individual basis, as the need arises, whilst reduction programmes must be organized into regular courses of treatment for effective results.

Concentrated plans of figure improvement prior to holidays, or in the spring season need a different format from those spaced out over many months. Clients wanting fast results and willing to spend time and money on achieving their wishes, are excellent salon business, but require special care and efficient organization to maintain well being.

The therapy clinic will need to be flexible in its treatment times if the full potential of figure improvement work is to be realized. Split sessions of working, so that staff are available to work evenings and lunch times are important in some situations – in city centres for instance. It is vital to be able to offer treatment at all times to meet the client's demands. Unprofitable areas will soon become evident, and the weekly routine can be adjusted, both through times of opening, and staff attendance. Permitted hours of opening should be used skilfully, so that no opportunity for business is turned away, or valuable staff stand idle. The busy times will become apparent and then measures can be taken to spread regular bookings over the weekly period, so that overcrowding does not result. Clients who prefer more privacy can then be directed to the quieter times in the week, so keeping staff fully occupied, and avoiding any hurried or frenzied clinic sessions. Good organization will show in client satisfaction and happy staff.

The purpose or reasons for clients having body treatment are very varied but include:

(*i*) **General reduction treatments** – linked with diet and exercise advice.

(*ii*) **Specific reduction or improvement** – which may or may not be diet linked.

(*iii*) **Relaxation therapy** – normally linked with advice on exercise for relaxation.

(*iv*) **Sports or toning massage** – for invigoration, with no diet normally needed.

(*v*) **Intensive figure improvement** – involving salon applications, diet, and exercise aspects.

(*vi*) **Post-natal improvement** – based on diet, postural improvement, exercise and salon applications.

GENERAL REDUCTION TREATMENTS

Based on a diet plan, these treatments form a large proportion of the therapist's business. The main improvement will come through weight loss, which, whilst it is actually achieved at home, is instigated and maintained within the salon, by the therapist. Slimming clients need encouragement and have to attend regularly for treatment to achieve results. Salon applications will speed the weight loss and inches reduction, and because clients feel their problem is being dealt with, they maintain their dietary intake correctly.

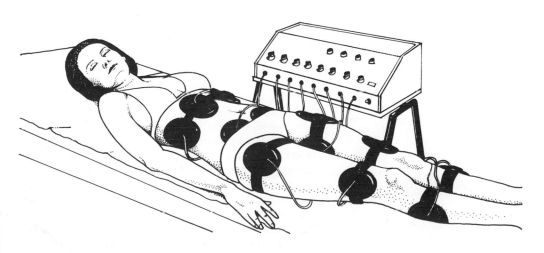

Electrical Muscle Contraction

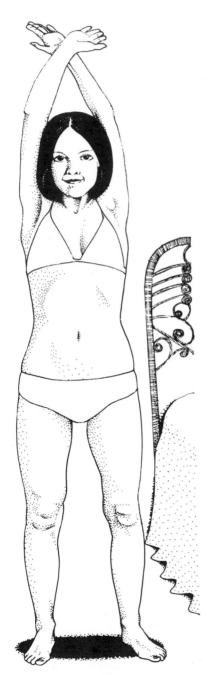

Home Exercise

Heat treatments, vibratory and vacuum massage, and muscle contraction may all play a part in the improvement. Home diet and exercise routines are vital for success, as there is no way a weight loss can be achieved without a reduction in food intake, or a very sustained increase in activity. The weight loss brings fast results and changes the figure shape, which, with salon applications forms the basis for the figure improvement.

The treatment would be sold as a pre-paid course, to encourage regular attendance, and might take the form of weekly treatments of one hour duration. Diet, posture improvement, and specific exercise advice would be given in addition. Some clients might benefit from more concentrated treatment initially, and may prefer to have two, or even three sessions the first week, slowly spacing them out over the following weeks. Whether the treatment course (usually twelve appointments) is taken within three months or only two, depends on the client's need for the therapist's support and guidance. The client may only actually need a weekly treatment whilst losing weight, to keep her in shape, but if she cares to have more, it will certainly improve her determination to succeed. That, after all, is the purpose of the *total plan*, and the therapist is not fulfilling her role of adviser if she only views her work from the standpoint of the actual treatments completed.

Most clients can be persuaded to achieve their own goals if organized correctly. Even those who rely heavily on salon treatment for results need a gentle form of encouragement, if only to ensure regular attendance. If health or restricted mobility problems limit their home efforts, or by temperament they need a lot of help, then consistent, concentrated attendance at the salon is necessary to achieve results. Although these results may never be as good as if there had been a personal effort involved, these usually mature clients are very valuable to the salon. Such clients may appear weak-willed to the younger therapist, but they can be the back-bone of the salon's trade. As therapists offer a service of body treatment, it should be willingly given when a client wishes to take advantage of that same service. If clients were able to obtain their own results without guidance and practical treatment, therapists would become unnecessary. It is giving a valuable service, particularly through reduction treatments, that makes the work so rewarding.

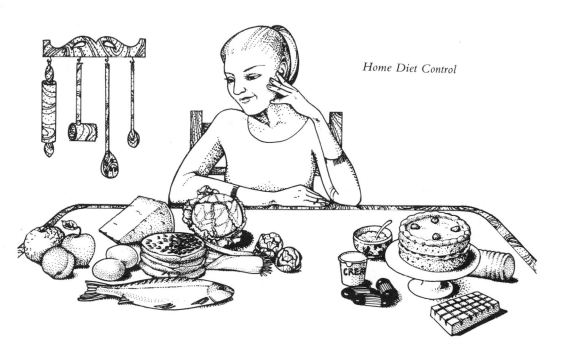

Home Diet Control

SPECIFIC REDUCTION TREATMENT

Where one area of the body needs improvement, a more concentrated approach to salon treatment is necessary. If weight loss is involved, the treatment plan has to ensure that the stored body fat is lost from the correct place. Diagnosis of the figure problem is especially important in this case to discover whether the condition is due to fatty deposits, muscular weakness, or postural faults. Without *correct* analysis of the fault, it cannot be remedied through treatment.

The plan should place treatments close together, two or three times a week, ideally every day in some cases (as in a health hydro). This allows a *build up* effect to develop at the same time as home guidance on posture and exercise is taking effect. Muscular problems particularly benefit from this approach, with postural and muscular re-education becoming a reality. Heavy areas of the body, out of proportion to the rest, can be treated by this method, possibly without diet adjustment, but with specific home exercise routines to reinforce the salon applications. Several areas out of proportion, however, point to a need for *total diet-linked reduction*, to achieve the improvement.

So the degree of the problem is a guide to the most suitable treatment. General weight charts can be used as a guide to tell whether the client is overweight for her height and build.

Conditions of muscular weakness, especially abdominally and for general contour improvement, are very suitable for specific reduction by electrical muscle contraction treatment. This is used for reduction of inches or toning up in an area of the body, and is effective in improving muscular strength and tone. Male and female clients can benefit from this treatment, as it emulates natural exercise, and can be applied without any effort on the part of the client.

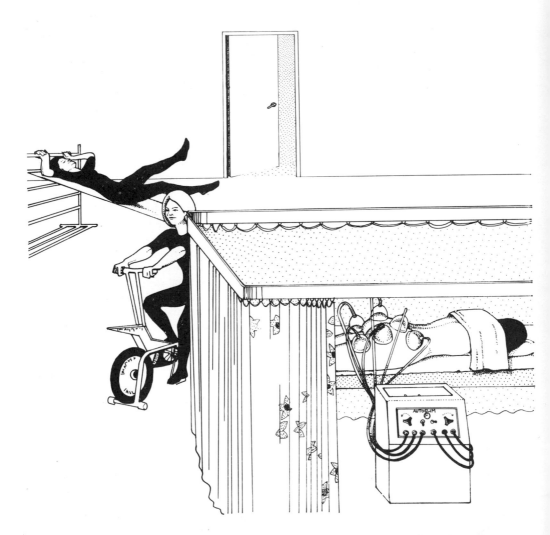

Specific Reduction Treatment

The specific reduction treatment may take the form of vacuum or vibratory massage for reduction of fatty tissue, in conjunction with diet control. All routines of reduction therapy can be applied in combination with heat therapy (sauna or steam baths, etc.) and manual massage, if time permits, in order to maximize results.

Depending on the degree of the problem, the treatment course can be planned in six, ten, or twelve, half hour practical sessions, with additional time required if sauna or another form of pre-heating is combined. As these treatments are popular with younger clients whose finances fluctuate, it is wise to offer treatment on an individual payment basis as well as in courses which are pre-paid. Whereas the the slightly older client likes the discount of the course charge, which reduces slightly the individual treatment cost, the younger client likes to pay as she goes. In this instance the younger woman's motivation to improve her appearance is sufficiently strong to keep her attending on a regular basis.

RELAXATION THERAPY

The treatment approach to relaxation therapy is quite different from that of figure improvement, if the client is to gain full benefit from the application – relief of nervous tension, stress, and total relaxation of muscular tissues, being the aim of the treatment. Normally no reduction in weight or inches is desired, and the treatment results are psychological, although based on physical effects produced through treatment.

Discovering that the client would benefit from this routine comes more from a sense of awareness between the client and the operator, than from actual facts discussed during the enquiry for treatment, or from the consultation. If a rapport exists, the need for a relaxation approach will be noticed in the client's attitude and conversation, and can be felt in the tension present in the muscular system. This is an example of the close affinity that ideally should exist in the treatment situation, giving maximum benefit to the client, and bringing job satisfaction to the therapist.

Organizing the treatment for full effects relies on maintaining the relaxation elements throughout. Heat treatments can be used for pre-heating the body and for relief of tension effects, and should be combined with manual massage, designed to relax rather than stimulate the system.

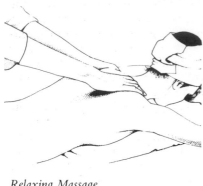

Relaxing Massage

The client may prefer to have manual massage without pre-heating, and would then need to be kept very warm to gain results. Treatment can be planned according to the client's needs, but ideally should be repeated regularly to prevent tension building up, and to help the client unwind. A one-hour body massage is necessary for full effect, and this may be linked with the sauna or steam bath routine (20 minutes), if thought beneficial. Regular clients may prefer to book a series of appointments to gain the cost reduction involved, and also to ensure their treatment time is available with the therapist of their choice. A quieter time in the week may be preferable or, after a period of stressful work, a treatment to restore the client to full vigour.

SPORTS OR TONING MASSAGE

The purpose of the treatment will be to invigorate, tone or stimulate the body systems. Active or highly toned individuals often prefer a more active or vigorous approach in treatment. They enjoy and are able to cope with the rigorous effects of hot saunas, cold showers, deep and effective massage, and heavy duty electrical therapy. Athletes in particular like this more active approach, and can benefit from manual massage designed to treat deeply the individual muscles.

The need for the sports massage should be decided prior to starting the treatment, as it changes the purpose and form of the total routine. The physical demands it places on the operator are extreme, and there is a move towards completing much of the body application electrically with heavy duty vibratory massage. This also answers the problems that female staff have if they are to be involved in working with male clients. As the mechanical massage is less intimate and lacks a personal touch, it is less likely that problems of a sexual nature will occur during the course of the treatment. This saves embarrassment on both sides, and is seen as the only solution to this common problem by the establishments where men are still treated by women.

The form the treatment may take will be pre-heating, cold showers or plunge pools, followed by manual massage or electrical therapy. Normally weight and inches reduction are not involved apart from maintenance of the figure and to avoid fatty deposits accumulating. Sports treatment may be booked individually, or block booked by a sports club or group wishing to use the facilities undisturbed by other clients. It is sometimes found simpler in these instances to charge a background rate for the sauna rooms, exercise equipment, and rest areas, etc., and charge on an individual basis for any actual treatment where a therapist is involved. Individually the treatment might take 45 minutes to one hour in total, depending on the effect desired. Costing on a time basis is helpful in these cases.

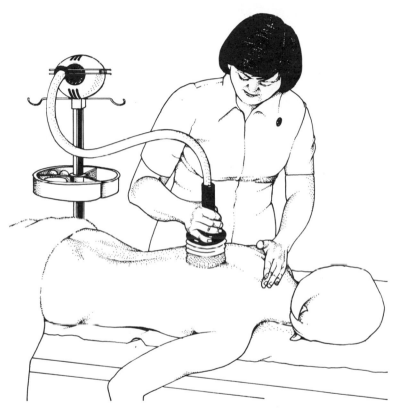

Vibratory Massage

INTENSIVE FIGURE IMPROVEMENT AND REDUCTION

Clients wishing to bring about a rapid improvement in their figure can be guided along an intensive programme of salon treatment, backed up by diet and exercise advice. If they are fit enough (and this point should be checked medically) then they may have the treatment daily. This form of therapy is undergone in the health hydro situation, where a severe reduction in food intake is also involved over the one or two week period.

As the diet given may be fairly stringent, treatment must be intensive, otherwise skin tone problems would result as a consequence of the subcutaneous fatty tissue loss. Acting as a support to the skin, the subcutaneous fatty tissue reduction leads to crepey loose skin, which, in the older woman, whose skin is less elastic, could be most unattractive. Exercise can be advised and supervised within the salon, and then practised at home to reinforce and speed results. Body building may be involved to reshape and firm contours, and this also requires supervision initially, to ensure that the progressive resistance exercises are being undertaken correctly.

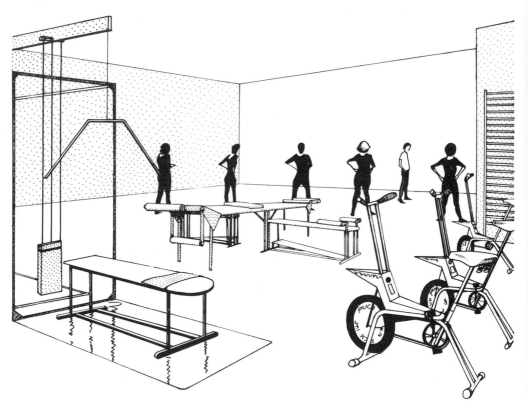

Figure Improvement

Salon treatments would include all forms of electrical therapy, chosen to speed results and reshape the figure. Muscle contraction, vacuum and vibratory massage, hydro massage, manual routines of massage, and cosmetic skin applications, may all be used in different combinations according to the figure problem and result desired.

Treatment may be undertaken daily, or three times a week with half hourly or hourly applications, depending on the client's tolerance and wishes. In this case the results are the main thing, rather than the enjoyment of the treatment; so the sooner the results are achieved the better. Client satisfaction will be assured if, with the therapist's help, she is quickly able to gain the figure improvement wanted. *Courses* of treatment are ideal, because they ensure the regular attendance on which the results depend. Younger clients will obtain results more quickly, due to their greater capacity for treatment, and lack of contra-indications to the salon applications (reasons why the treatment cannot be given). They also tend to be more vigilant about the home routines advised, and follow them with more interest.

POST-NATAL IMPROVEMENT

After childbirth the client needs a lot of help and encouragement to regain her figure. Medical approval must be given prior to treatment, and normally six to eight weeks after the birth is an ideal time to start salon work. Medically advised post-natal exercises can, of course, be followed between the actual birth and the start of salon work. The therapist can help by seeing that these *are* in fact followed, as a preparation for her work, and to get the womb back into the correct position.

The first stage of therapy will be full figure diagnosis, with postural and muscular checks, to ascertain the state of the body. Postural re-education to re-establish the correct standing position is important, and should be completed prior to advising specific exercises for figure correction. The figure problem is usually a combined one, of accumulated weight and muscular weakness. The strain on the abdominal muscles, causing them to be overstretched, has to be rectified. Breast tissue, if lactation is completed (breast feeding), or more normally these days never started, will still be extended. The breasts will lose size gradually without treatment, unless the client carries on feeding the baby whilst the figure correction is in progress. The breasts, like any other part of the body, however, will benefit from muscle toning and home exercise to avoid muscle sag. The appearance of being deflated is a surprise to many clients, and causes a lot of distress, particularly to younger mothers.

Weight loss is of the greatest importance, as the problem may not be due to one pregnancy but accumulated over several. Skin firmness can be regained with salon treatments, electrical therapy, and excellent cosmetic care. Oil massage and heat therapy (if not contra-indicated), will prove very beneficial to the tiny stretch marks apparent. Established skin rupture, from insufficient skin care in pregnancy or an excessive weight gain, can gain very little improvement from these measures unfortunately. Acquiring a tan, naturally or artificially in the salon, helps to disguise their presence and should be recommended to clients as part of their total post-natal plan for improvement.

Success in post-natal work relies on perseverence and regular attendance at the salon to ensure results. A course of treatment is the most effective way to get results for the busy mother with so many other demands on her time. Unless the treatments are pre-booked, the client might consider other elements in her life to be more important than her figure improvement and not feel able to spare the time. The relief from family demands at least once a week, acts as a tonic and reviver to mental and physical well being, quite apart from regaining the figure. Motivation to get back to the normal shape and fitness is usually strong, especially if few clothes fit, and a full wardrobe is waiting as an incentive.

Once or twice-weekly treatment is desirable, with attention to pre-heating, muscle contraction and specific reduction for heavy areas. Home diet and exercise advice are vital in this case for success. Time given during treatment for discussion of diet progress, problems, temptations, etc., will be well spent if it maintains adherence to the diet. A mother has many temptations and little time, and this fact should be considered when deciding the treatment plan and home guidance.

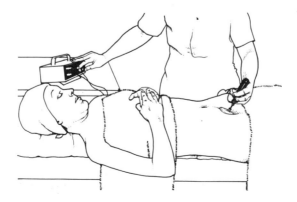

Muscle Contraction on Abdominal Muscles

CLIENT CO-OPERATION

Full client co-operation has to be obtained if effective results and total success in treatment is to be realized, particularly if weight reduction is involved. Interest and enjoyment in the routine advised is important, if regular attendance and home care advice is to be established. Therapists should try to avoid the attitude that clients could, and should, help themselves more with a bit of strong will. It may be true that clients could solve their own problems if they had no temptations, and could hide themselves away at a health hydro for several weeks. However, with family life, social temptations, and a seemingly endless public compulsion to force food on others, the pressures against the dieter are many, and the therapist's help is very necessary. Clients may in fact have made several vain attempts to solve weight or figure problems, and have given up in despair. Realizing from bitter experience how difficult it can be to achieve a consistent result, they may be rather disheartened and disinclined to believe in the plan you offer. So there may be this additional barrier of doubt to be overcome, by careful client handling, before co-operation can be gained.

The younger clients may co-operate very well with home routines, exercise, and diet plans. It is important to harness their strong motivation, to produce results based on the personally tailored total plan, worked out by the therapist. In this case the therapist's role of skilled adviser comes to the fore, and the actual applications become secondary. This will not result in *less* salon business, but *more* overall, as younger clients appreciate an effective result, and will turn to the therapist for all future figure help and treatment. The client who is allowed to do things her own way will often be a good advertisement for the salon, promoting treatments to friends and workmates. The younger client will also be prepared to spend more time and money overall on perfecting her figure, and is a good candidate for linked treatments and cosmetic sales. Once the client's co-operation has been established, and trust has been developed between the therapist and her younger clients, many extra treatments can be presented, which will be tried readily. Waxing (under-arm and leg), facial therapy, and suntanning routines are all complementary to body therapy, and increase business turnover.

Mature clients need the therapist's individual attention the most, and benefit from a personal approach to gaining results. Encouragement to come regularly for treatment, and a persuasive approach to salon applications, are the main ingredients for success. Co-operation is very necessary within the chosen treatment as well, to encourage the client to have the most effective range of applications that are suitable for her. Anxiety over electrical therapy, particularly muscle contraction, can limit the therapist's work with the older client, and often restricts results. With care, and attention to gaining client trust and co-operation, results can be achieved, although at a slower pace than in the younger person. By introducing the required system only when confidence is built up, the therapist can eventually gain the maximum result possible for her mature clients.

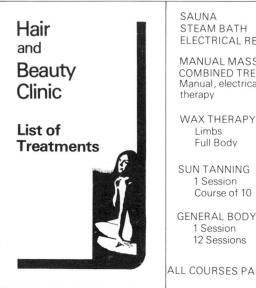

Hair
and
Beauty
Clinic

List of
Treatments

SAUNA
STEAM BATH   (20 Mins.)
ELECTRICAL REDUCTION
                                      (30 Mins.)
MANUAL MASSAGE   (1 Hour)
COMBINED TREATMENT
Manual, electrical and heat
therapy   (1¼ Hours)

WAX THERAPY (Paraffin)
    Limbs   (30 Mins.)
    Full Body   (1 Hour)

SUN TANNING
    1 Session
    Course of 10

GENERAL BODY TREATMENT
    1 Session   (1 Hour)
    12 Sessions

ALL COURSES PAID IN ADVANCE

There is great client satisfaction in having helped to obtain their personal improvement, and this spurs many clients to stick to diets and undergo home exercise. They can see that they are helping themselves, and it is very beneficial to general morale. This is real re-education in action, and truly shows the value of the therapist's work, helping people to have a better understanding of their body, and its needs. This also shows them how to keep in shape with the least effort. Some clients feel a strong need to suffer for their vanity as they see it, and feel cheated if they don't experience discomfort, or feel hunger whilst dieting. If these feelings can be turned into enthusiasm for effective home routines, they will be useful in speeding results, for improving the attitude to treatment, and for building interest in diet adjustment and posture correction. Then the client will be more able to solve her own problems, and they will be less likely to develop in the first place. With excellent client co-operation much of the therapist's work could be preventative, to avoid conditions occurring, rather than attempting to correct them once present.

MEDICAL LIAISON

Whilst figure improvement, weight reduction and general leisure forms of body therapy are still the major part of the beauty operator's work, there is a growing trend towards working in medical liaison. Experienced therapists will find themselves working under medical guidance in controlling obesity, for stress treatments, and post-cardiac routines, through treatment and background advice. This work will continue to grow in importance, as therapists increase their knowledge and experience to meet the new challenge.

Medical guidance is desirable for any client who has had recent medical treatment, has a known physical ailment, or is simply unaware of the state of her health. Before diet programmes, heat therapy, or any treatment designed to temporarily increase the pulse rate and alter the blood pressure, a check with the doctor for his approval is desirable.

Older clients may live a quite normal life with minor health problems, varicose veins, slightly high blood pressure, oedema (fluid retention), or mild anaemia. They appear to have no major problems until they are exposed to new experiences, which change their body's behaviour. Even before commencing cautious applications of manual or electrical therapy on the older client, it is worth having her check with her own doctor that all is well. Explain to the client the reason for the medical approval, and clearly state the treatments you plan to apply, so that these can be shown to the doctor. If it is understood why approval is needed – that it is for personal safety, well being, and to gain maximum results – then clients will respect your professional status, and have confidence in the treatments received.

CONTRA-INDICATIONS

Varying treatments have different effects on the body system, and so their contra-indications, or reasons why they should not be applied, also vary. Certain physical conditions, such as heart abnormalities, epilepsy, high blood pressure, diabeties, and asthma would be contra-indicated to many forms of therapy. Here medical approval would have to be obtained before any form of treatment, to avoid upsetting the body's balance or causing distress. Most individuals with severe conditions would know themselves to be unsuitable for treatment, and would only seek guidance on background factors such as diet.

There is a wide range of common health problems which would require careful adaptation of the treatments, but would not totally prohibit their application. Varicose veins, surface thread veins, scar tissue and skin disorders will all be noticed frequently, and will require particular care in the treatment choice to exclude them from the general application. Varying combinations of treatment can be used, based on the knowledge of their effects on the body, to plan the safest and most effective routines possible in the circumstances.

The importance of commencing a treatment plan with a figure diagnosis, and completing a record card becomes apparent as the effects of treatment on the body become evident. Even diet and exercise advice should be given with the client's physical health and general background in mind. Caution is the best rule to follow when starting therapy, to avoid mishaps. Commence with manual routines until more is known about the client and her health and physical condition. People's reactions to treatment vary considerably, and it is always wise to underestimate their tolerance level. The treatment can always be progressed for more effective results, but if damage is done, or confidence is lost, it is too late for it to be rectified. If there is even the slightest doubt as to the wisdom of completing a treatment routine, then further guidance should be sought before progressing.

Luckily the bulk of the clients will have no more than minor problems, which will only require careful choice of routine. Younger clients tend to have fewer contra-indications and also fewer figure faults. Older women need help the most, but tend to have more problems which restrict treatment. So skill and ingenuity is necessary in treatment choice, to combine successful therapy with safe and enjoyable routines.

PROFESSIONAL ETHICS

Having a sound knowledge of body anatomy and function does not make the therapist able to determine physical problems, which could alter or contra-indicate treatment. This must be left to the doctor, whose guidance will be very valuable to the therapist. Understanding what is within the therapist's field of reference is of the greatest importance, as it sets guidelines of suitable treatment, and guards against malpractice. Working thoroughly and consistently to achieve good results within the limits of the job also improves the status and professionalism of the therapy industry. Respect from the medical profession and ancillary workers is hard earned – and soon lost – if treatments are undertaken which could place individuals at risk.

The larger beauty therapy associations have a code of practice which they expect their members to follow, to promote good standards, and gain respect for their work. Advice is given regarding the limitations of the work, and suggestions given on treatment organization and general salon procedures. Beauty therapy still has a long way to go before it will have the professional status of para-medical staff, such as physiotherapists, etc., but a code of practice and growing standards of work will eventually lead the way to State Registration and more recognition of the value of beauty therapy generally.

Chapter 2

Figure Diagnosis

Care is taken in diagnosis of the figure so that all following treatment will produce effective results, without harm or discomfort to the client. From the figure assessment comes also recognition of faults outside the therapist's field of reference, or requiring medical referral prior to treatment. The majority of clients undertaking treatment or seeking advice, are perfectly healthy with simple figure problems, which, although a personal worry, are of no interest medically. However, where medical guidance is desirable, as in obesity or after childbirth, then it should be readily sought and willingly acted upon.

Figure diagnosis or assessment is a new field of therapy, where only guidelines can be given as to the best method of combining treatment to obtain results. Postural factors, diet, exercise and salon applications all have a part to play in the figure improvement. Choice will be based to a large extent on the figure diagnosis, with the knowledge and competence of the therapist being the main essentials for successful treatment.

ANALYSIS OF THE FIGURE

Posture

The first point to be noticed will be the *overall shape* of the client, and how she moves in normal daily life. This starts to form part of the **visual** assessment, which is then backed up by the **manual** and **verbal** aspects, gained later in the diagnosis. How the client looks when dressed, her posture, her general personality and interest in her improvement, all guide the therapist in forming the best improvement plan.

Visually, it has to be ascertained that poor posture is not causing figure faults, so the correct standing position should be checked before any other form of diagnosis is undertaken. The relevance of correct sitting, standing and walking, in attaining an attractive figure is fully covered in Chapter 4. Getting the client to observe her figure, and its faults, in a full length mirror, is of importance at the start of the diagnosis, and sets the professional tone of the treatment. A critical appraisal of the figure at this stage is of great value.

Attempts to disguise the faults present, by clever positioning or holding the muscles in to flatter the figure should be discouraged.

This provides an opportunity to explain what can be done, and the length and individual duration of planned treatment to create the desired result. It also shows what cannot be remedied by the beauty clinic, and may need plastic surgery. Some faults which cannot be changed, due to body type or habitual postural defects, can be made to appear less obvious with more mobility and suppleness in the general posture. Therapists should be knowledgeable about plastic surgery, and ideally will work in liaison with a surgeon of repute, to whom they can suggest clients for medical consultation, if embarrassment prevents clients confiding in their own doctor. Ideally the client should be advised to seek plastic surgery advice through the normal procedure of consulting her own doctor first, who will then recommend a plastic surgeon, who is known personally.

CORRECT STANDING POSTURE

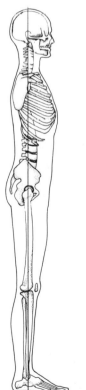

Line of Gravity

The visual diagnosis usually is completed within the initial body treatment, prior to the actual practical applications. The client should ideally retain only the minimum of clothing, or be naked under a towelling gown, so that the figure can be assessed. Modesty will dictate the most suitable method in the circumstances, and will often depend on the client's age and background.

The correct standing posture is considered to be when the person stands easily, with no strain, and can maintain a relaxed body posture without physically holding in any part of the body.

The head should be level and the chest slightly to the fore of the abdomen. The shoulders should be level and slightly squared.

The abdomen should be slightly retracted, and the buttocks tucked in, not protruding and causing a sway backed effect.

The knees should be slightly but not over extended, with the feet at a slight angle to each other, and not rolled inwards.

From the front the client should appear to be able to hold the posture with ease, and have an upright, but not stiff bearing. Viewed from the side, a check using the line of gravity, perhaps drawn on a full length mirror, will confirm the good or bad posture evident. A plumb line dropped down a wall, alongside a height measure, will achieve the same effect, and can be simply devised by weighting a piece of string and hanging it in a convenient position.

The figure would appear to have the line passing through first just the ear lobe, then the point of the shoulder, through or directly behind the hip joint, slightly in front of the knee joint axis, to end just in front of the ankle joint through the arch of the foot to the ground.

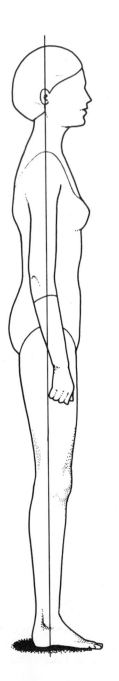
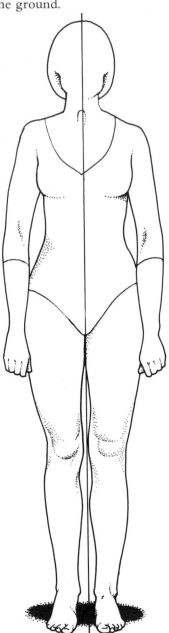

Correct Posture

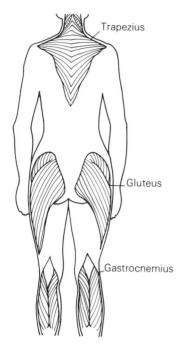

Trapezius

Gluteus

Gastrocnemius

Back

Anti-gravity Muscles

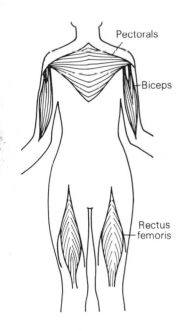

Pectorals

Biceps

Rectus femoris

Front

Anti-gravity Muscles

Considering posture only from this static position is of course incomplete, but it does show when postural re-education is necessary, before suggesting any other forms of exercise for the client.

The standing posture is maintained by reflex action on the part of the anti-gravity muscles, supported and supplemented by ligaments and fascia. So it is obvious that it must be correct before any other exercise will be effective in correcting any specific body fault. The downward pull of gravity is opposed in the body by these anti-gravity muscles, which maintain the upright position by being in a state of partial contraction at all times, except during sleep. The larger anti-gravity (or postural muscles) include the pectorals (chest), the trapezius (back), the gluteals (buttocks), and the quadriceps and gastrocnemius (legs), all of which in co-ordination with the joints and bones act to maintain movement. If the state of tone or contraction in these muscles is not present, as in sleep or unconsciousness during fainting, the person collapses, unable to maintain the erect and moving figure.

Evidence of poor posture, and figure problems linked with postural defects, may require that exercises are undertaken prior to, or alongside, the practical therapy and home advice given. Many common body problems such as round shoulders, a dropped bustline, protruding abdomen, pelvic tilt or a hollow back, are the result of habitual poor postural habits. If long established they may never be totally changed, but certainly can be improved through greater postural awareness and re-education of the muscles.

Clients who find it difficult to achieve and maintain the correct standing posture need to be trained to recognize the ideal posture, so that it gradually becomes established and seems the most natural position to them. Figure improvement through exercise is a vital part of total body improvement, and is covered fully in Chapter 4.

BODY TYPES

People come in all shapes and sizes, but for figure assessment purposes it is useful to consider whether they fall approximately into one body type or another. Body type, or *soma type*, from the Greek word for body (*soma*), was first thought of by an American physical anthropologist Dr. William H. Sheldon, as a convenient way of describing all main varieties of human physique. He considered that people were of several main types, the best known being endomorphs, mesomorphs, and ectomorphs, these terms being the accepted form of description to this day. These are three extreme body varieties or types, but most people exhibit characteristics of more than one type.

The Endomorph

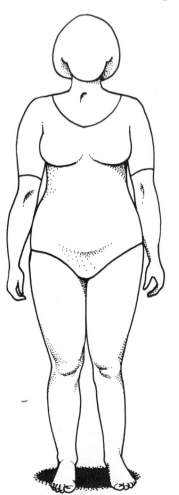

This type is rounded, often plump and with a heavy body. The contours are padded, the neck is short, and fatty deposits are in evidence around the hips, abdomen, neck and shoulders, and upper arms. The hands and feet may be small and delicate in appearance, whilst the limbs are short. Body movements may be slow and deliberate. Anyone who tends to this body shape either through hereditary factors or inherited eating habits, has a much greater problem achieving a slim figure, and may always be prone to weight accumulation.

The Mesomorph

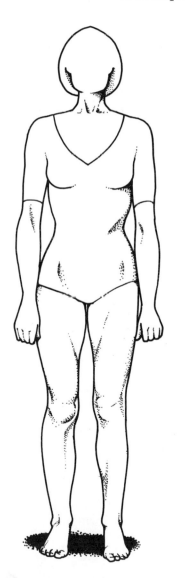

The shape here is determined by the muscular build of the individual, with well developed shoulders and slim boyish hips being the classic mesomorph type. The inverted triangular shape, and well toned musculature often point towards athletic interests, and this type usually has no weight problems whilst they remain active.

The Ectomorph

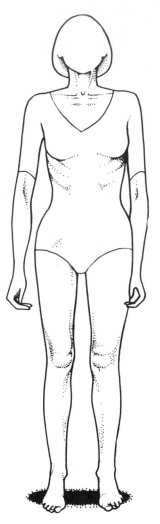

The long bones and slim pencil shape of the ectomorph are easy to recognize in both men and women. The long thin trunk is often associated with a bent over posture, and the person may appear lacking in vitality and energy. The ectomorph seems often to lack strength and stamina, and certainly does not have a lot of muscular bulk in the body for energy reserves. An underweight problem, with a lack of curves, may also be present.

In most clients there are elements of many body types, and few people will fit exactly into these extreme categories. Active individuals may be closer to the mesomorph, whilst the obese person may appear like an endomorph, due to the fatty deposits. Obesity changes the total appearance of both men and women, and is an added factor in deciding body type.

Recognizing the approximate group into which the client can be placed for assessment is helpful in deciding the correct size they could be, and judging how far from it they are. It also points out the genetic shape inherited, about which little in fact can be done. Like the bone structure and overall height of the person, the body type is set for life. Surface deposits of fat, which alter the body shape, and postural defects which present the figure badly to the world can, however, be altered, and the therapist is primarily concerned with these aspects of improvements.

Having considered the client's posture, and general body type, to determine any limitations in the planned improvement, the next step in the diagnosis is to assess specific faults present.

SPECIFIC FIGURE FAULTS

First in an upright position, following on from posture checking, the figure is observed tactfully and factors concerning various parts of the body are recorded on the client's card. The general body proportions are considered first; whether the upper and lower body are balanced in size, and in relation to each other. Common faults such as heavy hips, thighs, and buttocks, become evident even before measurements are taken. A heavy and dropped bustline will be obvious even when the client is dressed, but can be more accurately assessed with the client naked, and the chances of its improvement realistically judged. An excessively underweight client, with an underdeveloped bust and no curves to pad her contours, is also possible to assess by simply visual means. Therapists have to learn to use their visual senses, as well as their verbal ability to determine the extent of the figure problem, and understand what they are up against to effect an improvement.

A check list of specific body areas where problems might occur is useful initially whilst experience is growing in diagnosis techniques. It also provides a useful and thorough means of recording body faults, which require alteration, reduction or improvement.

The upright figure can be observed, first with regard to the shoulder girdle area of the body.

Shoulder Girdle

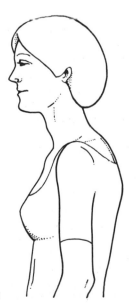

Head Tilt

Points that should be observed include: the position of the head in relation to the shoulders, with regard to a *forward angle of tilt*. It is a postural defect if a small degree of angle is present; this condition points to a need for postural re-education. The condition known as 'dowager's hump', where fatty deposits accumulate at the back of the neck at the base, over the spine, is often associated with a forward positioning of the head. The shoulders themselves, whether held normally in a round shouldered position, or high in relation to the head, indicating tightness or shortening of the muscles. If one shoulder is held higher than another, it may indicate muscular development, and as long as the difference is minor it may be ignored. However, extreme deviations from the normal require medical guidance before prescribing exercises, so recognition is important.

The shoulder blades (scapulae bones) may project like wings, or be abducted away from the midline (the spine). Although unsightly if extreme, the condition may be simply a combination of poor posture, and a lack of subcutaneous adipose (fatty) tissue to pad and round out the contours. Again, the degree of the condition guides the therapist, and if normal postural correction is difficult or painful to attain and maintain, then further help should be sought.

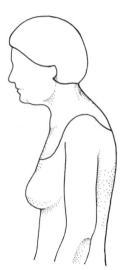

Dowager's Hump

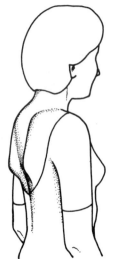

Scapula Abduction

Arms

The arms are a problem area for many women with conditions ranging from a solid muscular appearance, with fatty deposits, to the thin, scrawny arm, with loose crepey skin. The arms may be involved in a generalized overweight condition, or be out of proportion to the rest of the figure. Like the thighs, the upper arms are slow to reduce in size, due to the underlying muscular bulk, and need concentrated attention for good results.

THE BACK

Any deviations from the normal position of the spine, such as increases in the degree of spinal curvature, should be noted as these will limit or prohibit exercise and certain clinic treatments. These deviations take several forms which the therapist must be able to recognize even in their mildest forms.

Treatment of spinal curvature is obviously within the medical province and outside the therapists field of reference. However, recognition of posterior (backwards) anterior (forwards) and lateral (sideways) curvature of the spine, which is a diviation from the normal position will prevent incorrect treatment being applied.

KYPHOSIS

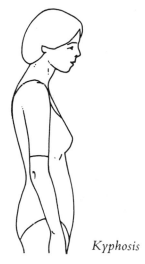

Kyphosis

Kyphosis is an increase of the normal posterior convex thoracic curve, which is often associated with tightness in the pectoral muscles. This condition is frequently linked with an abnormally large degree of concave (inwards) curve in the lumbar area of the spine (lordosis).

Lordosis normally refers to an exaggerated lumbar curve which may be associated with anterior pelvic tilt and shortened hip flexor muscles. Where a severe degree of kyphosis and lordosis is combined the condition is known as *kypholordosis*.

SCOLIOSIS

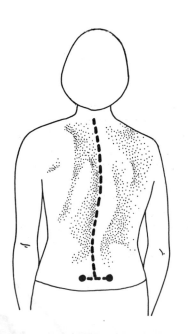

Scoliosis or lateral curvature of the spine may be to the right or left side, and will alter the total body alignment. The deviation from the spines normal position can be traced by following the spinous processes of the vertebral column, and comparing this line with a straight spine. An established degree of scoliosis may cause scapular diviation, slight horizontal rotation of the pelvic and shoulder girdles, uneven shoulder positions, and occasionally differences in leg lengths.

ROUND BACK

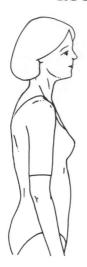

The condition termed *round back* is a rounding out of the spine in a posterior direction. The pelvis may be correctly positioned or have an anterior or posterior tilt. The condition may be clearly seen and felt with the client in a prone position.

FLAT BACK

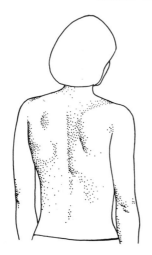

A *flat back* condition is a decrease or absence of the normal anteroposterior spinal curves. The back presents a rigid appearance.

Rib Cage and Breasts

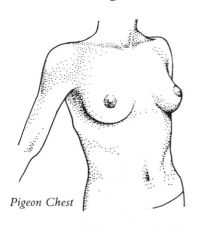

Pigeon Chest

The shape and position of the sternum and the rib cage is very involved with the way the breasts look and how they are positioned on the chest wall. Improving the general posture can have an immediate effect on the bustline, and general breast problems. Well supported breasts, positioned high on the rib cage, appear to have fewer faults, and less tendency to sag. The rib cage may be normal or expanded, boxy in shape, or may give the appearance of being long waisted.

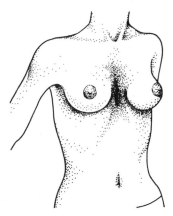

Hollow Chest

Deposits of adipose tissue, such as in midriff bulge, alter the general body shape and the relationship of the breasts to the rest of the trunk. Any unusual chest deformities should be noted including pigeon chest and hollow chest which, although rare, would alter exercise routines.

The breasts themselves should be noted for size, position, and any degree of sag in relation to the breasts' connection to the chest wall. The distance of the nipples from the clavicle should also be noted, particularly in post-natal work, or during general reduction on a client with a full bust. Underdevelopment should be noted, especially where a general underweight condition is not evident. Any abnormalities, such as superfluous hair, uneven breast size, or inverted nipples or lumps should also be recorded, to form a total picture to guide the therapist in her treatment choice.

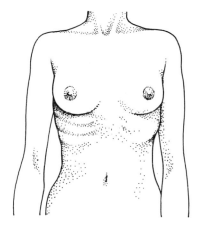

Boxy Rib Cage

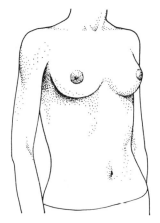

High Positioned Breasts

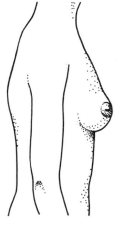

Breast Sag

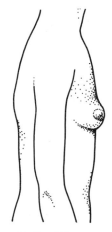

Deflated Breasts

The Waist, Abdomen and Buttocks

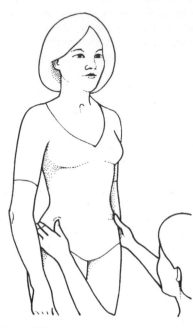

Pelvic Tilt

Muscular tone and the amount of adipose tissue deposits should be noted in these areas. Weak or elongated muscles in the abdominal area may result in a protruding abdomen, which will require salon muscle contraction and home exercises. Superficial fatty deposits over the buttocks, pelvic girdle, waist and lower abdomen, may indicate a need for general reduction, or specific reduction achieved electrically. Postural faults, such as a poor general posture due to leaning back, slouching or resting on one hip, rather than with the weight evenly distributed, may be implicated here. Pelvic tilt may be present, as a result of the weight carried during pregnancies where the centre of gravity alters due to the weight carried in front. The body's balance is displaced, and this has to be re-established.

The link between pregnancies and abdominal weakness also has to be recognized when assessing this area. The extension which occurs progressively over the course of the pregnancy (especially when an excessive weight gain is involved) is inevitably extremely difficult to rectify postnatally. Any operations, either gynaecological or general in this area, should also be noted; for they have effect on muscular strength, and subsequently fatty deposit levels.

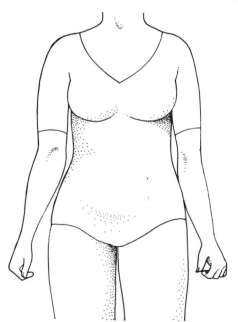

Thick Trunk Shape

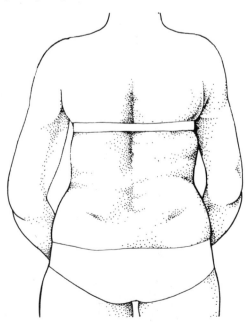

General Overweight

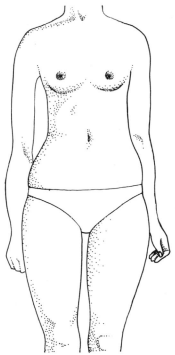

Out of Proportion Figure

The muscular bulk and fatty deposits of the buttocks are a common problem in figure diagnosis, and may indicate a weight loss is required. If no weight loss is needed or desirable, overall, then reduction of *inches* rather than *weight* is needed and may suggest a plan of salon treatment reinforced in its action by active home exercise routines. The actual shape of the buttocks should be noticed, whether hollow sided with the fullness of the buttocks indented, or simply over large. Whether the seat is rounded, low slung, or fuller towards the thighs, also gives guidance as to the best method of improvement.

An out-of-proportion figure, slight in the chest and midriff areas, but heavy from the waist downwards, is so common as to be considered an international figure shape. Fashion dictates that a very slim, long, lean shape is desirable; but nature tends to build women for their natural role in life, procreation, and provides the necessary equipment to fulfil that role. A wide pelvic girdle, though ideal for child bearing, also gives broad hips, and this will occur as a common figure fault seen often in the beauty clinic.

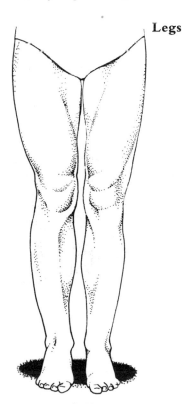

Legs

The general shape of the legs in relation to the rest of the figure and the body type should be noted. Heavy muscular legs, due to an inherited shape, or developed by sports, will be difficult to reduce, as the fatty tissue is present between muscle fibres as well as laid superficially over large muscle groups. This fat is often termed trapped, which, although not anatomically correct, is a convenient way to describe it for clients. It indicates it is less easy to remove, which indeed it is. The fatty tissues are in fact the same, they are simply not the first source of stored energy to be used up by the body, when on a reduced diet. Subcutaneous fat is lost first, and well established fat in heavy muscular areas tends to be lost last.

Muscular Legs

The shape of the legs, and any established faults such as knock knees, bow legs, hyper-extended knees, (back knees) or flat feet should be noted, for recognition purposes.

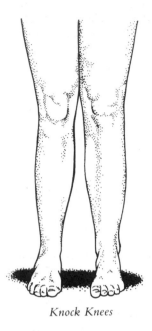

Knock Knees

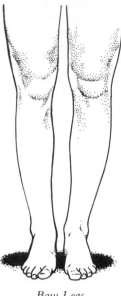

Bow Legs

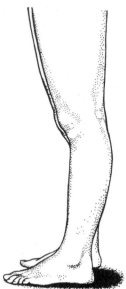

Hyper-extended Knees

Any conditions unable to be corrected by simple postural means are outside the therapist's field of reference, but they must be recognized as their presence alters exercise routines given for specific improvement.

Fatty deposits, areas of soft dimpled fat, (often termed cellulite) and areas of oedema, (swelling) should be noted. The circulation of the legs is also important, particularly for reduction treatments, and varicose veins, thread veins, and generally poor circulation should be observed, discussed, and recorded.

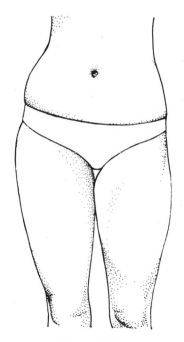

Heavy Thighs

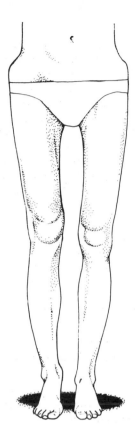

Very Thin Legs

Exceptionally thin legs, requiring shaping and building up to avoid space being evident between the thighs, may also be seen. Although a small proportion of the therapist's clients, the underweight individuals are a very rewarding aspect of treatment, and can obtain very successful results with careful figure diagnosis.

To complete the upright figure diagnosis the client should be viewed from the side, to obtain a total picture. Faults will be more evident from the side than from the front or back, and as this is the profile often presented to the world, it is important. Bust sag, protruding midriff and abdomen, and the position and size of the buttocks and thighs, can be confirmed from the side view, to give an overall picture.

A test for excessive subcutaneous adipose (fatty) tissue in any area of the body can be made by using a *skin fold test*. If loose surface tissues can be held away from the underlying muscles, and are sufficient to fill a finger and thumb without discomfort, the client is generally or locally overweight. When undertaken for medical purposes the skin fold test is given with calipers for accurate measurement, but for beauty purposes a simple pinch test is adequate, usually given on the upper arm, inside thigh, or back. As therapists use so many different forms of body assessment to gain a full figure diagnosis, including manual massage, the pinch test is often superfluous.

This list of figure points completes the initial diagnosis, and permits the treatment to progress. Although it appears complex, it is often assessed in a few minutes visually, checking through the list of possible faults, and only recording those present. Most clients benefit from simple posture correction and find it makes general exercise easier to perform.

Further information is obtained about the figure during a manual treatment, where muscle tone, adipose tissue distribution, and circulatory factors are noted. Until further knowledge is gained of the client's health and tolerance to electrical therapy, the treatment should be carefully chosen for safety.

ANATOMICAL POSITIONS

In all analysis and treatment of the body a descriptive plan of its architecture will be found useful, so that it is clearly understood what part of the body is involved in treatment. These descriptive terms indicate the anatomical positions and aspects of the body, and form a guide to all applications of body therapy, salon applications and exercise routines. They also indicate the muscle position and used in conjunction with joint movements, provide helpful guidance on muscular actions and locations within the total muscular system.

The term 'anatomical position' refers to an erect standing position, with the arms at the sides and the palms turned forward. It is a similar position to the correct standing position used in posture checks and from it can be seen the following directional descriptive terms.

Superior – upper – towards the head end of the body (the shoulder girdle is within the superior part of the body).

Inferior – lower – away from the head (the foot is part of the inferior extremity).

Anterior or **ventral** – front (the knee cap is located on the anterior side of the leg).

Posterior or **dorsal** – back (the spine and shoulder blades are located on the posterior side of the body).

Medial – towards the midline (centre) of the body (the big toe is located on the medial aspect of the foot).

Lateral – away from the midline (the outside thigh is on the lateral surface of the leg).

Proximal – nearest to the trunk, or point of origin of a part (the knee is located at the proximal end of the lower leg).

Distal – farthest away from the trunk, or point of origin of a part (the hand is located at the distal end of the forearm).

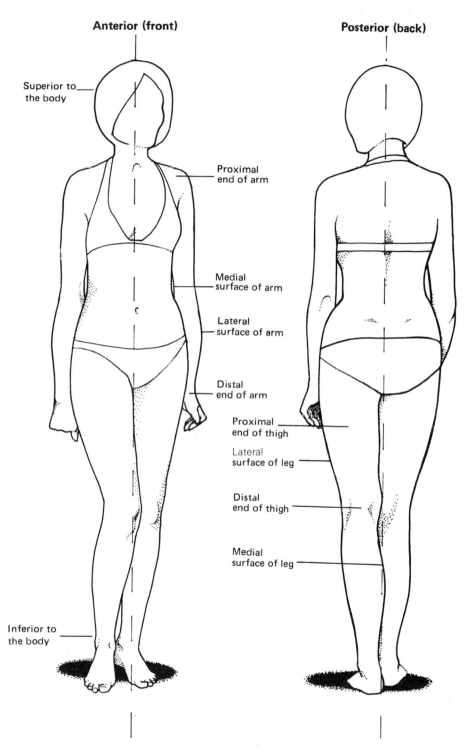

Anatomical Positions

MANUAL BODY ASSESSMENT

After the initial figure diagnosis is completed much additional knowledge can be gained by manually treating the body and assessing its condition. Initially, whilst building up an overall picture of the client's health and her figure needs, it is wise to concentrate on *manual* massage, until possible contra-indications have been checked.

The massage adds to the visual figure diagnosis in several ways, as the therapist discovers the state of the client's muscular and circulatory systems, and assesses the figure faults in relation to the client's age.

Skin Conditions

The age of the client, and her general health, will have affected her skin texture and its elasticity. A crepey, or loose skin may be the result of weight loss, poor health, incorrect care, or simply ageing in process.

Stretch marks, from pregnancy or a large weight loss, may also be present. Soft, puckered skin in the abdominal area should also be noted.

Dry or greasy skin texture will determine the best treatment medium – talc, cream or oil – to improve the skin texture.

Poorly textured skin, easily stimulated skin, and poor circulation will all need to be recognised, as their presence will affect the plan of treatment.

Varicose veins, thread veins and bruises will contra-indicate many forms of *electrical* therapy.

Muscular Condition

The tone or tension present in the muscles will act as a guide to the client's physical state. A muscular build will often indicate that the client will be able and willing to help her figure problems through personal efforts rather than from salon applications. A well toned body will be less likely to accumulate fatty deposits, and should normally have few figure problems. If the level of activity decreases however, weight can accumulate, and be felt overlying strong muscle groups.

Loss of muscle tone, particularly in the abdominal area can be felt (palpated) during massage, and will indicate the amount of rehabilitation of the waistline and abdomen that is needed. Linked with pregnancies, operations, and simply overweight and postural problems, this condition is very common. An accumulation of weight (adipose tissue) in the area, makes the problem worse, and gives a protruding abdominal shape.

Tension present in the muscles to an excessive degree, may cause pain and stiffness to be evident. Hard muscles, where relaxation appears difficult to obtain, may be due to nervous tension, pain in the area, or incorrect postural stance. If pain is felt during manual applications, medical guidance should be sought by the client to determine the cause.

Some clients are simply tense individuals who need help to relax their muscles and minds. Relaxation therapy and soothing elements in massage can then be used to good effect.

Areas of tension building up, which could develop into fibrositis nodules, can be dispersed through massage, associated with heat. Noticed on the manual assessment, their presence will indicate a need for preventive measures to avoid pain, and stiffness becoming established.

Weight Deposits

Where weight reduction is involved the distribution of adipose tissue in the body is important in order to determine the best means of its elimination. Generalized subcutaneous (surface) fat covering the trunk and proximal parts of the limbs, will make certain treatments less effective, and will point to the need for a diet. Localized fatty deposits over muscular areas may benefit from deep massage and electrical therapy applied specifically in that one area, and diet may not be involved.

Fatty deposits and their underlying muscular support, (whether weak or strong) will determine the safest and most effective method of obtaining figure improvement.

The form the fatty deposit takes will be determined by its location on the body, how recently acquired, or long established it is. Superficial fat is quickly gained, and quickly lost, through diet. Localized deposits may be long established, and feel solid or hard to the touch. They are more difficult to remove through diet, as the fat is present between muscle fibres, and tends to be the last area to reduce. Fatty deposits in between the knees, thighs, and over the upper arms, tend to feel less solid, and appear soft to the touch. The fatty condition termed cellulite is another example of the form adipose tissue can take, where a dimpled skin condition is present, which appears like orange peel.

When considering adipose tissue and its removal from the body it is important to remember that fat cells *are* 'fat cells', wherever they are in the body, and whatever we like to call them for convenience and in client discussion. They do appear to take a different form when associated with weak muscular areas, as compared to heavy muscular groups. Certain areas of the body are fat depots, common to many men and women, where fat is usually lost last, making it resistant to diet reduction. Hips and thighs are common in women, the abdomen, waist and lower back in men.

So there is no reason why fatty deposits cannot be accepted as being different and more difficult to remove in certain areas of the body. Once its position and cause is known, however, the plan for its removal can commence.

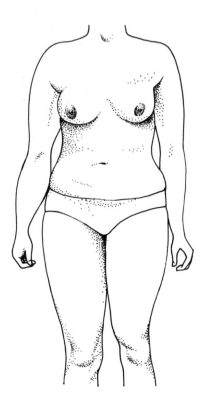

General Overweight Condition

TESTS FOR MUSCLE STRENGTH

Simple tests can be performed on the massage plinth or by the bedside to give an initial guide to the client's strength and general mobility. A need for postural exercises, relaxation routines or specific active exercise work will become evident if a few simple exercises are undertaken. The need for electrical muscle contraction applications is also decided at this stage, based on the knowledge gained of the muscle's strength.

Abdominal Area

With the client lying supine (face up) on the couch, the strength of the abdominal muscles can be determined if the following exercises are completed.

1   Sitting up from a lying down position. Tests the rectus abdominus and obliques.
2   Touching the toes, with the head inclined towards or touching the knees, which also tests for mobility in the back – and muscle shortening in the hamstrings.

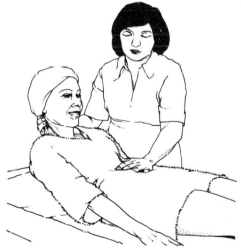 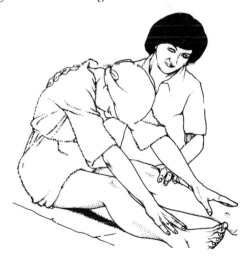

Legs

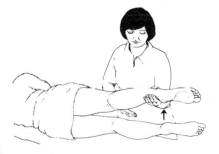

With the client lying on her side the legs can be tested, just by raising the upper leg, and bringing the lower one to meet it, then lowering both slowly.

With the client sitting or semi-reclining, the strength of the thighs can be tested by making the muscles contract against resistance by holding the foot in full extension, and asking the client to pull the toes up, against the operator's resistance, whilst holding the calf and then the thigh, with the other hand, to test the muscles' strength. The movement can be altered with the toes pulled up, and the client attempting to hold the position against the operator's even, controlled pressure to bring the foot into extension.

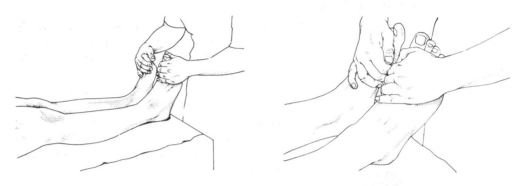

Testing Against Resistance

Arms

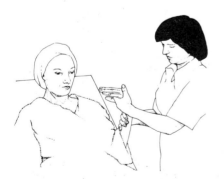

The same eccentric (extension) and concentric (contraction) muscle work can be performed on the arms to gain the same knowledge. The client can be advised to hold her hand to her shoulder, and attempt to keep it there, against the operator's pressure to extend the arm. In reverse, also with the arm extended, and held by the operator, the client attempts to return the hand to the shoulder against the operator's resistance.

All movements where the client is helped to perform exercises, or has joints extended, are undertaken by the operator using first *passive* movements. These guide the client, carefully place her limbs, support her during exercise, or work to give her joints full mobility, by extending them to their limits but not beyond.

These passive movements are followed by *active* movements, where the exercise may be a free movement (without assistance), an *assisted* movement (the operator guiding and assisting), or *resisted* movements, (against operator's or client's resistance).

Following the passive and assisted muscle work, the client may be asked to perform a few free exercises by the bedside, to extend knowledge of muscle strength, and general posture.

Toe touching – to test mobility in the back and hamstrings (upper back thighs).

Waist bending – to judge balance, strength and suppleness in the trunk.

Arm swinging and rotation – gives guidance as to posture and mobility in the shoulder girdle.

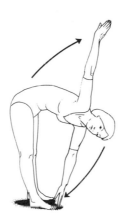

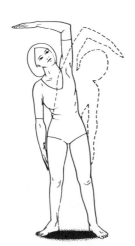

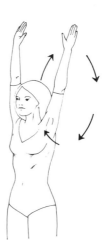

CELLULITE

Cellulite (pronounced cell-u-leet) is a convenient name given to areas of fat that are hard to lose, and assume a dimpled, lumpy appearance under the skin. This condition of fatty deposits was first termed 'cellulite' by the Swedes, and the name was quickly adopted by the French as being a convenient title for difficult areas of weight. To suffer from cellulite seems far more acceptable than to be simply fat, and the name persists to this day.

As a convenient title for a form of weight condition it does have some use, and as it is well known and liked by clients, it is acceptable to use the term in client discussion. The fact that it is a form of fat should be remembered however, when planning its removal, or trying to prevent its formation. Few very slim women are to be seen suffering from cellulite, although some of normal build do appear to have weight of this type on the upper outside thigh, buttocks and inside knee.

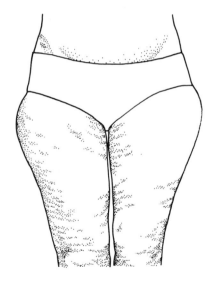

Medical opinion is that cellulite as a special condition does not exist, and that it is simply the form fat takes when it settles in certain areas of the body. Just as individuals have fat depots – areas where weight accumulates if input outstrips output – it is considered that people can be predisposed to retaining fluid and so appear to have cellulite. The sad fact is that to have cellulite is socially acceptable; being fat is not: and so cures for cellulite are eagerly taken up by the public.

Cellulite is always a controversial subject, and therapists must make themselves aware of both sides of the argument, and to be knowledgeable without appearing foolish in the light of respected medical research.

In beauty circles, cellulite is considered the type of fat that does not disappear when the client diets. It needs special help to be removed, usually through an elimination diet, deep and effective massage, and an improvement in the circulation brought about by faradic type and galvanic currents, used in treatments. The problem is considered to be associated with fluid retention, and a build up of toxins in the body, caused by incorrect diet, and inactivity. Contributory factors are considered to be insufficient water intake, fatigue, tension and altogether an unhealthy life: these problems resulting in sluggish digestion, constipation and poor circulation.

An over-abundance of fatty foods, high alcohol intake, and insufficient sleep contribute to overweight and poor health, as well as to cellulite. Many of the reasons for formation of cellulite would contribute to a general overweight problem, so nothing is exclusive to its appearance.

Clients predisposed to fluid retention will find their problem aggravated by increased levels of hormones in the body. The pill, pregnancy, hormone therapy in the menopause, all favour fluid retention, and can result in areas of the body seeming to have cellulite. Changes in the diet can bring about constipation, and body toxins are retained, which in turn affects the body's normal elimination process.

Nothing so far stated really gives reason to think cellulite is a special condition, only a certain form of fat, which responds better to certain forms of treatment than others.

As all the therapist's body work is concerned with determining the figure or weight problem, and deciding the best cure, cellulite can join the list of conditions needing special care and treatment.

The fat condition 'cellulite' is seen as being present due to a strong slowing down of elimination, an accumulation of wastes in the body, and a change in the formation of the connective tissue in the subcutaneous layers of the skin. Its presence is recognized by its location and appearance, and the feel it has on treating the problem. The flesh may seem loose, easy to move around, or solid, hard and difficult to manipulate. The skin may seem tightly stretched over the distended areas, and actual rupture (stretch marks) may be apparent.

A severe loss of weight can result in loose hanging folds of flesh and skin, and this is sometimes termed 'soft cellulite'. It is of course simply due to a loss of supporting fatty tissue, lost too quickly for the skin to snap back into position. This is a special problem with older clients whose skin elasticity is poor.

Solid areas of cellulite-type weight, usually on thighs and buttocks, look distended, and can feel sensitive to the touch, probably due to pressure on nerve endings and fibres in the skin. Specific 'cellulite' routines which combine peeling, muscle contraction and multi-pad galvanic applications help disperse the problem, and ensure weight goes from the correct areas. For success, increased natural exercise and fundamental changes in diet and lifestyle are necessary. It is possible to find small areas of fatty deposits on really slim individuals, but this is unusual and normally a client considered to have solid cellulite is overweight and needs a total figure improvement plan. This would then encompass the normal elements of diet, exercise and salon applications suited to her health and figure problem.

Learning to eat well, to get the most from the food, whilst cutting down on fatty and carbohydrate elements, is something of benefit to all. Cutting down on salt, highly seasoned food, and alcohol likewise must be beneficial whether it is fat or cellulite that is the problem. Purification and elimination are considered the main aims of a cellulite biased diet, but as these are important elements in any reduction plan, if good health is to be maintained, they don't call for any radical changes in diet thinking. Fresh fruits, vegetables and fluids all help elimination, and are most important when fluid retention is involved.

Special diuretic teas, taken as part of the normal fluid intake, increase the amount of urine passed, and aid the fluid retention problem.

Sauna and steam bath therapy stimulate the circulation, and if combined with a friction rub or deep kneading massage, really help to disperse fatty areas.

Exercise for all parts of the body, to tone and invigorate the system, should be advised, and for success needs to be followed regularly. Deep breathing exercises play a particularly important part in eliminating and preventing cellulite.

BREAST CONDITIONS

One of the most important apsects of figure beauty to the client is the shape and position of the breasts. Unfortunately it is also the least freely discussed of all figure problems, due to modesty, embarrassment, or a puritanical attitude on the part of the therapist. As it is an aspect of figure beauty which suffers greatly in the course of normal life, it is worth special consideration. It is closely involved in both pregnancy and lactation, and changes in size and structure to meet physical demands, so it is likely to suffer in the process, without adequate care from exercise support and skin care routines.

In order to know what can be helped by the therapist or what cannot be altered, due to a long standing problem, it is vital to have an understanding of breast structure and function. The size of the breasts is to a large extent a genetic thing, just as height, colouring, etc., are. The overall size and shape of the individual's build also plays a part. The quantity of surface fat present on the body alters the breast size and shape and thin people often have small underdeveloped breasts, due to a lack of body fat.

The breasts themselves are positioned on top of large muscles which cover the chest like breast plates, stretching from the breast bone to the arm (pectoralis major). The actual breasts, therefore, do not contain muscular tissues, but their shape in youth is upheld by powerful suspensory ligaments (Coopers ligaments) which hold the breasts forward, and act against gravity to give the much sought-after support.

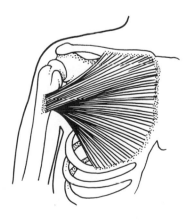

Pectoralis Muscle of Breasts

If the development and function of the breasts throughout life is considered, then the possibility of correction or improvement at these different stages will become apparent. The age of the client, her medical history, and number of children will provide background reasons for the breast condition present. In youth the breasts should be firmly supported, the skin elastic and clear from stretch marks. In the childbearing years, the effects of the distension and strain placed upon the breasts from pregnancy and lactation (breast feeding) may be evident. During menopause normal ageing processes cause a change to occur which alters the firmness and shape of the breasts. So age, body weight, health and the effects of normal life are the main points which have to be considered in the figure diagnosis.

Any deviation from the normal development – such as inverted nipples, underdevelopment, superfluous hair on the breasts, excessively heavy breasts on a slim figure – would all benefit from medical scrutiny to determine the cause of the problem, and find a solution.

In Youth

In a young woman the breasts – or mammary glands – are rounded, firmly supported by strong tendinous fibres, and have a firm, upright appearance. They should be supported on strong chest muscles, and be at the most perfect stage of development, prior to childbearing. Their size and shape will be determined by genetic factors, and the amount of body fat generally present. The nipple – or mammary papilla – is pale pink or light brown in colour, and has 15—20 lactiferous ducts opening on to its surface, these being the milk ducts which will come into action after childbirth when the child suckles on the nipple and is breast fed. The breasts consist of glandular and fibrous tissue with adipose (fatty) tissue interspaced throughout. The actual gland of the breast is covered by subcutaneous tissue which on the upper surface of the breast forms suspensory ligaments, which hold the breast in its upright position in youth.

In youth few problems should be evident apart from underdevelopment, or those associated with postural defects. A poor carriage, round shoulders, protruding shoulder blades, all contribute to a low dropped bustline. Young women with larger breasts occasionally adopt this posture, to disguise their size. A reduction plan and exercise routine for improving the position of the shoulder girdle

muscles may be indicated. Severe underdevelopment, particularly if associated with late
arrival of monthly periods, or presence of body
hair in the male sexual pattern, should be directed
for medical attention. *Recognition*, not treatment, is
the therapist's role in this case.

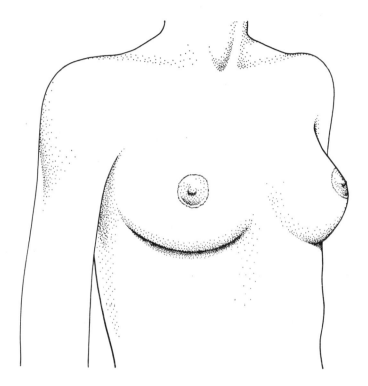

Breasts in Youth

Likewise, any abnormality of the nipples,
inverted, or full and puffy in appearance, although
it may guide the therapist in her overall body
treatment plan, is not within her field of treatment.
Adolescence is a time of much change physically,
and usually not until maturity is reached do minor
imperfections, such as uneven or small breasts,
warrant medical attention. However, if linked
with other problems, like excessive body or facial
hair, erratic periods, fluctuating weight, and so on,
then clients should be advised to seek medical
guidance.

Assuming a healthy body, the younger woman
can be encouraged to care for her figure generally,
and include exercises for the breasts amongst her
daily routine.

Childbearing Role

The breasts are structured for breast feeding, that being their role in the body anatomy, and are ideally fitted for the task. Even small breasts are capable of the extension and development required to breast feed successfully, as it is the ability of the glandular matter in the breast that determines the milk flow.

In the early stages of pregnancy the breasts enlarge slightly, and the coloured skin around the nipple (the areola) darkens from pale pink to dark brown, depending on colouring. The colour fades a little after childbirth, but will always indicate it has occurred. This change is directly associated with changes in the hormone levels in the body at this time.

The actual structure of the breasts starts to change under the influence of increasing amounts of oestrogen and progesterone secreted from the placenta. The gland of the breast consists of 15—20 lobes, these being formed of lobules connected together by areolar tissue, blood vessels, and ducts. Each lobe of the gland is drained by a lactiferous duct which converges towards the areola, where they form lactiferous sinuses, which act as milk reservoirs in pregnancy and lactation. These potential alveoli formed in youth, change into secreting alveoli, in readiness for their milk secreting role in lactation. The amount of adipose tissue in the breasts increases, as does the blood circulation, and the breasts appear full and heavy.

Cross Section of Mammary Glands

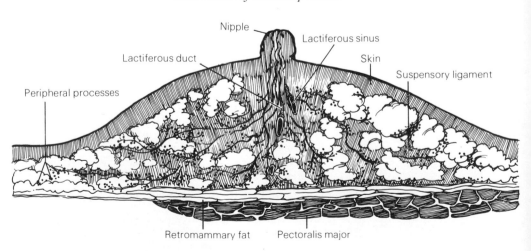

Nipple

Lactiferous sinus

Lactiferous duct

Skin

Suspensory ligament

Peripheral processes

Retromammary fat   Pectoralis major

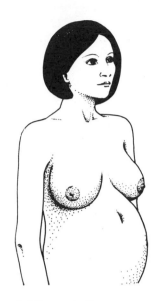

Distended Breasts in Pregnancy

Latter stages of pregnancy bring about a distension of the breast tissue, with the breasts seeming swollen, and traced by evident veins. Much of the skin stretching, which leaves evident striations on the surface, occurs during the latter months of the pregnancy. It could be guarded against by checking overall body weight, ensuring well supported breasts, and increased cosmetic care, use of oils, tissue building creams, and regenerating ampoules, or pre-natal products.

The flow of milk after the birth is initiated by suckling, which stimulates the abundant nerves in the papilla and areola. Without suckling the flow of milk soon ceases, but the breasts are distended with milk for some time, causing discomfort. Lactation is normally possible for 5—6 months after the birth, then diminishes as the child is weaned. Some women do not develop enough glandular tissue to feed their baby, some can breast feed for a few weeks only, and many choose not to feed their babies themselves. Reasons whether to breast feed or not are based on personal feelings, convenience factors and social opinion dominant at the time. Therapists should be knowledgeable about the effects of breast feeding on the figure, and guide their clients accordingly.

Breast Feeding

Many myths persist regarding the damage caused to the breasts' appearance by prolonged breast feeding. Few women know or are told that it is the changes occurring during the pregnancy itself that bring about the greatest difference in breast structure and appearance, this being through hormonal stimulation, over which they have no control. Most women are willing to accept small changes in appearance for the sake of a desired child, and with care can minimize the damage to the figure beauty.

Breast feeding is a natural process and does act to return the womb to its original size and position in readiness for future childbearing. This effect, aided by effective post-natal exercises for the lower abdomen, help to reduce the risk of prolapse of the womb in later life. The whole process of childbearing and lactation co-ordinates well in healthy women, and the stimulation of the child sucking on the nipple exerts a strong pulling effect on the womb muscles, helping the figure to regain its former shape and strength.

On the conclusion of natural lactation the breasts resume a resting condition, any remaining milk is absorbed, and the alveoli shrink. Changes occur in the adipose tissue, and it may reduce or be used up by the body for its food needs. The body tends to retain body fat and fluid, to protect the feeding child's milk supply, whilst lactating is in process. This, combined with an increased need for fluids to keep the milk supply going, makes weight reduction difficult for the feeding mother. After breast feeding is naturally concluded, the breasts undergo a change in their connective tissue and collagenous fibres, which can result in a soft flaccid appearance. The suspensory ligaments may be less supporting to the breasts and a dropped appearance can result. Even if the mother does not breast feed, her figure still has to recover from the extension it has undergone, and the same general care is indicated.

It is through these childbearing years that the therapist can be of greatest value to her clients, by helping them maintain and regain an attractive figure. Without adequate care, pregnancy and lactation can be very disfiguring to the body, both through muscle and skin distension. Luckily much help can be advised, both pre-natal (before the birth) and post-natal (after the birth).

Pre-natal Care

Guidance on diet, to avoid an excessive weight gain, can be given, or support and encouragement used, to keep a client to her medical diet advice. Good support for the breasts during pregnancy, particularly for the fuller breasted woman, with a well fitting bra, chosen for its support effects rather than for fashion, will pay dividends in maintaining an attractive shape. Advice on skin care to reduce the risks of skin stretching, which is a result of the distension experienced: treatment for relaxation, including adapted forms of massage, to help circulation, avoid cramp and backache, so common in pregnancy: facial and body treatment for keeping spirits high – all help to keep morale at its best.

Post-natal Care

Recovery of the figure, rehabilitation of the waistline and refirming and uplifting the breasts are all aspects of post-natal body treatment. Muscle contraction (electrical work, linked with post-natal, and specific improvement exercises, all work to regain the youthful figure. Weight reduction, if linked with figure reshaping and exercise,

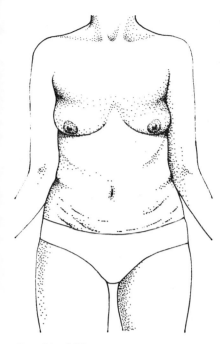

Post Natal Figure

will ensure that the client regains her original figure and gets back to full health. Tissue bracer creams, nourishing oils and regenerating products to tighten and firm the softened skin texture are all effective in improving skin appearance.

Both in pre- and post-natal work the breasts are treated as part of the total body improvement or maintenance. They cannot be successfully considered or treated in isolation from the body as a whole. Weight facts, health, muscle tone, and postural considerations all have a bearing on the shape of the breasts, as they do on all parts of the figure. As the breasts suffer the most change of all figure aspects over the course of the woman's reproductive life, they are most affected at adolescence, pregnancy, in lactation, and finally during the menopause.

Menopause

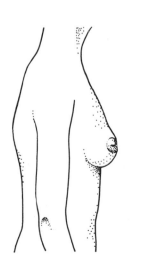

In menopause the role of the breasts as mammary glands is finished and the actual gland atrophies (decreases), and the ducts of breasts degenerate and disappear almost completely. If childbearing has taken place the breasts will have suffered the wear and tear of life, and unless well supported with underlying strong muscles and sufficient adipose tissue, may have a dropped appearance. The breasts' attachment to the chest wall may be narrow, and the actual breasts may hang down below this attachment level. From the side the breasts may appear as fallen empty pockets, and from the front the nipples may be completely below the breasts attachment level.

Whether the breasts are full or thin, the problem remains the same, that is the degree of drop or loss of support. With simple exercises to determine the power of the breasts' attachment to the chest wall, and the breasts' support from suspensory ligaments, the problem can be easily assessed. If on lifting the arms, upwards, from a front position to above the head, the breasts do not change position, with the nipples remaining static, the problem is beyond the therapist's help. Plastic surgery to improve the actual appearance, or good bra support to create an illusion of an uplifted figure are the two alternatives.

Of course, not all young women have good figures, some are very underdeveloped, if they are extremely slim. Likewise, not all mature women have a dropped bustline, and many take great care to exercise and maintain a trim and attractive shape. Body weight, posture and health all directly relate to the figure potential.

Much of the work of the beauty therapist in dealing with breast conditions will revolve round educating the client on the function of the breasts, and the care they require if firm, well supported, well shaped breasts are to be maintained throughout life. As a professional the therapist should be able to achieve this without embarrassment to her client or herself.

PLASTIC SURGERY
Breasts

If the shape and position of the breasts cannot be improved by natural means, such as altering the body weight, or improving muscular support, then plastic surgery might be considered. If a client is the correct body weight for height, and still suffers from having too small, large or pendulous a bustline, then mammaplasty (plastic surgery on the breasts) should be considered.

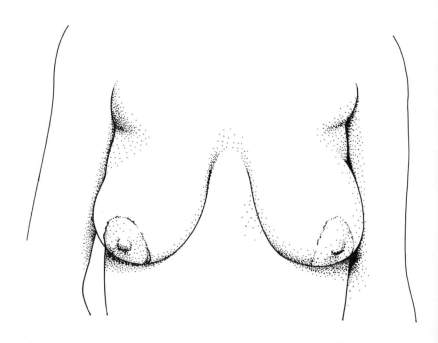

Pendulous Breasts

Therapists should have an awareness of the advantages and drawbacks to improving the figure by surgical means. The risks, as with any operation, have to be thought of, and unless the problem seems of immense importance to the client, the therapist is best advised to be knowledgeable but neutral with her advice.

There are two main aspects of mammaplasty – breast reduction, and breast augmentation (enlargement), although much of the plastic surgeon's work is involved with reshaping pendulous breasts as well.

Breast Reduction

Breast reduction may be performed through the National Health Service if the problem is acute, and the weight of the breasts is causing pain and distress. The body weight may be a contributory factor here, and any excess fat may need to be lost prior to the operation.

The excess weight is removed by the surgeon, who keeps the nipple and areola (surrounding pigment) intact, to retain the sensitivity and feeling of the breast. The fat is removed after first a circular incision is made around the areola, then from the areola to the fold below the breast, and lastly at right angles to this incision, so that a flap

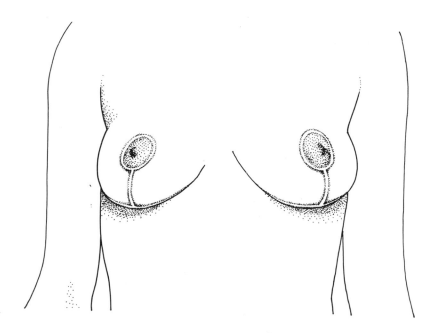

Reshaping of the Breasts

is formed. This is loosened from the underlying breast tissue, and folded back so that the unwanted weight can be removed surgically. Once the correct size has been reached, the skin is fitted back into the new breast shape, and the excess trimmed away. A new position has to be cut in the skin for the original nipple and areola, and these are then stitched in place. The incisions under the breast are closed up and, with time, the scars fade away until hardly visible.

In reducing the breasts, the surgeon also accomplishes an uplift effect, and endeavours to keep the breast in proportion, so that if weight is regained, the breasts will not become distorted, or too pendulous.

Breast reduction or major reshaping is a major operation, and is carried out under general anaesthetic. A great deal of medical after-care is needed, and the cost, if paid for privately, would be £600–£800, depending on surgeon and residential facilities.

The success of the operation though, can save women years of misery, either if they are young and have very large breasts, or older women, after childbirth has spoiled a youthful shape. Scars are a feature of all mammaplasty, but are considered a worthwhile price to pay for regaining the figure. The improvement tends to be permanent unless an excessive amount of weight is gained. As some women have about 1.30—1.80 kg (3—4 lb) of weight removed from each breast, it becomes evident that in severe cases it is well worth the discomfort, the recovery period, and the cost. If available through the National Health Service, the wait might be lengthy.

Breast Uplifting

Breast uplifting is another very popular and successful operation which, as it does not involve as much overall reduction, has a shorter recovery period. Pendulous breasts can be reshaped, loose skin removed, and a more youthful bust line created.

Breast Augmentation

Adding to small underdeveloped or virtually non-existent breasts is another area where plastic surgery may be the only answer. If, even with exercises to build the underlying muscles, the chest is still flat, augmentation may be considered. Some surgeons are loath to undertake the operation until childbearing and lactation are finished

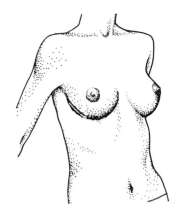

Breast Augmentation

with, due to the changes in breast tissue at these times. Lactation, though possible after breast enlargement, can be uncomfortable, with the breasts becoming heavy and taut. So milk may have to be dried up to avoid discomfort.

After an implant operation, also, the breasts do not feel quite the same, although visually the effects are excellent. In a lying position the breasts tend to stay in an upright, more conical, position, rather than sloping to the sides like a natural bosom. So unless the women who require enlargement have found a permanent partner, who is in accord with their desire for a larger bosom, they should think hard before embarking on the operation.

There are two methods of augmentation, both based on the same principles of implants to give the breasts the bulk they lack. One method uses pre-formed silicone prosthesis of a firm but flexible consistency which is inserted through an incision on the underside of the breast, into the cavity between the breast and chest wall. A more recent advance is use of flat silicone envelopes, which are inserted and then filled with special liquid or gel. These balloon-like implants give greater flexibility to forming an attractive shape, and are useful to equalise uneven sized breasts.

Older methods of grafting fat from the buttocks have now been superseded by these silicone prosthesis and 'balloons'. Silicone injections are no longer used to increase breast size, due to the potential danger of entering a vein, with serious complications.

Breast augmentation can be done at any age, but is most effective if childbearing has spoiled an attractive figure, or if the woman has always lacked full breasts, as the difference is then so immediate. A smallish or deflated breast condition is the most successful, as it has enough padding to disguise the addition. The scars are small, with a 3.8 cm (1½ in.) incision line by the envelopes implant method, and a 6—7.5 cm (2½—3 in.) scar left by the prosthesis method. Lying low at the side of the breasts, the scars are scarcely visible, and recovery is normally very good. Cost is high at £350–£550, with patients being in hospital for 7–10 days. The cost of the 'envelopes' or prosthesis is over £100, accounting for a good proportion of this high cost.

Most clients who have received expert advice on improving their breast conditions through surgery seem to decide in its favour, and are usually delighted with the results.

DIAGNOSIS OF THE UNDERWEIGHT CLIENT

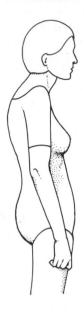

Kyphosis

The underweight client, though unusual, has particular problems, which, when recognized on the initial diagnosis, can be improved through treatment. A lack of body fat, angular and protruding bones, and general underdevelopment of muscles, all indicate an underweight problem. However appealing a *slim* figure may be, an *underweight* figure is not, and often appears a real worry to the client. To be too thin is not attractive or feminine, although normally perfectly healthy.

Often a total development programme is indicated if the figure generally is underdeveloped, with the chest flat and skinny, and the shoulder blades abducted. This ectomorph body type is often an example of **kyphosis**, with the rounded shoulders and sunken appearance of this condition. Light exercises can be advised to increase mobility in the shoulder girdle (see Chapter 4) and help the round shoulders.

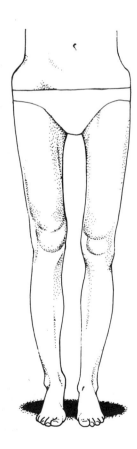

Very Thin Legs

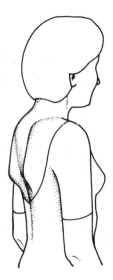

Shoulder Blades
Protruding

The thin person uses up food more efficiently than a larger individual, and will find it difficult to acquire body fat to pad the contours. If a diet planned to gain weight is not successful an alternative method of improving the figure shape (see Chapter 4) is through building muscular tissue to pad the angular nature of the bones. The diet should therefore be biased to contain foods for energy and tissue building, as well as to gain weight to help the muscle bulk to develop.

The weight and muscle has to be gained slowly and naturally so that it becomes permanent, and slowly builds a more attractive figure. By specific exercise and by eating body building proteins, curves can be developed where they are needed. In this way unwanted fat does not accumulate, and the attractive slim areas of the body can be retained, and built into the more rounded figure shape.

The exercises should not be too vigorous, so that they do not consume all the energy intake (food), but they must be specific enough to develop muscles in local areas. That means that strenuous exercise of the large muscle groups, particularly of the thighs and buttocks, must be avoided, but shape making muscles can be concentrated on. Chest muscles (pectorals and serratus anterior), those tapering the neck to the shoulders (trapezius and sterno mastoid), the postural muscles of the back, and if necessary calf and thigh muscles, can be built up.

Progressive resistance exercises are used to build the muscle bulk in these areas, so giving curves where none existed before. This form of exercise performed, using body weight, or dumbells as the resistance force, is very effective in building muscle fibres. As the strength of the muscles increase, so does the size, and this can be used to advantage, to give support to the breasts, round out the shoulder line, and give shape to the legs. When muscles are exercised systematically against gradually increasing weights the narrower fibres develop until they are as broad as the others. Wherever shapely curves are needed, strengthening exercises are essential, and form the only long term answer to the really underweight client.

Gaining Weight

As with all forms of correction however, other factors play their part, including diet for weight gain and vitality, and a relaxation programme to improve general respiratory and circulatory factors (see Chapter 3 **Gaining Weight**).

COMMON FIGURE
FAULTS

From careful diagnosis it becomes apparent that certain figure faults which are commonly seen, stem from life itself, and are as a result of natural events occurring throughout the life cycle. In women, childbearing, breast feeding, and the general domestic situation of family life, all take their toll on the youthful figure. Some figure conditions are so common they can hardly be termed faults, but are normal, however much disliked, at certain stages of life.

A chart showing several of the typical figure problems with which the therapist will have to deal daily may prove useful as an aid to diagnosis and choice of treatment.

Young Healthy Women

1. **Good figure,** but with out-of-proportion hips and thighs.

Controlled weight loss (diet), with specific reduction on heavy areas (with vacuum, plus faradism), backed up by active exercise.

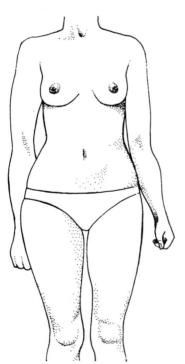

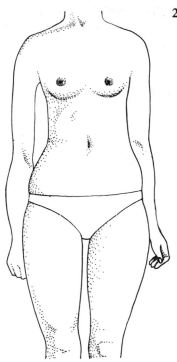

2. **Poor posture,** round shoulders, small bust, heavy hips, thighs, overall correct weight, figure out of proportion.

Posture correction, shoulder mobility exercises. Muscle building exercise, plus electrical contraction (faradism) for pectoralis major (chest).
Reduction of inches on hips and thighs, using vacuum, vibratory and faradism treatment. Sauna or heat therapy. (Local not general reduction.)

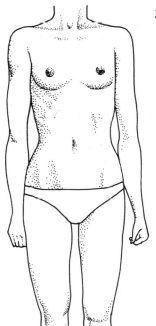

3. **Underweight client,** small breasts, angular bones, tense, highly strung disposition.

Relaxation therapy, breathing exercises. Modified diet, high fat and carbohydrate additions. Muscle development with natural progressive resistance exercises, and faradic contractions to build muscles. Isometric (static) muscle contraction work to build strength and stamina.

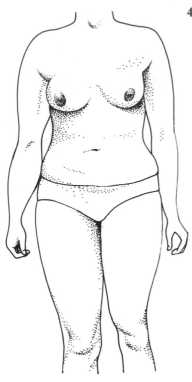

4. **General overweight condition,** with adipose deposits on hips, thighs and upper arms particularly.

General reduction diet, suited to life style, encouragement from salon treatment, supported by increased activity from sports and leisure activities.
Once weight loss is progressing, specific reduction treatments will increase results and help figure shaping. Faradism, vacuum, vibrating treatment and preheating.

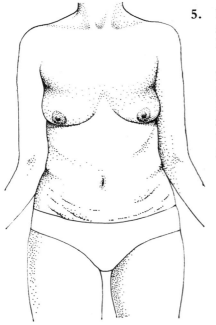

5. **Post-natal condition,** with distended abdominal area, bustline dropped, excess weight on hips, lower back and thighs.

Following medical post-natal care advise exercise to firm, tone and shorten abdominal muscles. Reduction diet suited to circumstances (modified if lactating). Muscle contraction for trunk and thighs and breasts. Vibratory and pulsed plus gliding vacuum for stubborn fat deposits.

Middle Age Clients

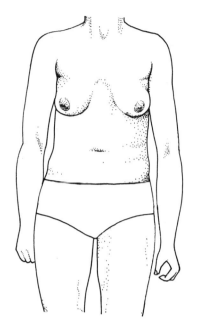

6. **Slightly overweight client,** about 2.70—3.60 kg (6—8 lb) – breasts becoming pendulous, middle trunk thickening, legs becoming varicosed, fluid retention problem on legs and abdominal area.

Modify diet, and encourage natural exercise to increase mobility and improve posture. Improve circulation with faradism, modified heat therapy, steam baths, and manual massage. Specific natural exercise for reduction of waistline, and uplift of bustline, reinforced by muscle contraction (faradism) to achieve fast results.

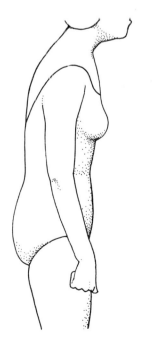

7. **Poor postural stance,** stooped, causing 'dowager's hump', forward head position, and low bustline, on client of correct weight. Out-of-proportion hips and thighs, with soft fat deposits.

Postural re-education required, plus specific local reduction on hips, and thighs.
Shoulder mobility exercises, bust improvement exercises, deep breathing and relaxation therapy advised for background support.
If not contra-indicated, vacuum massage plus faradism for hips and thighs. If contra-indicated, heat therapy (locally applied, lamps or paraffin wax) or generally given sauna or steam bath, followed by deep massage to improve circulation, and eliminate waste products.

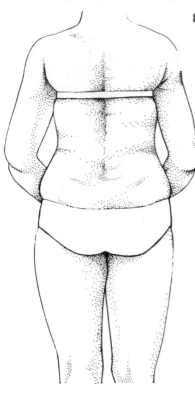

8. **General obesity,** with reduced mobility, weight on joints, causing stiffness, breathlessness and lack of vitality.

Medical consultation prior to beauty therapy treatment, to ascertain health. Medical or clinic reduction diet. As weight decreases, natural exercise, and postural exercises should be increased to tone and firm muscles.
Weight loss of about 1 kg (2lb) weekly aimed for.
Choosing treatments to speed results, and maintain morale, including vacuum and vibratory treatment initially, progressing to muscle contraction later.

Chapter 3

Diet – The First Step to Figure Improvement

It is not necessary for beauty therapists to be dieticians, nor should they try to be. However, a basic knowledge of nutrition is essential as part of the *total approach* to figure improvement, when reduction is required. It also makes it possible to interpret diet information for the client, in such a way that a plan can be individually tailored for her needs. The therapist has the time and opportunity to discuss diet problems during treatment, and is in a unique position to offer informed help and guidance.

Most reduction diets provide all the necessary food elements for good health, and would be successful if followed consistently. Many are not adhered to, however, and there are many reasons for this, including a low motivation to reduce, usually wrongly considered weak will power. Failure may be due to a feeling of being deprived, or stem from a dislike of the food ingredients contained in the diet. Many factors are involved, most of which can be overcome by a strong wish to succeed, and the encouragement of a caring and skilful therapist. From a greater knowledge of the client's life style, eating habits, and possible areas of temptation, the therapist can act as a reference point, guiding and encouraging along the path to the ideal weight. Although the actual weight loss has to be achieved through personal restraint, it is often instigated and maintained by the therapist, who acts as a pivot point for the overall improvement plan.

The study of dietetics, which uses food and drink to maintain health, can be utilized by the therapist to produce diet results for the clients. Understanding the value of different foods will enable a diet to be planned to include as many familiar well-liked foods as possible, without exceeding the total calorific value. Likes and dislikes in food are very important, as they restrict what can be planned into a diet; for few people will eat foods they have an aversion to, however good they may be for them. Changes in eating habits can be achieved slowly, particularly if associated with an evident improvement in looks and vitality. As man is a creature of habit, his way of living and eating cannot be changed instantly, but it can be modified and certain fattening elements replaced.

Illness often requires that a totally different diet is followed, and when medically prescribed will normally be adhered to, as the motivation to succeed is strong. Temptations for the dieter are many, with familiar patterns of eating, established over many years, being very difficult to break. Some are even handed down over the generations from family to family, until ill health or economies force a change. No wonder then, that the repetitious and limited diet plan, when offered, seems uninteresting and calculated to make the individual suffer.

Variety and adaptation are the keynotes to success in dieting, with the food chosen for its nutritional value, but also with regard to personal taste and the individual life style followed. Through conversation the therapist is able to learn a lot about the client's food tastes, and it is then possible to put this knowledge to good use in planning the diet.

It is a fact that people can differ in weight considerably, yet be on similar calorie intakes, and have similar build, occupation and interests. Accepting this fact it becomes important to know the client's actual food intake over a day or period, to determine the approximate calorific value. Then this total can be reduced or altered by a diet, or the body made to use it more efficiently through exercise and salon treatment. Both methods can produce a weight loss. Either decreasing the amount of food taken in, or increasing the amount of energy given out, will result in a more balanced weight level; for it is only when the needs of the body are over-supplied that the excess is stored as fat, and an overweight or obese condition results. If the needs or demands of the body are increased through greater activity, the stored fat is used up, utilized by the body for energy, heat and other vital processes.

Basics of a Sound Diet

The food consumed in the daily diet must be capable of providing an adequate supply of energy for the body's physical needs. It has also to permit the growth and maintenance of tissue, in its body building capacity, and be able to regulate body processes to maintain health.

Basically all the things needed for a healthy existence fall into six groups, the first four making up the bulk of the requirements.

Carbohydrates – which are essential for the production of heat and energy, and which help maintain body temperature

Fats – which constitute a reserve of heat and energy, and can be stored by the body.

Proteins – vital for growth and repair of body tissue.

Water – an essential constituent, forming 70% of body weight, involved with digestion, absorption, and circulatory systems.

Mineral Elements/Vitamins – Minute elements which, although having no energy value, are vital for good health as they control and regulate the processes in the body.

Energy Measurements

Until recently the energy content of food and fuels, and the energy output of the body and machines was measured by the same heat unit – the calorie. Now for nutritional purposes the *joule*, which is a unit of energy, replaces the *calorie*, which is a unit of heat. As this recommendation was adopted fairly recently, in 1972, the two measurements will continue to be used side by side for some time. In the case of the therapist's interpreting diet information for her client, it will be more convenient to continue to use calories for food measurement during discussion, for the time being. But as with many aspects of treatment, the information is converted into client language, which is easily understood and recognized.

The new measurements can be termed *energy values*, and the expression, *the energy content of foods* will replace *calorie content*. The body's needs likewise will be known as *energy intake*, rather than *calorie intake*. If the two forms of measurement are compared, it becomes easier to see how one will gradually supersede the other, in the therapist's calculations for her client's diet plans.

Calories

A calorie is the unit used for the measurement of the heat producing power of food. It is defined as the amount of heat required to raise one gram of water 1 degree centigrade.

1000 calories are represented as a kilocalorie, shown as kcal or Calories, with a large C.

Nutritionalists working in larger amounts will use this measurement more frequently, to calculate diet needs.

Joules

The joule (pronounced jool) is derived from the small calorie, by multiplying by 4.18.

So   4.18 J = 1 cal
4.18 kJ (kilo joules) = 1 kcal
4.18 mJ (megajoules) = 1000 kcal

As with other new measurements gradually being adopted in the weighing and measurement of clients, i.e., metric, using grams and kilograms, and centimetres and metres, it is preferable not to try to convert, but to try to *think in the new measurement.*

Approaching the new energy measurement in this way it is helpful to know the total energy needs of the individual, say 2500 kcal or 10 mJ, and work back from that point using it as a scale.

FOOD SOURCES OF ENERGY

Fats and carbohydrates are the main sources of energy in the body, and are also the most implicated in overweight problems. The amount and availability of food's energy or fuel-giving properties are shown as calories or joules per the gram(g). Fats are high at nine calories or 37 kJ per g, with carbohydrates and proteins being four calories per gram or 15 kJ/g and 17 kJ/g respectively.

Other food elements and water, although they have no calorific or energy value, add special effects to the body's digestion and metabolism. The balance of fats to proteins and carbohydrates in the diet should be carefully considered, and determined in relation to the person's age and occupation when deciding the total calorie or joule level. Individual needs can differ very widely, and if a large weight loss is required the client must be advised to consult her own doctor before starting the reduction plan.

It is not within the therapist's province to recommend diets for any purpose other than simple weight reduction, or addition, but rather to use her knowledge to reinforce readily available diet information for her clients. Whatever form the diet takes, it will always relate ultimately to energy or calorie levels, as these form a universal and easy form of measurement. Discovering what is the correct food intake can be difficult, but wherever an overweight condition exists, it is safe to assume energy intake is exceeding bodily output, and a reduction in food consumption (particularly in the so-called empty calories), is indicated. Sugars, fats and starchy foods, although so enjoyable to eat, can be cut from the diet, without any loss to health, if the basic diet is sound.

The body's needs differ throughout life, and at certain times more calories are needed to replace energy expended, or to meet a growth need. Childhood adolescence, and pregnancy are peak times for growth, and body building foods are required in larger quantities at these times. Periods of intense activity, training, stress, or increased responsibilities require a high calorific or energy level to be available in the food intake, otherwise a weight loss would result.

In reverse, there is the more common situation, where the body stores food that is in excess of its needs for present consumption. Because food is eaten not only for survival, but also because it is enjoyable, it is very easy to overeat and thus gain weight. This point is an important one for therapists, as simple over-indulgence is the major cause of overweight problems. Self-restraint is the only long term answer.

WEIGHT REDUCTION

Weight reduction, to be successful, relies on achieving a balance of all essential elements for health, whilst reducing total consumption of food. The diet has to ensure that the individual's calorific needs are not fully met by the food allowed, otherwise the weight would remain static. The object is to make the body burn up its own fat to meet its energy needs. Fat is stored mainly as a layer under the skin, padding body contours, and forming folds of *unattractive* flesh. It is also deposited between the body's organs, in excessive amounts, causing congestion and often resulting in poor digestion. Body fat is not lost quickly, and there has to be a considerable reduction in food intake to achieve a weight loss of approximately a kilo (2 lb), a week, and often half a kilo (1 lb) is a more realistic figure to aim for.

By reducing only certain foods in the diet, it is possible to ensure that only adipose (fatty) tissue is lost. Vital body building and tissue maintenance factors must be kept constant for good health, and this can be achieved by using a knowledge of the function of food in the body, to plan the diet. Food elements can be combined in the diet, so that they provide the most energy and nutritional value to the body, whilst speeding the reduction process.

Simply to stop eating so much would seem such an easy solution to make the unwanted weight disappear and, in a few cases, that is exactly what happens, and the therapist's job is done for her. Normally, however, the reduction is very hard to achieve, because of deeply ingrained attitudes to food and its preparation, as part of family and social life. In many countries hospitality is closely linked with food, and the practice of offering guests some refreshment is age old, and a serious hazard to the slimmer. Clients sometimes feel the restriction in their social life more keenly than restrictions in their diet, but it is possible to help them towards a programme which permits social eating and prevents them seeming a diet bore when in company. Such small points can decide the success or failure of a diet, particularly for women who enjoy an active social life.

The reduction diet has to gradually re-educate the eating habits of the client, and attempt to establish new tastes to replace the familiar fattening pattern. Protein foods should take the place of carbohydrate foods as much as possible, with as little fat as is possible used in cooking. Cravings for sweet foods can be satisfied by fruits and low calorie beverages, with artificial sweeteners used in tea and coffee. The client should be encouraged to spread out her food intake over the day, and to take as much exercise as possible to balance her weight. Any sport, or general activity such as walking is useful, as long as the extra appetite it creates is not satisfied by carbohydrate elements. This vicious circle effect often happens with young women if they become over zealous in their activity programmes, and they can experience real hunger.

Overall, the aim is to create a sound diet that will bring about a weight loss, without feelings of fatigue, hunger or being deprived in any way. In fact a well-balanced diet should not seem deficient, but appear to be offering a wider choice of foods. This does rely on more careful choice and preparation of food, and here the client's interest has to be encouraged to obtain the degree of involvement necessary for diet success. Some women, particularly busy mothers, do not feel they warrant this amount of attention, or are justified in having different meals from their families. With a therapist's advice and personal interest in their progress, they will soon develop a different outlook, and see the advantages of improved looks and increased vitality to the whole family unit.

Guidance on food choice, preparation, and adaptation to fit diet and social needs, *does* come within the therapist's field of reference, and it will be a major factor in achieving diet success. The therapist has a valuable contribution to make through diet guidance, as part of the total approach to figure improvement.

NUTRITION

A full study of nutrition, being extremely complex, is outside the scope of this book, and it will only be possible to touch briefly on the main points of importance. However, some guidance of how nutritional knowledge can be employed for diet planning should prove useful. This may also give insight into reasons for diet success or failure, which is of tremendous practical relevance to the therapist's work.

Nutrition is the process whereby the body absorbs food and converts it into substances needed for life. A normal varied diet should provide all the substances needed for health, apart from increased mineral and vitamin requirements during pregnancy (particularly iron and calcium). Clients on a very restricted food range, or who dislike certain important food sources, such as fruit or vegetables or meat, may also suffer from deficiences in their diet. Appetite normally ensures enough food is taken in: unfortunately it does not also act to tell when food needs are being oversupplied, and a weight surplus will result. When overweight conditions arise, carbohydrates are the first food element to be restricted in the diet, as they are often consumed in larger amounts than required.

Many foods consist of more than one element: for example, cheese, which contains protein, for body building, mineral elements (calcium and phosphorus), is also a first class source of energy. Easily available and suitable for a wide range of dishes, cheese is an excellent food for the slimmer. In fact milk, cheese, eggs, meat, and fish all have good dietary value, but surprisingly it is difficult to get them all accepted as part of a normal diet; for the study of nutrition is very involved with taste and what people will accept in their diet. The liking for starchy and sweet foods in the advanced countries of the world is a major factor in the overweight conditions that are so common at the present time. Apart from being unattractive, obesity constitutes a hazard to health, and is implicated in many diseases.

Carbohydrates

Carbohydrate foods – sugar, bread, potatoes, cereals, cakes and sweets, are so well-liked and easy to eat. They are enjoyable in taste, but unfortunately short term in energy giving power, and very inclined to be stored as adipose (fatty) tissues in the body. Carbohydrates do have an important role as suppliers of readily available energy, and for some very active occupations are needed in large quantities, as they are quickly burnt up to meet physical demands. If carbohydrates were used as a major source of calories or energy in the slimmer's food intake, severe problems of hunger or fatigue would result, and the diet would be broken.

Apart from obvious sources of carbohydrates, there are several other ways it can be obtained, including vegetables, fruits, liver, shellfish, and a small amount in meat. So if sweet elements were omitted from the slimmer's diet, there would still remain an adaquate amount to supply all the carbohydrate needs of the body. By using fruits and vegetables rather than sweet, starchy foods, the digestion as well as the weight loss would benefit. Plant cell wall products, often called cellulose, although having no energy value, speed food substances through the body, keeping the system regular and preventing constipation. Dieters who are unused to eating natural fruits, should have this benefit explained to them, as constipation can be a problem in diet regimes, when the system is adjusting to less food bulk.

Summary   Carbohydrates are organic foods and foodstuffs, composed of the elements carbon, hydrogen, and oxygen, with an energy or fuel value of 4 kcal/g (16 kJ/g). They are:

1   Essential for the production of heat and energy, and help to maintain body temperature.

2   Necessary for the metabolism of fat, and full utilization of proteins. If too little carbohydrates are taken, fats are only partly broken down and the result is toxic substances being excreted by the kidneys. Carbohydrate taken with protein increases its body building capacities.

3   Plant cell wall products (cellulose), stimulate the bowel and help prevent constipation.

Proteins

Proteins are essential for maintenance of the cells which make up the body. They also supply long-lasting forms of energy, and manufacture hormones – chemical messengers which regulate the activities of the body. There are many forms of proteins, and it is ideal nutritional practice that these should be mixed in the diet, for variety, their food value and general economy. On digestion with enzymes in the gastric, pancreatic and intestinal juices, proteins are broken down into their components parts and are known as amino acids.

Proteins are generally known as first class, being the proteins of milk, eggs, meat, fish and cheese: second class being that obtained from cereals, nuts and vegetables. This classification does, however, present a false picture, as in fact the protein value or quality stays constant, though the percentage present in certain foods is less, so a greater quantity of the food would have to be consumed to gain the same protein quota. It is possible to obtain sufficient protein value from these so called second class proteins only, as in the case of vegetarians or vegans, but the sheer bulk of food needed might cause overweight problems.

High protein diets are very popular, and do seem to sustain the slimmer from suffering real hunger. When examined closely these diets are in fact more low carbohydrate, than high protein, as the actual amount of protein present and able to be used by the body is fairly low in many foods. Eggs have 11%, hard cheese 25—35%, and cooked fish and meat 17—24% and 20—32% respectively. It can be easily seen why these foods play such a large part in the slimmer's diet, being palatable, sustaining, and socially acceptable.

However, it is essential that some of the protein, a quarter at least, should be eaten with a carbohydrate food source, otherwise it cannot fulfil its body building capacity, due to its digestion in the body. Without the carbohydrate link, the protein would be used by the body purely as an energy source, and would be used up wastefully, with detriment to physical health.

To choose foods which are made up of both protein and carbohydrate seems ideal for reduction, so it is useful to discover the chemical composition of as many popular foods as possible.

Summary   Proteins are organic foods and are extremely complex in structure. All are composed of carbon, nitrogen, oxygen, hydrogen, and sulphur, with some containing phosphorous in addition. Proteins yield 4 kcal/g (17 kJ/g), this being the level the body is able to utilize safely, although when measured scientifically outside the body, its heat or energy power is much higher. Protein is available as first or second class, and is essential for:

1   Growth and repair of body tissue, particularly in childhood, and after illness.

2 Formation of hormones, which regulate the secretions of the body, sweat, tears, etc.

3 Maintaining body temperature, through its stimulating effect on metabolism.

4 Sustaining energy levels.

Fats

Fats are the most readily available and cheap form of energy giving foods, with a high calorific or energy value. Eaten in moderation they give taste and flavour to a diet, and when restricted from the food intake, are badly missed. This is not only because of habit, but due also to the fact that the amount of fat in the food determines the feeling of satisfaction experienced at the end of a meal. This lasting effect of the food consumed is an important point for slimmers, and is one reason why very low fat diets can give the feeling of not having eaten enough. The appetite is not satisfied, even if the body's actual needs are! It is foolhardy to disregard this problem, as it is often the slimmer's downfall. Planning a certain amount of fat into the diet, therefore, has a dual purpose: that of energy provision, and to avoid hunger pangs, imaginary or otherwise.

Fat can be stored in the body and, like carbohydrate, when digested is converted into fatty acids which can be used by the body, like a reserve. A certain amount of body fat is essential, as it insulates and reduces heat loss, and acts to protect vital organs from injury. When a client commences a reduction diet, the reserves of fatty tissue are reduced, and if these are not replaced, a change in weight and shape will result.

The correct quantities of fat in the diet are necessary to aid general digestion, and help the absorption of vitamins. Due to the very large amounts of fats taken in the diet, it is possible to reduce the total for weight reduction without detriment to health. Foods containing a high fat percentage, or cooked in fat, or the actual dairy foods themselves are so popular that a deficiency is seldom likely to occur. Changing the method by which food is cooked, for example grilling instead of frying fish, drastically reduces the fat content of the diet. Severely fat free diets are not recommended however, unless on medical advice, as problems of fatigue, and poor skin healing and dryness could result. Practical considerations such as these are of importance to the therapist, as it is her responsibility to ensure her client's skin is supple enough to cope with the inches reduction, without becoming slack and wrinkled. Drastic reduction in the mature woman presents this problem very frequently, and little can be done to remedy the condition once established.

Fats are obtained from butter, margerine, oils, suet, milk, cream cheese and bacon, and yield a high calorific or energy value for very little bulk. Meat is also an important source of fat, though it is usually considered for its protein value.

Summary

Fats are composed of carbon, hydrogen, and oxygen and are of organic origin. They have the highest yield of calories, 9 kcal/g (37 kJ/g), making them twice as effective as an energy source as proteins or carbohydrates. Fats are mainly available as dairy produce, and are essential when large demands for energy are placed on the body. They plan an important part even in the slimmer's diet, in moderate amounts because they:

1   Are the most valuable form of heat (energy) and can be stored in the body for future use.
2   Protect and support various tissues and organs in the body, i.e., kidneys, and nerves.
3   Help vitamins to be absorbed.
4   Help prevent the loss of body heat.
5   Act to prevent a feeling of hunger, as they are slow to be digested and absorbed.
6   Add calories (joules) without adding bulk to the diet.

Water

Although not a food element, the importance of water as a factor in the diet should be considered to maintain the body's hydric balance. The body has the capacity to balance its total amount of fluid, keeping it constant by retaining sufficient fluid from the food and drink consumed. Most foods have a high percentage of water, which the body is able to use in this way.

Some two-thirds of the body weight in adults is water with, surprisingly, fat having the lowest percentage of water of all the body tissues, at only 10%. In fat people the proportion of water in the body is lower than in thin people, because fat contains so little water. Fluid lost in turkish or sauna baths (around ½—1 kg (1—2 lb) a session), is soon recouped by the body, but does help to encourage the dieter, and acts to make her adhere to the diet that will really achieve the weight reduction.

In a reduction diet clients should not be encouraged to restrict their fluid intake unless it is coupled with an excessive consumption of tea or coffee, taken with milk and sugar. Half size cups can be suggested, and use of artificial sweeteners. This normally cuts down the total consumed, as when they are not enjoyed, only the quantity required to answer thirst needs is consumed. Thirst acts naturally to keep the body's fluid level correct, and as long as the urge to drink is not satisfied with carbohydrate beverages, all will be well.

MINERAL ELEMENTS AND VITAMINS

Although these produce no energy value, they are important for maintaining health and are vital for existence. In a normal varied diet there should be no deficiency, apart from possibly iron and calcium during pregnancy and lactation.

A brief look at their effects in the body rounds out the picture presented of a sound diet, because without their inclusion many normal body processes would not occur. Both the mineral elements and vitamins aid in catalysing the reactions of the body, and their presence can be seen at work in a wide range of body processes. Deficiences can result in the food consumed not being fully utilized by the body, so that nutrient values are not extracted. So a successful reduction diet must be checked to see that it does contain sufficient of these elements, to make full use of the smaller total quota of food permitted.

The careful choice of foods in the reduction diet should ensure that all mineral elements and vitamins are present in the right quantities, and no artifical supplements are needed. Only in the case of individual aversion to particularly rich sources of mineral elements or vitamins, such as fish, fruit or milk, will vitamin pills be necessary. Most vitamins taken in this form are excreted in the urine, if they are in excess to the body's needs, so if clients want to take them, there is no reason why they should not.

With the lack of carbohydrates and fats in normal quantities in the slimmer's diet, the food is likely to taste more bland and unpalatable. So it is possible to use known sources of minerals and vitamins to add flavour and variety to the diet. Some of the tastes may have to be acquired, but can be very valuable if accepted, not only to help affect a weight loss, but as part of the total re-education of the eating pattern. Fresh fruits, vegetables, and peppers in salads are some examples, as they give bulk to the diet, have low calorie levels and supply many of the body's mineral and vitamin needs.

Both mineral elements and vitamins are extremely complex in structure and function, and have widely differing sources, being scattered throughout the whole food range. A brief survey completes the knowledge of a sound diet and includes:

MINERAL ELEMENTS
(often referred to as salts)

Calcium

Required by the body in conjunction with phosphorus for the formation of bones and teeth, it is also important for muscular activity. Calcium can only be absorbed in the body in the presence of Vitamin D, without which the calcium, although taken in through food, is unable to be used and passes through the body. Calcium is a good example of a mineral element important for both structure and function of the body. The normal levels of calcium required, usually obtained from milk, would need to be supplemented in pregnancy and lactation. This could take the form of cheese, cabbage, and bread (fortified with chalk).

Phosphorus

Phosphorus is an essential constituent of all cells, and enters into the composition of bone minerals. Foods taken for their calcium content will also ensure that the phosphorus level will be adaquate. Milk, cheese, and fish all have a high phosphorus content, and a deficiency in this element would be very rare.

Iron

Necessary for all tissues in the body, and essential for the formation of red blood cells, in combination with haemoglobin. Women require more iron in their diet, through inevitable losses from the menstrual flow of blood. Iron deficiency anaemia is a fairly common problem in women, and should be considered particularly when planning diet regimes for women of childbearing years. The demands for iron from the foetus during pregnancy, and the blood loss associated with the actual birth, are very difficult to make up by dietary means. The body takes a long time to make up any iron loss, and functions on a very small store, so every opportunity to add iron rich foods to the diet should be used. Found in liver, red meat, green vegetables, dried fruits and fish, iron has an important contribution to make to overall health and vitality.

Iodine

Acts as a controlling force on the thyroid gland, forming thyroxine through a complicated series of processes. It is stored in the thyroid gland, and exerts an influence on the metabolic rate. Its presence in the diet prevents goitre, and associated thyroid deficiency conditions. Available from sea foods, watercress, onions, and vegetables grown on soils containing iodine.

Sodium

Sodium in the form of common salt regulates the water content of the body. Excess sodium is excreted in the urine and sweat, and a deficiency, as with excessive sweating in a hot country or through heavy work, can be corrected by drinking salt water, or taking salt tablets.

Potassium

Potassium is essential for the functioning of striated and unstriated muscle tissue and for nervous tissue. Without its presence the heart could not beat. The balance of potassium in the body is regulated by the kidneys, and as most foods contain an abundance of this element, a deficiency is unlikely.

Trace Elements

Present in minute quantities in the body, their actions on the body processes range from cellular function, to helping food taken in to be fully utilized and absorbed within the digestion process. Some elements appear to be unnecessary to humans, whilst others are important. Further research may reveal the purpose of these elements, which include: aluminium, arsenic, boron, cobalt, copper, fluorine, molybdenum, nickel, selenium, silicon, and zinc.

VITAMINS

There are at least 13 vitamins concerned with human nutrition, and these are available from a wide variety of foods. Some are fat soluble, others water soluble, but a varied diet should contain all the known vitamins needed for health, unless they are destroyed by poor cooking.

A brief outline of those vitamins, which are of practical importance in diet plans, include:

Vitamin A

Vitamin A is available from liver, liver oils, dairy produce, and as carotene from carrots and green vegetables. Vitamin A and carotene are fat soluble, and are not lost through boiling in water, or through most methods of cooking, so a deficiency is unlikely. An actual deficiency would be detectable as night blindness, or poor vision in dim light. Vitamin A is very important for skin health, and for maintaining the epithelial tissue in the respiratory and urogenital tracts. It is also involved with the growth of bone tissue, and the regulation of the nervous system.

Vitamin A helps the body in its fight against disease, and used to be known as the anti-infective vitamin, because of its effects.

Vitamin B (group)

This group of vitamins has widely differing tasks, the most important being its ability to free the energy from foods, making it available and able to be used by the body. Three of the group are of interest to the therapist, Vitamin B_1 or Thiamin, B_2 or Riboflavin and Niacin or Nicotinic Acid.

Vitamin B_1 or Thiamin

Vitamin B_1 is widely distributed among foods, nearly always in small amounts. Main sources are pork, offal, cod roe, wheat germ and oatmeal. Without thiamin the body is unable to completely oxidise glucose to carbon dioxide and water, where its energy is liberated. Muscular weakness and degeneration of the nerves results, into the condition termed beri-beri, which is still evident in some eastern parts of the world.

Vitamin B_2 or Riboflavin

Essential for human metabolism as it plays a part in the oxidation of glucose in the cell. The amount required relates to the amount of carbohydrate consumed, and a deficiency could result if the bulk of the energy requirements were being met by a carbohydrate source. As this is the case with some overweight individuals eating sugary, starchy foods, some provision should be made to ensure an adequate supply. When the diet is replanned to eliminate the high carbohydrate intake, the problem will disappear, like the excess weight. Sources of Riboflavin include liver, milk, butter, egg yolk, cheese, and skimmed milk powder. A weekly portion of liver goes a long way to supply Vitamin B_2 requirements, and should be built into a reduction diet if at all possible.

Niacin or Nicotinic Acid

Like Thiamin and Riboflavin it plays a part in the release of energy from food. A shortage leads to muscular weakness, mental and digestive disorders, and the condition known as Pellagra. Sources of Niacin are bread, meat, nuts, liver, yeast, meat extracts and whole grain cereals.

Vitamin C or Ascorbic Acid

This vitamin is perhaps best known of all the vitamins, from its history of preventing scurvy, during the sailors' undertaking of long sea voyages, when they obtained it from lemons, oranges and other fresh fruits. It is indeed a most important vitamin, as it assists in the formation of the connective tissue in the body, and helps the absorption of iron from food in the intestine. Available from new potatoes, blackcurrants, soft fruits (raspberries, etc.) citrus fruits, certain apples (Bramleys seedling), gooseberries, and raw cabbage and peppers (a good source in diet salads). It is necessary to have a regular intake of Vitamin C, and to make sure that foods chosen for their Vitamin C content do not lose that beneficial element by poor cooking. Vitamin C is very sensitive to losses through cooking, particularly in water, and food should be cooked for the minimum time possible, ideally in small batches at a high temperature. Foods cooked in fat do not lose the Vitamin C content so badly, but of course the ideal is to eat as many foods raw as possible.

Vitamin D

Important for the formation of sound bones and teeth, in combination with calcium. Shortage of Vitamin D and the effects of poor diet can cause rickets, a condition of improper calcification (hardening) of the bones in children. Rickets is a result of defective intake of calcium and phosphorus, and faulty deposition of these elements in the bones, owing to a lack of Vitamin D. Even adaquate supplies of calcium will not be effective, without the presence of Vitamin D.

Vitamin D is available from

two sources ⟨ Food / Sunlight

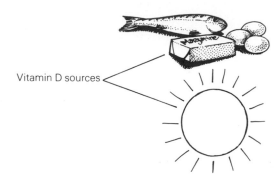

Vitamin D sources

From food it is obtained from fatty fish, cod liver oil, eggs, and enriched margarine. It is not easily lost in cooking or food storage, but needs to be protected from heat to prevent the oils turning rancid. The body is able to store Vitamin D in the liver, so the correct amount required can be arranged into a weekly diet plan, unlike Vitamin C which has to be obtained in daily doses.

The body is able to produce its own form of Vitamin D from the sun through a complicated series of processes, on the skin's surface. This means that the skin has to be exposed to sunlight for the Vitamin D to be produced. Housebound women, or those who from religious dictates have to keep their skin covered, are unable to gain in this way, and cases of rickets have been found in present times, particularly amongst the children of Hindu and Moslem families. Artificial forms of sunlight (ultra violet exposure) produce the same effects.

METABOLISM AND DIGESTION

The way the body is able to make use of the food it takes in and utilize it for energy, growth, and general health is termed *metabolism*. The process by which the food is actually broken down from its complete and complex form, into a state by which it can be absorbed into the blood stream is known as *digestion*. The two processes are bound to be inter-related, with any change in the digestion being reflected in the metabolism of the body. Strains placed upon the digestion, due to excessive food consumption or an unbalanced diet, will quickly alter the way in which the body can make use of the food eaten. An overweight person can also be poorly nourished, due to faulty metabolism caused by the excessive weight gained.

A fuller knowledge will show that it is not only important to have a well-balanced diet, but it is also necessary for the food to be eaten in the right combinations for diet success. The process of digestion shows clearly as well the value of eating a little and often, if the system is not to be overloaded. The manner in which foods act together to release their energy or nutrient value is important for diet guidance, and to ensure maximum benefit is gained nutritionally from the reduced food intake. This makes sure the client gets the most out of the food allowed on her diet.

To know something as well of how the body stores fat as a reserve, is to have the key to reversing the process, through a modified diet. The greater the understanding of how the body deals with the food taken in, the more easily the therapist will be able to plan successful diets, suited to the client's needs.

The body uses or metabolizes basic food elements in two general ways: it **catabolizes** them to release their stored energy for work, and **anabolizes** them for building protoplasm (cellular growth and maintenance), and to manufacture enzymes, hormones and other essential body compounds. Anabolism is dependent on catabolism, and relies on it for the energy to accomplish its own vital role. Cell growth, repair, and reproduction (mitosis) are achieved through the process of anabolism. The body has to supply energy from food for work activity, muscular actions, and to produce heat; but to sustain adequate general health, these other background processes have also to be maintained.

Carbohydrates are the body's preferred fuel, and only when glucose (a final stage of digestion) is not available in sufficient quantities, will the body cells turn to fats, and then lastly protein. This prevents the body from using up its own muscular strength when on a restricted food intake. Stored fat is used up (subcutaneous adipose tissue) rather than muscle fibres. Only in cases of illness or starvation (enforced or self-inflicted as in anorexia nervosa) will actual wasting of muscles and body tissues result, due to this inbuilt safeguard.

When the body's needs have been met, excess glucose in the blood is converted to fat (mainly by liver cells) and is stored in the body's fat depots as adipose tissue. Unfortunately the amount that can be stored by the body is almost limitless, and as obesity does not totally incapacitate the individual, its risks to health are often underestimated.

METABOLISM

The body needs a nutritious and varied diet to meet its living and working requirements and, depending on the person's size and way of life, it is possible to calculate their energy needs. Individuals vary considerably in how they expend energy, and the slim, highly strung client is one example of this difference: taking in far more than her fair share of food, yet staying in energy balance (at a constant weight). Unfortunately most people do not have such an efficient metabolism, able to move on unwanted calories, to be excreted by the body or used up in nervous tension. Most clients store any additional calories not needed immediately by the body as fat under the skin, ready for future use. Without an increase in activity or reduction of food intake, an overweight problem quickly results.

Basal Metabolic Rate (BMR)

The amount of fuel (food) needed to fulfil the daily activities can be calculated, based on the surface area of the body. The calculation is based on normal living requirements (BMR) and the energy needed for work. The BMR is defined as the energy output when the body is at complete rest (not asleep), 12 hours after a meal (so no digestion is taking place) and in a warm room (so no energy is used keeping warm). This rather artificial definition is useful, however, as it gives guidance as to the food required for background living or existence. Surprisingly two-thirds of the body's total dietary needs are to meet the demands of this background living activity in most people. Apart from extremely active workers who expend a large part of their food intake in physical work, the average person uses only about a third of total food intake in work calories or joules. So increasing activity in work is only going to have a small effect on body weight. If exercise is to be involved with reduction, to burn up stored fat, it will need to be sustained with every aspect of daily life increased in activity.

An average BMR can be calculated from a person's height and weight, with regard to their sex, age, and environment. As people grow older their BMR falls by about 5% every 10 years. In the same way food energy needed for work decreases as movements become more efficient and the work is accomplished more economically in terms of energy expenditure. Unless there is a corresponding decrease in food intake, an overweight problem or obesity will result.

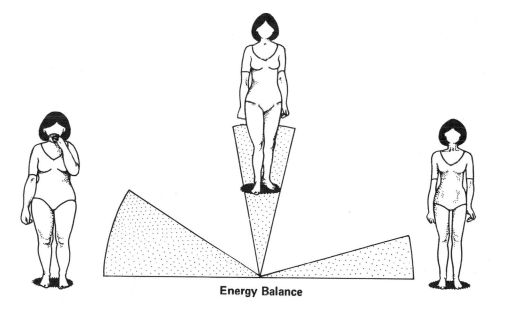

Energy Balance

Individual metabolism varies considerably, with certain people being prone to surplus weight, whilst others have a job to maintain sufficient body weight. Sometimes obesity itself causes metabolic malfunction, due to the strain placed upon the body's systems. Certain illnesses affect metabolism, and so alter body weight, sometimes drastically. A noticeable increase or loss of body weight which occurs *without* a change in food intake, indicates the need for medical attention.

This point is of importance to therapists when dealing with overweight clients, as very rarely the obesity may be due to a physical condition or disease such as a thyroid abnormality or endocrine disorder.

Most weight problems, however, are connected with an excess of food over the needs of the body, whatever they might be. Having a metabolism which stores rather than burns up fat is unfortunate, but rather than bemoaning the fact clients should be helped towards realizing a solution. Eating little and often, to stir the metabolism into action, is one useful eating pattern found beneficial to the overweight. Reducing the 'empty' calories content of a diet, (the carbohydrates, sugars, etc.) and replacing these with proteins and moderate amounts of fat is another way to increase metabolism. It also ensures that the best value is obtained from the food eaten, in nutritional terms.

Generally increased activity in all forms of daily life will also help the reduction programme, and get a lethargic system into action. Improved digestion and more regular bowel movements will increase the feelings of general fitness and vitality and should encourage a more positive approach to controlling and reducing the weight programme.

DIGESTION

Food used to supply the body's needs comes in a wide variety of forms, some readily available to the tissues, others requiring further digestive action to make them useful for growth or energy. Food classes such as proteins and carbohydrates must be broken down (hydrolised) into a form small enough to be absorbed into the blood stream. Digestion is the process where complex food structures are broken down into their simple forms and made available to the body.

THE DIGESTIVE SYSTEM

The digestive system consists of:

1   The alimentary canal.

2   Glands secreting digestive juices that act upon the food matter.

The Alimentary Canal

The alimentary canal is a passage over 9 m (30 ft) long leading from the mouth to the rectum. It is lined throughout with mucous membrane which lubricates the system. Muscular walls act upon the foodstuff eaten, and help its passage along the alimentary canal. The alimentary canal consists of:

the **mouth,** the **pharynx,** the **oesophagus,** the **stomach,** the **small intestine,** the **large intestine.**

The glands are:

(*i*)   **The Salivary glands** – secreting saliva in the mouth.

(*ii*)   **The Gastric glands** – secreting gastric juices in the stomach.

(*iii*)   **The Pancreas** – secreting pancreatic juice in the duodenum.

(*iv*)   **The Liver** – secreting bile in the duodenum.

(*v*)   **Intestinal glands** – secreting intestinal juice in the small intestine.

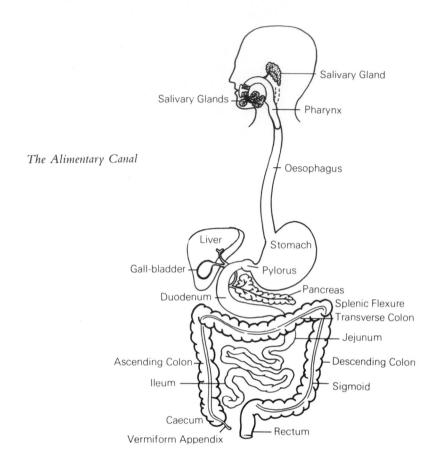

The Alimentary Canal

Salivary Gland

Salivary Glands

Pharynx

Oesophagus

Liver

Stomach

Gall-bladder

Pylorus

Duodenum

Pancreas

Splenic Flexure

Transverse Colon

Jejunum

Ascending Colon

Descending Colon

Ileum

Sigmoid

Caecum

Rectum

Vermiform Appendix

STRUCTURE OF THE DIGESTIVE SYSTEM

The Mouth

The digestive system commences at the mouth, where food is ground up, masticated, and diluted with saliva. Together the teeth and tongue break up the food into smaller portions, ready to move further down the alimentary canal. Present within the saliva is an enzyme called **ptyalin**, which commences the process of starch digestion, into sugar. Saliva also moistens the food and makes it alkaline in reaction. Appetite and hunger both provoke saliva to be secreted in the mouth, aiding the digestion process. Unappetizing food may seem more difficult to get down, due to this lack of natural salivary juices, normally induced in response to taste buds in the mouth.

The 32 teeth of an adult are arranged in two sets, 16 in the upper jaw (maxilla), and the lower jaw (mandible). There are four types of teeth: incisors (chisel shaped), canine (pointed crown), premolars (two projections) and molars (four or five projections).

The set consists of an arrangement so:

Molars	Premolars	Canines	Incisors	Canines	Premolars	Molars
3	2	1	4	1	2	3

This being the jaw formation on the top and bottom.

Each tooth is made up of three parts, the crown, the root, and the neck. The crown protrudes from the gum, whilst the roots are like fangs embedded in the gum. The neck area joins the crown and the root. Each tooth is made up of dentine – the hard bony substance, enamel – an even harder substance which covers the dentine in the crown, and dental pulp – which fills the centre of each tooth. The dental pulp also contains the nerve endings and blood vessels which nourish the tooth.

Teeth are extremely important as part of the digestion process, permitting a wide range of differing food textures to be consumed and prepared for later stages of absorption. Clients who wear dentures may find it more difficult to cope with hard foods and their digestion may suffer from a lack of roughage in the diet. Constipation may become a problem if only soft, easily swallowed foods make up the bulk of the diet.

The Pharynx

At the back of the mouth lies the pharynx, which is about 13 cm (5 in.) long and leads backwards from the mouth. It has three areas – the naso-pharynx, which lies mostly behind the nose and has nothing to do with digestion: the oral-pharynx, shared by both air and food, at the back of which lie the tonsils which are two masses of lymphatic tissue and which help to fight bacteria present in food: and the larygeal pharynx, which merges with the oesophagus.

When food is swallowed the pharynx contracts, forcing the food downwards into the oesophagus. At the same time the nasal passages are blocked, the soft palate rises, and the larynx rises up under the epiglottis, closing the trachea (windpipe). Choking occurs when these processes are not co-ordinated.

The Oesophagus

This is a collapsible muscular tube about 25—30 cm (10—12 in.) long, leading from the pharynx to the stomach, behind the trachea and heart, through the diaphragm. The muscular tube is made up of voluntary and involuntary muscle fibres, with the outer layers laid longitudinally and the inner layers placed in a circular fashion. Through this muscular formation a wave-like movement is formed (termed peristaltic movement) which drives the food into the stomach.

The Stomach

A muscular, bag-like, organ, placed high on the left side of the abdominal cavity, beneath the diaphragm. Its size and shape adjusts according to its contents. At either end of the stomach are control mechanisms which permit or restrict the movement of food into or out of the stomach. The upper part is guarded by a valve called the cardiac sphincter, and the lower end, which narrows to lead to the duodenum has the pyloric sphincter to control the exit of the food matter.

The stomach is made up of several coats, outermost being the peritoneum, which prevents friction between the organs of the abdominal cavity. Next a muscular layer, then a submucous layer, which is made up of connective tissue and is rich in blood vessels. Then, forming the stomach lining, is the mucous layer which has the capacity to expand and contract, according to the food consumed. The convoluted surface of the inner stomach provides a greater surface area for the secretion of acid gastric juices to work on the food, until it becomes liquid in consistency and has been neutralized.

Protein digestion commences in the stomach, with proteins becoming peptones. The gastric juice contains the ferments pepsin, rennin, and hydrochloric acid, which is antiseptic in action, and provides the correct medium (atmosphere) for the digestive juices to work in. The food is churned with strong muscular movements and leaves the stomach in a series of gushes. Certain foodstuffs are absorbed directly from the stomach, including water, alcohol, and glucose.

The stomach also has another important task, that of producing the anti anaemic factor, which controls the formation of blood cells in the bone marrow.

Small Intestine

This part of the digestive tract leads from the stomach to the large intestine and is between 6—7.4 m (20—24 ft) in length, all of which has to fit in the abdominal area. It has three distinct parts, the duodenum, the jejunum and the ileum.

The duodenum is the first part of the small intestine and is fixed to the back of the abdominal wall by peritoneum. It is approximately 24 cm (10 in.) long and curves like a letter C. Lying within the curve of the C is a large gland called the pancreas. The jejunum and the ileum make up most of the total length and lie to the front of the abdominal cavity. The structure of the walls of the small intestine is similar to the stomach walls, but internally its formation is different. This is in order to equip it to carry out its job of digestion and absorbtion of food more efficiently. The internal lining is puckered and covered with hair-like projections which are called villi.

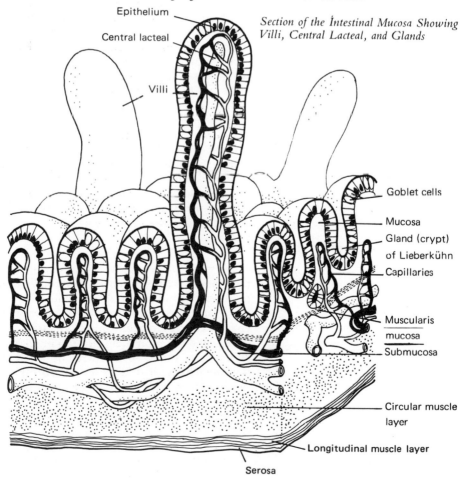

Section of the Intestinal Mucosa Showing Villi, Central Lacteal, and Glands

Epithelium

Central lacteal

Villi

Goblet cells

Mucosa

Gland (crypt) of Lieberkühn

Capillaries

Muscularis mucosa

Submucosa

Circular muscle layer

Longitudinal muscle layer

Serosa

These are concerned with the absorption of food and contain minute blood and lymphatic vessels, and small glands which secrete intestinal juices.

Within the small intestine digestion takes place of protein, carbohydrate, and fats. This is accomplished under the influence of three forms of digestive juice, namely *pancreatic juice* from the pancreas, *bile* from the liver, and a juice from the small intestine called *succus entericus*. The digestion which occurs is absorbed into the blood stream lower down the small intestine. Protein continues its process of digestion down to amino acids, carbohydrates finally into simple sugars (glucose), and fats become glycerine and fatty acids, which after absorption travel to the liver. Here they may be oxidized for energy, used by the muscles in activity, or stored in the body as fat tissue (adipose tissue).

The Large Intestine

The last stage of the alimentary tract begins at the ileum and ends at the rectum. It is about 1.5 m (5 ft) in length and has three parts, the ascending, transverse, and descending colon. The first part consists of a lined pouch called the ceacum from which extends the vermiform appendix.

The remainder of food undigested, plus roughage and unabsorbed digestive juices pass into the large intestine in a liquid form. Water is absorbed in the large intestine, and the faeces are formed. In the large intestine are a lot of resident bacteria which normally do not cause disease (bacillus coli). In cases of constipation or diarrhoea the residual food matter passes too slowly or quickly through the largest intestine, and too much or little water is absorbed.

The Digestive Juices

Enzymes present in the substances secreted by the glands of the alimentary tract have the power to convert food material into a simple form, able to be absorbed into the blood stream. Different enzymes have different digestive tasks to accomplish, depending on their location in relation to the alimentary canal. They accomplish their role without changing their own form, but can only work effectively if in the right medium or atmosphere.

Each part of the alimentary tract has different enzymes within its digestive juices:

ENZYMES WITHIN THE DIGESTIVE TRACT

Location	Secretion	Enzyme	Aspect of Digestion
Mouth	Saliva	Amylase	Cooked starch → maltose
Stomach	Gastric juice	Pepsin Rennin Hydrochloric acid	Protein → peptones
Liver	Bile salts	Assists lipase (from pancreas)	Fats (first stage of digestion)

Pancreas	Pancreatic juice	Lipase
		
		Trypsin
		Chymotrypsin
		Amylase
			Fats → mono and di-
			glycerides
			  and fatty acids
			Peptones (protein) →
			  poly peptides
			Starch (carbohydrate) →
			Maltose

Small intestine		Succus entericus Peptidase Maltase Lactase Sucrase	Poly peptides → amino acids Maltose → glucose Lactose → glucose and galactose Sucrose → glucose and fructose

OBESITY

Obesity is a bodily condition marked by excessive generalized disposition and storage of fat. It ranks as a major health hazard in many developed countries, as it is a heavy burden in itself, physically and emotionally, and makes the individual more prone to other illnesses. There are many possible reasons for obesity, several connected to psychological disturbances, with problems occurring particularly in adolescence, during pregnancy, and through the menopause in women.

Internal signals that tell a slim person when she has eaten enough seem to be faulty in the overweight or obese person. In this case it is not hunger alone that prompts a desire to eat, but rather outside influences, the smell or availability of food, or simply habit. This internal factor appears very hard to control, and for diet success some strong will is involved to overcome the desire to eat appetizing foods in excess of the body's needs.

It does seem that certain people are prone to gaining weight and have a pre-disposition to obesity. Their problem is not in fact different in principle from the slimmer person's, although their battle to achieve and maintain an ideal body weight will be harder. Research has shown that the *fat* person's *fat* cells have a greater capacity to store body fat, and less is mobilized in the body for energy or heat production. It is felt that this tendency is determined during pregnancy or early infancy, by incorrect feeding or dietary practice with the baby. A fat baby is far more likely to become a fat adult, or will find it much harder to remain slim in adult life.

Research on a substance (a hormone) such as FMS (fat mobilizing substance) seem to show that if the fat could be prevented from being deposited, then overweight problems could be eliminated without reduction diets. This work is still in its infancy, but its principle is similar in action to the effect of adrenalin on the body, which stimulates the sympathetic nervous system. Finding substances which are not harmful, non addictive, and help individuals towards a more sensible pattern of eating, are the subject of considerable medical research due to the associated health hazards of obesity.

There are many secondary diseases associated with obesity which make the condition a public health problem. There is a greater incidence of varicose veins amongst the obese, also of hernias, due to the infiltration of fat deposits in the abdominal area. Flat feet, bronchial disorders and arthritis are also more common.

Causes of Obesity

1   Genetic factors seem to be very involved in the incidence of obesity, where overweight seems to 'run in families'. Exactly what the connection is has not been clearly ascertained, as family customs and social eating habits are difficult to separate from the real issue of the tendency to obesity.

2   The economic status of individuals does seem to have a bearing on obesity, with a much higher proportion in the so called working classes or poor people. This is because the cheaper foods also tend to be the more fattening, like bread and potatoes, and these are used to fill up large appetites. This group are also felt to care less about their obesity, and tend to view it as a fact of life, about which little can be done.

3   Poor eating habits, with nibbling between meals, and a desire for there to be something continually in the mouth. Sometimes, however, obese people are found to eat less than thin people, but their metabolism does not use the food effectively and overweight still occurs.

4   Changes in physical activity, like a change of job, retirement, or becoming a housewife. Retirement after a very active occupation is particularly bad, unless a sport of some kind is maintained. There is the tendency to continue eating in the same pattern, even though the body's needs have diminished.

5   Psychological factors have a great bearing on obesity, with many overweight people seeming to eat for comfort or as a substitute for affection or love in their personal life.

6   Endocrine factors are involved in a very small percentage of cases, although too often the 'glands' are blamed as an excuse for over indulgence. As the storage and utilization of nutrients is closely controlled by hormones, an imbalance could lead to excessive storage or loss of fat.

7   Pregnancy frequently starts off a pattern of obesity that is difficult to cure. Weight gained over several pregnancies is hard to lose, and the

old myth of needing to eat for two throughout the pregnancy still persists. Now it is known that the body is able to use its resources more effectively in pregnancy, so a larger quantity of food is not needed, only different proportions of the basic food elements.

8   A person's age and sex does seem to make them more likely to be overweight, with the female being more prone to the problem than the male, with puberty, during pregnancy and at the menopause being the worst periods for the condition to be present. This would suggest that the sex hormones have some relationship to overweight problems, a fact which would appear reinforced by the weight gain many women experience when using 'the pill'.

Treatment for Obesity

The aim of any treatment for obesity is to dispose of the large stores of fatty tissue in the body. To do this the energy expenditure of the body must be increased over the energy intake from food. The slimmer must also have a strong wish to lose weight, or a reason that motivates the effort involved and makes it seem worthwhile. An obese person who has no strong desire or will to lose weight, however much they may need to, will be a reluctant and unsuccessful slimmer.

Various chemical means of increasing energy expenditure are theoretically possible, including stimulatory agents, and chemical substances which alter the food metabolism. Many of these methods have unfortunate side effects, and all have to be medically prescribed. Obviously it is preferable to treat obesity without the use of drugs, by re-educating the diet, and taking in fewer calories (or joules). Also any diet is made more effective by regular exercising, as this increases energy output.

WEIGHT CONTROL

The Yo-Yo Syndrome

Clients who experience real difficulty in losing weight, and maintaining the loss, may suffer from a condition known as the Yo-Yo Syndrome. Here body weight fluctuates, and adipose tissue is lost and regained many times over. If it has been medically ascertained that there is no abnormality in the basal metabolism, and they suffer from no medical condition such as hyperthyroidism, then an eating re-education programme can be tried.

It appears that the appetite controller situated in the hypothalmus at the base of the brain does not work very efficiently in the obese person. So if the satiation mechanism cannot be relied on, then the food intake has to be readjusted from newly acquired eating habits. These being designed initially to lose the stored weight, then to maintain a constant weight, without any weight gains.

Strong will, and motivation to succeed play a large part in obesity control. Encouragement in any form is welcome and slimming clubs, health hydros, therapy treatment, and the guidance of a caring therapist all serve to reinforce the doctor's recommendations to achieve the desired weight loss.

OBESITY THROUGHOUT LIFE

Obesity can be present throughout life, but appears with depressing frequency at certain stages: in infancy, adolescence, during pregnancy, at the menopause and in old age. In all cases taking in more food than the body needs is the prime cause of the weight problem. It may not seem more than the body *wants* or *desires*, but it must be more than it *needs*, otherwise the excess energy would not be stored as fat.

Knowing how much food is necessary for healthy life is difficult for anyone, but particularly for the housewife feeding a family, or the mother involved with child feeding. Evidence of excess body fat forms a good guide, showing that surplus food, not needed immediately by the body, is being stored, usually as surface fat. This indicates that many energy producing foods, such as carbohydrates, can be cut down, leaving proteins and fats (in moderate amounts) for growth and health. Each individual's need is different, and two very similar people will be found to eat totally different amounts of food, and yet stay a constant weight. One may have to watch everything that is eaten, whilst another may never have to give it a second thought. So watching for body fat accumulations, using the skin fold test, is the best method of assessing whether the food intake needs to be reduced.

Pregnancy

The problem of obesity in pregnancy is very real and stems often from a misunderstanding of the body's needs at this time. Certainly the quality of food taken in must be chosen with the unborn child's needs in mind, and protein foods for growth are very important. There is no need however to eat for two, and as long as a sufficient increase of calories (joules) is present to cope with the strains placed on the mother's resources, a healthy baby will result, at less risk to the mother. Overeating during pregnancy is often over-indulgence, a release from the normal strain of having to attempt to remain slim at all costs. It is a chance to eat favourite foods without the normal feelings of guilt and subsequent recriminations. The pregnancy is made to take the blame for the weight increase, and provides a convenient excuse.

Modern ante-natal practice is to keep a strict eye on weight gains, as excess weight increases the risks of the pregnancy to the mother, and can affect the unborn child. In the later stages of pregnancy, obesity increases the chances of developing toxaemia, which can be fatal to the baby. A combination of high blood pressure and an accumulation of extra cellular fluid, with the resulting oedema (swelling) can result in the condition occurring. A sudden increase in weight in the last weeks of pregnancy often gives warning of its onset, and this is watched for very vigilantly in ante-natal care. The only cure for toxaemia is for the baby to be born as soon as possible, to safeguard its survival and the mother's health.

Obese women have a greater risk of miscarriage (natural abortion) at all stages of the pregnancy. They also find it more difficult to conceive, with infertility being a special problem of the younger obese woman. The occurrence of still-born babies to obese women is greater, and if operative treatment is necessary, such as *Caeserean section*, then complications are more likely to develop. Recovery after the birth is slower in overweight women, and they take longer to return to full strength and vigour than their slimmer counterparts. Weight gained over subsequent pregnancies, and not lost between them, tends to accumulate until a real problem is established needing diet, exercise and salon treatments to achieve a remedy.

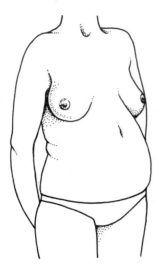

Obesity in Pregnancy

Childhood Obesity

It is in childhood that the obesity pattern starts for many, with overfeeding making the body's fat cells enlarge and multiply, starting a trend which will be a problem throughout later life. Eating habits, using food to placate or reward a difficult child, are prime causes of infant overnutrition.

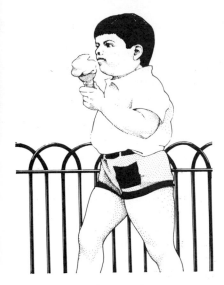

Food becomes intrinsically linked with reward, and this connection is the downfall of many obese adults attempting to reduce through a diet plan.

Also encouraging children 'to eat up', 'to grow big and strong', is another mistake of anxious parents, causing the child to go beyond its appetite's needs. The body is then less able to recognize when it has eaten enough, and is simply eating from habit or enjoyment of the food, rather than from need. It now seems evident that an obese child is far more likely to be obese in adult life, or will have a harder time avoiding weight problems, than an individual fed the correct dietary needs in early life. Very rarely is the cause of childhood obesity due to anything but excess food consumption. However, medical advice should always be sought before advising a diet, just to check this point.

Adolescence

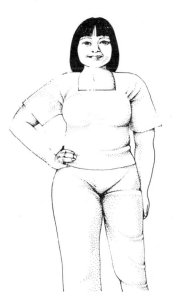

Weight problems in adolescence add additional embarrassment to the worries of gaining maturity and forming relationships with the opposite sex. To be held in esteem or to be simply accepted as the same as companions, is very important in adolescence. The overweight youngster appears different, and this can increase shyness and bring distress at a crucial stage in the development of personality. Maturity and overall growth do reduce the overweight problem in many cases, the individual seeming to grow out of it. As relationships develop and more confidence is gained, the dependence on food diminishes and other interests grow in importance. The value of a slim and attractive personal appearance becomes recognized, and the obesity problem can disappear spontaneously as the opposite sex, rather than food, becomes the major interest.

A diet for reduction in adolescence must be palatable, high in proteins and nutrients, but low in wasteful carbohydrate values. Foods enjoyed at this stage of life are often very carbohydrate biased, and include sweets, buns, fizzy drinks, crisps, chips, chocolate, and bread. Removing these elements would bring about a weight loss, but lack of co-operation from the young person often makes this the least successful stage of obesity to control.

Menopause

Changes occurring in the woman's body during menopause can affect body metabolism and cause weight problems. The regression (reduction) of

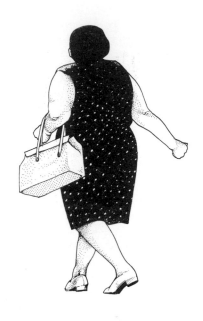

female hormones at this time, allowing the male hormones to become more dominant, would seem to be involved in the weight irregularity. Women taking the female contraceptive 'pill' also experience difficulty in weight control, and this would seem to reinforce the connection that sex hormones have with food metabolism.

Depression experienced during the menopause is also a factor in overeating and weight accumulation. The woman may eat for comfort or from boredom, and when weight begins to alter the appearance she may feel there is little point in bothering anyway. It can become a vicious circle unless a positive approach to rectifying the figure problem is made. The therapist can make a valuable contribution in this instance, helping the client to take an interest in her appearance, whilst removing the weight gained.

The pattern of weight control may be erratic until the client has settled after the change of life, and monthly periods are gone for good. Health and spirits should then improve and weight will be easier to control. Slim women seem to experience less depression and discomfort during the menopause than overweight ones because their bodies are fitter, and they are less prone to the associated health hazards of obesity. Varicose veins, arthritis, shortness of breath, aches and pains, high blood pressure and constipation are all possible problems of middle aged women. Obesity increases their incidence and severity in the menopause.

Retirement and Old Age

Obesity in old age, particularly after retirement, is a common problem and may be linked with undernutrition of the individual. Food taken in is not always of the right type, and lacks variety, essential protein and minerals, and makes elderly people a vulnerable group dietwise. As people grow older they expend less energy, do their work more efficiently with economy of movement and effort, and their basal metabolism decreases. So they do in fact need to eat less, if they are not to gain unwanted weight. But the food must be of the right type. Habit and eating patterns established over many years tend to maintain the food intake at a certain level, above bodily needs, and obesity can result.

Obesity brings forward many health problems, which the individuals could avoid for longer if they were lighter. Strains placed on physical systems of the body bring about pain and swelling in the joints, cardiovascular disorders, and kidney and liver malfunction earlier than need be. Diabetes can develop as a result of being overweight, with the body unable to cope with the demands placed upon it.

HEALTH HAZARDS OF OBESITY

It is now recognized that long term obesity decreases life expectation, and is prematurely ageing. This fact is seen in action when life assurance is sought, with obese people having to pay increased premiums, as they are seen as at greater risk, due to their weight.

The fact is that the physical systems are designed to cope with a normal weight body, and when overloaded show signs of strain. An obese person has to make a greater effort to complete any task, placing additional stress on the heart and vascular system. The heart enlarges to cope better with its task, and the blood pressure increases as blood is pumped more swiftly around the body to meet its demands.

Finding physical movement such an effort, there is more tendency to sit and not burn up calories through exercise. Lassitude, breathlessness and irritability are all minor problems common to the obese person, which normally disappear as the weight is lost. In fact the obese person may seldom feel really well, because of aches and pains throughout the body caused by strain on the weight bearing joints. Pain in ageing joints will be present prematurely, as will varicose veins, again as a result of excess body weight.

Certain diseases appear more frequently in the obese person, particularly diabetes and kidney disorders. Long standing obesity, with its associated dietary habits, is implicated in many diseases, if not as a prime cause, certainly as a contributory factor. Gall bladder disease and actual damage to the liver (cirrhosis) is more common among fat people. Luckily loss of weight quickly reduces the health risks and in many cases no damage is done. The manner in which the body can recover from obesity is an example of its resilience and complexity. Pain on damaged joints decreases, general health and vitality return and the individual appears to lose pounds and years together. Even serious diseases are improved, as the strain of the body weight is removed, and the dietary intake improves. High blood pressure, bowel disorders, and indigestion, which can cause personal misery, are all improved and may no longer need medication for relief.

These health factors can act as tremendous encouragement to the overweight client, and their relationship to obesity can be exploited to the full by an experienced therapist, well used to the problems of dealing with obesity. The list of health hazards in obesity is enormous, as it affects most of the body processes. It includes:

(*i*)   Premature ageing of the body.

(*ii*)   Cardio-vascular disorders.

(*iii*)   Kidney disorders.

(*iv*)   Cirrhosis of the liver.

(*v*)   Gall bladder disease.

(*vi*)   Abdominal hernia.

(*vii*)   Increased risk of diabetes.

(*viii*) Varicose veins.

(*ix*)   Arthritis of weight bearing joints.

The obese person will also be more prone to fatigue, lassitude, and aches and pains, all directly related to the presence of adipose tissue in excessive amounts.

WEIGHT CHARTS

Weight charts are useful to give clients some guidance as to their aim in weight reduction. However, they should not be adhered to too rigidly, as once a person has reached a reasonable weight, say within 6 kg (1 stone) of their ideal size, the final shape should be a personal matter. Although the therapist can advise, it is better not to dictate to the client how she wants to look.

Once the individual is satisfied with her figure, and knows how to maintain the lost weight, the therapist has been successful and should be content with the achievement she has helped her client towards. For an attractive body is not necessarily one that matches the ideal weight-for-height figures shown on a weight chart. These figures have been put together for life insurance and medical nutritional purposes, and they are not always applicable in therapy, where figure beauty, rather than pure low body weight, is the aim. Once the problem of being really overweight is gone, then an attractive feminine figure is sought. Attractive proportions are desirable, a firm bust-line, trim waist and seat, and well shaped legs.

A mature figure may need to be up to 2.72 kg (6 lb) above the weight chart guide if the breasts are not to be completely deflated, and the neck and face lined and scraggy. In middle age particularly, the extremes of weight loss should not be followed unless an intensive programme of salon treatment and home care for toning purposes is commenced. The thinner figure may look much better when dressed, but can be very unattractive when naked, with loose hanging flesh unsupported by adipose tissue. The skin fold test is useful in deciding when an individual has reached a satisfactory weight through the diet plan. Then figure reshaping may need to be introduced to continue the inches loss without a further reduction of weight. This avoids shapely curves being lost, and ensures an overall more attractive figure.

Younger women with firm muscles, elastic skin and good general health who are prior to childbearing, should be encouraged towards their ideal weight, with diet, exercise and salon treatment. For them loose skin and stretched or weakened muscles are not going to be a problem. The older woman will have to adjust her aims in figure improvement with factors of health and age in mind. Good health has to be maintained whatever the wish for an ultra slim figure. The weight loss should be more gradual, and perhaps acceptance of a less than perfect figure is realistic in middle age. Excess weight alone is not usually the whole problem in any case, with unattractive leg veins, a dropped bustline, soft crepey skin or stretch marks being a far bigger disfigurement.

So when advising clients on their correct weight consider all the factors, and be realistic. Clients may not achieve an ideal weight, but may be perfectly content with a substantial loss. Don't set clients an impossible target with the weight guidance – set them to a loss they can achieve easily, to spur them on. Provide a target weight loss that seems possible. For example, giving a 90 kg (14 st) client a goal of 50 kg (approximately 8 st), would demoralize the most determined slimmer. A loss of 13 kg (2 st) seems possible and within the capabilities of the dieter, and once achieved, can be progressed till the correct weight is reached.

Always set slimmers a task which they will or can succeed with, put their target within their reach, give strong and enthusiastic support, and success is assured.

Weight Guidance Charts

Most clients still like to recognize their measurements in stones and pounds, and these will be in use for some time yet. Therapists, however, should be using the metric measurements, and will work in kilograms, and centimetres. One kilogram equates to 2.2 of a pound, and 5 cm equals approximately 2 inches, although when rounded up and multiplied these figures become rather inaccurate. Instead, therapists should try to *think* in the new measurements, but *be happy to convert* the figures into a form the client can appreciate. A simple conversion chart for weight, based on a graph will be adequate for most therapy purposes. Tape measures are printed with both inches and centimetres, so it is a simple matter to obtain both types of size measurements. This will make it simpler eventually to change over completely to metric measurements, when clients have become used to them in everyday life.

A set of simple weight, distance, fluid, and heat conversion charts will be found at the back of the book, and should prove useful in this transitionary period.

A conversion graph giving approximate weights in stones and pounds and kilograms should help the therapist in client guidance (see illustration weight conversion), and for more accurate conversion the detailed graph gives weights in the most commonly found weight areas.

WEIGHT CHART AND CONVERSION GRAPHS

Height – without shoes.   **Weight** – naked. If clothed add 2.27 (5 lb) extra.

Height		Women		Men	
1.47 m	4' 10"	49.5 kg	7 st 12 lb		
1.50 m	4' 11"	51.7 kg	8 st 2 lb		
1.52 m	5' 0"	52.6 kg	8 st 4 lb		
1.55 m	5' 1"	53.9 kg	8 st 7 lb		
1.57 m	5' 2"	55.3 kg	8 st 10 lb	57.1 kg	9 st 0 lb
1.60 m	5' 3"	57.1 kg	9 st 0 lb	58.5 kg	9 st 3 lb
1.63 m	5' 4"	58.5 kg	9 st 3 lb	60.3 kg	9 st 7 lb
1.65 m	5' 5"	60.3 kg	9 st 7 lb	63.0 kg	9 st 13 lb
1.68 m	5' 6"	61.7 kg	9 st 10 lb	64.4 kg	10 st 2 lb
1.70 m	5" 7"	63.0 kg	9 st 13 lb	65.8 kg	10st 5 lb
1.73 m	5' 8"	64.0 kg	10 st 1 lb	67.9 kg	10 st 10 lb
1.75 m	5' 9"	65.3 kg	10 st 4 lb	69.4 kg	10 st 13 lb
1.78 m	5' 10"	66.7 kg	10 st 7 lb	71.5 kg	11 st 4 lb
1.80 m	5' 11"	69.4 kg	10 st 13 lb	73.8 kg	11 st 9 lb
1.83 m	6' 0"			76.3 kg	12 st 0 lb
1.85 m	6' 1"			77.9 kg	12 st 4 lb
1.88 m	6' 2"			82.3 kg	12 st 13 lb
1.90 m	6' 3"			85.8 kg	13 st 3 lb

These are average weights. Individuals with a small frame should deduct 2.27 kg (5 lb).
Those with a large frame add 3.18—3.63 kg (7—8 lb).

A weight loss of about 1 kg (2 lb) weekly is a sensible amount. A downward trend is the
main aim and is more important than achieving a rigid loss weekly.

Approximate weight conversion graph

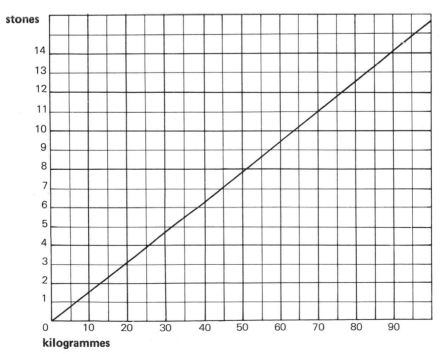

Common weight levels: Conversion graph

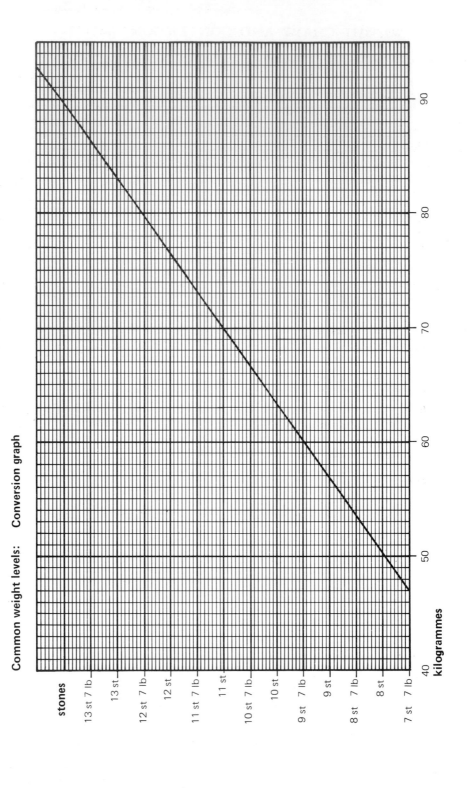

stones

13 st 7 lb
13 st
12 st 7 lb
12 st
11 st 7 lb
11 st
10 st 7 lb
10 st
9 st 7 lb
9 st
8 st 7 lb
8 st
7 st 7 lb

40   50   60   70   80   90

kilogrammes

REDUCTION DIETS

Weight Reduction by Dieting

The range of diets available is immense and still continually growing. Public interest has increased the amount of fad or crash diets being promoted, mainly based on severe restriction and a repetitious command to eat only one or a very few foods, usually fruit, vegetables or meat. Slimming foods, biscuits, soups, crispbreads, and low starch bread have become a large industry, and all set out to capture the interest of the slimmer. These products will appeal to inconsistent dieters, who view them as an easy means of achieving weight loss. They do provide an exact amount of calories (joules) and guard against the temptations of normal food, but do not help to establish a normal reduced pattern of eating. As slimmers will not wish to live for ever on special diet foods, they must learn to judge their dietary needs from the wide range of ordinary foods available.

The therapist has to guide her clients through the maze of confusing and often conflicting information available, in order to find the best path to weight reduction and subsequent control. If the client is obese, it has been seen that a need for medical guidance is necessary before commencing any diet plan. This ensures there is no reason other than overeating to account for the weight gained. If a medical diet is given, the client can be helped to follow it conscientiously, and can be helped by salon treatment.

If the problem is simple overweight, caused by overindulgence, then a diet suited to the client's likes and dislikes can be suggested to achieve a weight loss. By assessing the degree of willpower likely, a diet can be chosen that will suit the client's temperament, and not leave her subject to temptation. A liking for certain classes of food should be carefully considered in the diet choice, if success is to be achieved and the diet maintained. Some people are capable of simply cutting down the food they eat, whilst others need a very disciplined approach, with the food intake strictly dictated, and no flexibility which could lead to temptation.

Through discussion, the need for a bulky or moderate fat content diet can be discovered, to guard against constipation, or a dry skin condition forming. Longing for sweet elements can be coped with on calorie controlled diets, with calories being deducted from the total, and the slimmer having to do without elsewhere. Calorie counting can cause hunger unless well organized however, as with too much taken in carbohydrate form, it will not sustain the slimmer and provide energy and food for growth and tissue maintenance. Lists of the calorie content of common foods are also widely available, or can be provided pre-printed by the therapist as a service to the clients. From this the client can work out total consumption, 1000 or 1200 calories, or whatever level is considered necessary to bring about a weight reduction. Calorie counting will make life simpler for working women, who may find it difficult to obtain suitable lunch time diet food, and who prefer to take the bulk of their daily calorie intake in the evening meal with their families. Though not the ideal way to slim nutritionally, it works for many women as it suits their way of life, and does not require a change in the social habits.

Calorie Controlled Diets

Still one of the most popular effective diets, it is designed to reduce the stored fat content of the body, and remove the surplus weight. All foods and drink have an energy value, and so the calorie or joule value of different items will give guidance as to how much they are related to obesity. By restricting the food intake to 1000 or 1200 calories, the body will be forced to burn up its fat deposits. High calorie foods will use the total allowance wastefully, and low calorie foods give better value by giving bigger portions, adding bulk to the diet and providing variety of tastes and textures.

Low Carbohydrate Diets, or Carbohydrate Exclusion System

As we have seen, the body can be forced to convert into carbohydrate, and vice versa, and then use up the available carbohydrate to metabolize fat. Professor John Yudkin has worked out the carbohydrate content of all foods and has given each a value – the Carbohydrate Unit, known as CU.

It is suggested that a healthy balanced diet can only be achieved by eating foods from the following four groups twice a day:

1 **Milk and cheese.**
2 **Meat, fish and eggs.**
3 **Fruit and vegetables.**
4 **Butter and margarine.**

A pint of milk should also be taken daily. As meat, poultry, fish, eggs, cheese, butter, margarine, and fats contain no carbohydrate units they can be eaten freely on this diet. Each CU is the equivalent of 5 g of carbohydrate (20 calories).

The therapist should acquaint herself with this carbohydrate exclusion system, as although not as well known as calorie counting it has certain advantages for some clients. By knowing the client's tastes and life style, there may be many who would find it more agreeable to lose weight by this system. 10—15 CU can be consumed daily, and can be taken as food or in alcoholic form, which would appeal to social drinkers. Although a waste of the CUs it might mean that clients might stick to this diet plan, even though they have been previously unsuccessful with others that prohibit drinks even in moderation. The quantity of carbohydrate units can be adjusted up or down, if not enough or too much weight is being lost, 1 kg (2 lb) a week being the ideal loss. (*See* **Food Value Chart** *for CUs of food.*)

Fad Diets

These are currently popular crash diets, usually based on one or more types of food, i.e. steak and orange, or banana and milk diets. They often exclude the other nutrients necessary for maintaining a healthy body whilst losing weight. Vitamin supplements are an essential element, even if the diet is short term. These diets are turned to because of the high weight loss they offer, rather than the steady 1—1.5 kg/M (2—3 lb) recommended in sensible dieting. Magazines and the media generally promote this type of diet, so therapists must have a sensible alternative, and should be capable of persuading clients that theirs is the better way, and just as effective long term.

Of course, for a small weight loss on healthy young people, there is no reason why the fad diet cannot be put to use to get the diet plan started, but it has a few problems for the more seriously overweight. It is very difficult to maintain a long term weight loss this way, because of boredom, aversion to the food contents and a lack of variety to stimulate the palate. It also gives no sound guidelines to establish a new eating pattern for the future.

The limitations on the food range tend to throw the system out of balance, and constipation and bad breath result. Weight is lost but is regained very quickly. Fat may not be being burned up properly, and essential body building elements lost, causing fatigue, listlessness, and headaches. The dieter may be eating up her own body strength and power. Luckily people quickly become fed up with their fad diets, and give up.

The Banana and Milk Diet

This is one example of a fad diet that is very popular because it is so easy to follow and needs no preparation, weighing of food, etc. It is low in calories, at less than 1000, and consists of 2 bananas and a glass of ordinary milk taken three times a day. Meat extracts taken in the form of hot drinks can be taken in addition, as they have no calorie value.

The diet can be useful to get a dieter started, or used for a light diet day once a week to maintain a weight loss, instead of a fruit only day. It can be alternated with ordinary low calorie food days to relieve boredom, and used if clients appear to have got stuck at a certain weight. However, it does not establish a sensible eating pattern for the future, and so has a limited use in diet re-education.

High Protein Diets

These are not fad diets, but have a high proportion of protein to carbohydrate, and are still well balanced, containing all necessary minerals and general food elements. Many medical diets are high protein, and low carbohydrate, and work very well in a large range of circumstances. Some high protein diets are a bit extreme however, and the dieter is advised to eat practically nothing but meat, cheese and eggs. If the client has a history of kidney infection, care must be taken to see that the body can adequately rid itself of the protein intake, otherwise overloading occurs and the kidneys could retain urea, leading to complications. Apart from being a wasteful diet, as the body does not need that amount of protein, it also could be a harmful one, if the protein is not balanced with other food elements in moderate quantities.

Well balanced, the high protein, low carbohydrate diet is one the therapist will find very useful in client guidance, and as it helps in re-education of the diet, will be a long term answer for many overweight people.

Having looked at how the body digestion works, it is now easier to see the shortcomings, or even dangers, of many diet plans, particularly if they are given without medical supervision.

SLIMMING OR DIET CLUBS

Moral support is desperately needed by certain slimmers, and diet or slimmers' clubs offer one solution to the problem of diet failure. Group therapy does seem to work for many, and appears successful often after many other attempts to stick to a diet have failed. Therapists should encourage their clients to join a diet club if they feel it would be beneficial to their reduction efforts. Many clients will find a therapist's attentive supervision just as effective however, particularly if a pleasant but fairly firm attitude to the weight control programme is adopted. Clients seeking advice about slimming clubs should be advised to consult their own doctor first, to ascertain their obesity is not connected with any metabolic malfunction or physical illness. Checks for blood pressure, anaemia, diabetes mellitus and thyroid abnormality are necessary before embarking on a large weight loss programme. In most cases a weight loss is very beneficial, but the doctor may prefer the diet to be medically prescribed.

Slimming clubs vary in their approach, but most expect regular weekly attendance, and rely on group morale to prevent individuals breaking their diet plan. Diets do tend to be all of one type, which is rather restricted, and they cannot be personally tailored to the individual because of time restrictions. Well balanced, high protein, and low carbohydrate diets are most in favour. Lists of permitted and forbidden foods guide the slimmer towards her goal weight. Success is rewarded by admiration and envy from the rest of the group, and the presentation of a badge or similar sign to show the weight loss achieved.

Many clients will be attending slimming clubs and, like medical diets, these form a useful background to the therapist's work and are complementary to it. Not all clients maintain their weight loss, and are unable to accept new eating habits as advised by the clubs. Their obesity may mask some underlying psychological problem, and they may need medical help rather than a different system of dieting for their success.

GAINING WEIGHT

So much attention is centred on the overweight person, and solving her problems, that the client who is too thin tends to be neglected. It can be just as depressing to lack curves as it is to have an overabundance. Excessive thinness can be unsightly, and is seen by the individual as unfeminine and unattractive to the opposite sex.

Thin clients can be helped to improve their figures through diet, relaxation therapy and a different approach to their life style. The reasons for the underweight condition may be due to body type and individual temperament. The body shape, regardless of height, is of the Ectomorph type, with long slim limbs and muscles. The torso is normally slight, and the client usually can only cope with a small food intake, due to a small digestive system.

There is one simple rule in diet to which there are no exceptions – weight is gained when more energy (food) is taken in to the body, than is needed by the body for work or living requirements. So by taking in more energy than is given out, weight will be gained. The thin person is often highly strung, and burns off fat very efficiently through bouts of activity throughout the day. Body movements are fast and the daily life is accomplished at high speed. The thin person is everything the obese person should be, and is not. However, when nervous tension shows itself in excessive weight loss, the client has to be helped to break the vicious circle of anxiety, and adopt different eating and living habits.

Diet plays an important part in the therapy, with the client being advised to eat three meals a day of well-balanced, high protein, and moderate fat and carbohydrate content. Fats have the greatest fattening capacity, but are sometimes upsetting to the digestion of the slim person, causing bilious attacks. The food should be attractively presented to tempt the small appetite, and diet supplements such as 'Complan' used as meal substitutes if necessary to keep up the calorie intake when the desire for food is low. The manner in which the food is eaten will alter its effectiveness, and the client should be advised to eat slowly and allow time for digestion. Many thin people eat on the run, hence the lack of fat deposits and the slender body shape.

Supporting the diet should be relaxation therapy, with heat and manual massage, to help the client to unwind and recognize her own tensions (see Chapter 5). Building confidence in the thin person is difficult, and requires much reassurance and encouragement to achieve figure improvement through a weight gain. 200—300 grams a week is an ideal gain to be aimed for until the correct body weight is reached. Foods of high energy concentration, such as fats, sugars, cream, starches, butter, honey, salad dressings and nuts, are extremely useful for gaining weight. There should be a good proportion of first class protein, to help build muscles, and an abundant supply of vitamins, particularly Vitamin A, D, and the B group.

Remembering the body type and natural disposition of the person, it may never be possible to achieve the average weight for the height, as shown on weight charts. However, any improvement is usually welcome, to cover bony areas and so form a more attractive figure.

FOOD VALUES

	Normal Portion	Calories	CU
Apple			
raw	100 g (4 oz)	40	2
sweet stewed	100 g (4 oz)	100	3
pie	200 g (8 oz)	400	4
Apricots			
fresh	100 g (4 oz)	30	2
canned	100 g (4 oz)	70	5
dried	25 g (1 oz)	50	2
Asparagus	100 g (4 oz)	10	$\frac{1}{2}$
Avocado Pear	75 g (3 oz)	75	1
Ale (strong)	250 ml ($\frac{1}{2}$ pt)	210	5
Almonds	30	170	$\frac{1}{2}$
Bacon			
fat grilled	50 g (2 oz)	350	0
lean grilled	50 g (2 oz)	185	0
Banana	100 g (4 oz)	50	5
Beans			
baked	100 g (4 oz)	100	4
broad	100 g (4 oz)	50	3
butter (boiled)	100 g (4 oz)	100	4
french or runner	100 g (4 oz)	10	$\frac{1}{2}$
Beef			
steak grilled	100 g (4 oz)	345	0
roast (fat)	100 g (4 oz)	435	0
roast (lean)	100 g (4 oz)	255	0
corned beef	100 g (4 oz)	265	0
beefburger	100 g (4 oz)	415	0
stew (with veg)	150 g (6 oz)	240	0

	Normal Portion	Calories	CU
Beer			
light	250 ml (½ pt)	80	5
stout	250 ml (½ pt)	100	7
Beetroot	50 g (2 oz)	15	1
Biscuits			
plain	3 medium	125	3
sweet	2 small	160	3
chocolate	2 medium	290	5
Blackberries			
fresh (no sugar)	100 g (4 oz)	30	2
tinned	100 g (4 oz)	100	4
Blackcurrants			
fresh	50 g (2 oz)	15	1
Blancmange	100 g (4 oz)	140	4
Brandy			
one measure	a measure	65	4
Brazil nuts	5 only	180	¼
Bread			
all, types, ordinary and			
starch reduced	1 slice	70	3
bread and butter pudding	100 g (4 oz)	185	8
sauce	25 g (1 oz)	30	7
Broccoli	100 g (4 oz)	15	0
Brussels sprouts	100 g (4 oz)	20	0
Butter	25 g (1 oz)	220	0
Buns			
currant	one	175	4
Cabbage			
raw or boiled	100 g (4 oz)	10	0
Cake			
plain sponge	50 g (2 oz)	175	5
fruit or cream	50 g (2 oz)	400	8
Carrots			
boiled	75 g (3 oz)	15	1
Cauliflower	100 g (4 oz)	10	½
Cereals	18 g (¾ oz)	75	4
Celery	100 g (4 oz)	10	0
Cheese			
cheddar	25 g (1 oz)	120	0
cream	25 g (1 oz)	230	0
Danish blue	25 g (1 oz)	100	0
Dutch	25 g (1 oz)	90	0
Cheese omelette	100 g (4 oz)	410	0
Chicken			
roast	100 g (4 oz)	215	0
Chocolate	50 g (2 oz)	330	5
Chop Suey	100 g (4 oz)	250	4
Cocoa Cola	1 glass	80	3
Cider	250 ml (½ pt)	110	7
Cocoa (½ milk and with sugar)	1 cup	145	3

	Normal Portion		Calories	CU
Cod fillets				
steamed	100 g	(4 oz)	90	0
Coffee				
black, no sugar	1 cup		5	0
milk added, no sugar	1 cup		25	0
Crabmeat	50 g	(2 oz)	75	0
Cream				
double	25 g	(1 oz)	130	0
single	25 g	(1 oz)	60	0
Cucumber	50 g	(2 oz)	5	0
Custard	50 g	(2 oz)	65	1
Damsons	50 g	(2 oz)	17	1
Dates				
dried	25 g	(1 oz)	70	4
Doughnut	50 g	(2 oz)	200	6
Duck	100 g	(4 oz)	355	0
Dumpling	100 g	(4 oz)	240	5
Egg				
poached or boiled	50 g	(2 oz)	90	0
fried	50 g	(2 oz)	155	0
Figs				
dried	25 g	(1 oz)	60	3
Fat				
cooking	25 g	(1 oz)	260	0
Fish cakes	100 g	(4 oz)	250	4
Flour	25 g	(1 oz)	100	4
Fruit Pie	100 g	(4 oz)	210	10
Fruit Salad				
tinned	100 g	(4 oz)	80	10
Gin	25 g	(1 oz measure)	65	4
Goose	100 g	(4 oz)	370	0
Gooseberries	100 g	(4 oz)	40	2
Grapefruit	100 g	(4 oz)	10	1
Grapes	100 g	(4 oz)	60	3
Greens	100 g	(4 oz)	15	1
Haddock				
fresh, steamed or smoked	100 g	(4 oz)	110	0
Halibut	100 g	(4 oz)	150	0
Ham				
fat	100 g	(4 oz)	490	0
lean	100 g	(4 oz)	250	0
Herring				
fried	100 g	(4 oz)	270	0
Honey	25 g	(1 oz)	80	5
Ice cream	50 g	(2 oz)	110	3
Jam	13 g	(½ oz)	325	2
Jam roll				
baked	100 g	(4 oz)	460	6
Jam tart	50 g	(2 oz)	220	6

	Normal Portion	Calories	CU
Jelly	50 g (2 oz)	45	2
Kidneys fried	100 g (4 oz)	230	0
Kippers	100 g (4 oz)	230	0
Lamb chop, grilled			
fat	100 g (4 oz)	570	0
lean	100 g (4 oz)	310	0
Lamb			
roast	100 g (4 oz)	330	0
Lard	13 g ($\frac{1}{2}$ oz)	120	0
Leeks	100 g (4 oz)	30	1
Lettuce	50 g (2 oz)	5	0
Liver			
fried	100 g (4 oz)	310	0
Lobster	100 g (4 oz)	135	0
Loganberries			
fresh	100 g (4 oz)	20	1
tinned	100 g (4 oz)	115	6
Macaroni cooked	75 g (3 oz)	100	5
Mackerel			
fried	100 g (4 oz)	210	0
Mandarin oranges	100 g (4 oz)	70	2
Margarine	13 g ($\frac{1}{2}$ oz)	110	0
Marmalade	13 g ($\frac{1}{2}$ oz)	35	2
Marrow	100 g (4 oz)	10	0
Mayonnaise	13 g ($\frac{1}{2}$ oz)	90	0
Meat paste	25 g (1 oz)	60	0
Melon	150 g (6 oz)	25	2
Milk			
skimmed	1 cup	70	0
whole, ordinary	250 ml ($\frac{1}{2}$ pt)	175	3
Mincemeat	25 g (1 oz)	35	2
Mince pies	50 g (2 oz)	220	5
Mushrooms			
raw	50 g (2 oz)	5	0
fried	50 g (2 oz)	125	0
Oatmeal	75 g (3 oz)	345	3
Olive oil	13 g ($\frac{1}{2}$ oz)	130	0
Omelette			
plain	100 g (4 oz)	230	0
Onions			
boiled	100 g (4 oz)	15	0
fried	100 g (4 oz)	110	0
Orange			
raw	75 g (3 oz)	25	$1\frac{1}{2}$
Pancakes	100 g (4 oz)	340	8
Parsnips	100 g (4 oz)	60	2
Pastry			
short	50 g (2 oz)	325	5
Peaches			
fresh	100 g (4 oz)	35	2
·tinned	100 g (4 oz)	75	4

	Normal Portion		Calories	CU
Peanuts	30		170	1
Pears				
fresh	100 g	(4 oz)	55	2
tinned	100 g	(4 oz)	110	4
Peas	50 g	(2 oz)	35	1
Peppers	100 g	(4 oz)	25	0
Pilchards	100 g	(4 oz)	215	0
Pineapple				
fresh	100 g	(4 oz)	55	2
tinned	100 g	(4 oz)	80	5
Plaice				
steamed	100 g	(4 oz)	105	0
Plums				
fresh	100 g	(4 oz)	40	2
tinned	100 g	(4 oz)	85	4
Pork				
fat	100 g	(4 oz)	515	0
lean	100 g	(4 oz)	325	0
Port	50 g	(2 oz)	90	$4\frac{1}{2}$
Potatoes				
boiled	100 g	(4 oz)	120	4
chips	100 g	(4 oz)	270	4
crisps	50 g	(2 oz)	320	2
Prawns	50 g	(2 oz)	60	0
Prunes				
dried, raw	50 g	(2 oz)	75	2
Radishes	50 g	(2 oz)	10	0
Raisins	25 g	(1 oz)	70	4
Raspberries				
fresh	100 g	(4 oz)	30	4
tinned	100 g	(4 oz)	120	6
Rhubarb				
cooked	100 g	(4 oz)	15	0
Rice pudding	100 g	(4 oz)	170	4
Rum	25 g	(1 oz)	65	4
Salad oil	1 tablesp.		125	0
Salmon				
fresh steamed	100 g	(4 oz)	230	0
tinned	100 g	(4 oz)	155	0
Sardines	50 g	(2 oz)	170	0
Sausages	75 g	(3 oz)	240	2
Scones	25 g	(1 oz)	105	3
Scotch egg	100 g	(4 oz)	300	2
Shepherds pie	100 g	(4 oz)	130	3
Sherry	50 g	(2 oz)	70	4
Shrimps	50 g	(2 oz)	65	0
Sole				
steamed	100 g	(4 oz)	95	0

	Normal Portion	Calories	CU
Soup			
cream	200 g (8 oz)	200	0–2 depending on thickness
consomme	200 g (8 oz)	10	0
Spaghetti			
cooked	150 g (6 oz)	400	10
Spinach	100 g (4 oz)	30	0
Steak and kidney pie	100 g (4 oz)	345	5
Sugar			
brown or white	1 tablesp.	110	4
Syrup			
golden	13 g ($\frac{1}{2}$ oz)	45	2
Sweets			
boiled	25 g (1 oz)	95	4
Tangerines	100 g (4 oz)	30	2
Tartare sauce	1 tablesp.	70	1
Tea			
lemon no sugar	(1 cup)	1	0
milk only	(1 cup)	20	1
milk and sugar	(1 cup)	75	2
Toad-in-the-hole	100 g (4 oz)	330	7
Tomatoes			
fresh	100 g (4 oz)	15	0
Tongue	100 g (4 oz)	345	0
Trifle	100 g (4 oz)	170	7
Tuna fish	100 g (4 oz)	200	0
Turkey	100 g (4 oz)	225	0
Turnips			
boiled	100 g (4 oz)	10	1
Veal	100 g (4 oz)	124	0
Vita wheat	1 piece	100	1$\frac{1}{2}$
Whisky	1 measure	65	4
Wine			
red	75 g (3 oz)	60	4
white dry	75 g (3 oz)	50	3
Yorkshire pudding	50 g (2 oz)	125	3

Butter and all other fats are rated at nought on the carbohydrate exclusion diet, but rate very high on the calorie counting diet. Sweet elements are found to carry a lot of weight-producing elements in both forms of diet. Certain elements of food use the calories or joules so wastefully that they should be excluded from the diet if possible. Dumplings, fruit pie, fizzy drinks and sugar in all its forms, are examples.

Chapter 4

Figure Improvement Through Exercise

THE VALUE OF EXERCISE

The way the client looks depends not only on weight, but on shape, altered by the muscular bulk and tone of the body, and on postural factors. So figure improvement through exercise becomes a necessary part of the therapist's skill, in order that figures can be maintained or improved. Where weight loss is involved, muscle toning becomes vital to firm the contours and avoid loose skin forming, particularly in the older client. This can be achieved naturally, using the client's own efforts, or electrically, with muscle contraction treatments applied within the clinic. No amount of salon treatment can compare with natural exercise for toning the whole body's system, and increasing respiration and arterial flow. However, muscle contraction treatment is an effective substitute, or can act to reinforce and speed personal efforts when used in combination with natural exercise.

The co-ordination of mind and body experienced with well chosen exercises is very effective in improving a client's morale, and can bring about renewed vitality. Well performed exercises strengthen muscles, improve posture, and act as a defence against injury or strain. All forms of exercise can be utilized by the therapist when planning the client's home advice, to increase the effect of the salon treatment and diet. Any activity that is enjoyable and brings about an increase in energy expenditure – walking, sports, swimming, and specific exercise – all speed weight and inches reduction within an overall treatment programme.

As exercises can be viewed unfavourably by some clients, they must be made effective, simple, and varied to maintain interest. They should also be within the client's capabilities to perform without strain, or breathlessness. Personal instruction, group sessions of exercise or yoga, or use of exercise equipment, all help the reluctant client to participate. Continuing support and interest from the therapist in planning new exercises, and re-assessing progress is also very effective encouragement.

Before being able to plan an effective routine of exercises that will not strain individual resources it is important to understand how the body works and achieves movement. The two main systems involved are the skeletal and muscular, under the control of the nervous system. Understanding the effects that the physical laws of gravity, leverage, motion and balance have on maintaining a healthy and supple body, will also prove useful when devising exercise plans.

THE SKELETAL SYSTEM

The skeletal system has several important functions – giving the body its height, support, movement and posture. It also protects delicate areas with its bony formation, for example the skull and rib-cage, and is responsible for blood cell formation and calcium storage.

Bones come in four types, long, short, flat and irregularly shaped, and they are joined to each other by joints in several ways permitting movement. There are three main types of joints, **synarthroses**, (fixed, fibrous joints), **amphiarthroses** (cartilaginous, slightly movable joints) and **diarthroses** (synovial, freely moveable joints).

The majority of joints in the body are of the freely moving type, and take many different forms, permitting a wide range of movements. These fall into four main groups, gliding and angular movements, circumduction and rotation, which between them encompass most everyday activities of the body. The shape and action of joints are normally classified into seven groups, but modern research favours the principle of classifying joints according to movement, and the curvature of the articulating surfaces, terming these ovoid and sellar. Ovoid articular surfaces are curved inward (concave) or outward (convex, egg shaped), and the corresponding surface into which it fits is known as sellar or saddle-shaped.

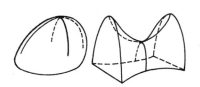

Ovoid and Sellar

The traditional method of classification of diarthroses, or freely movable joints, divides them into:

1 **Plane or sliding.**
2 **Hinge.**
3 **Pivot.**
4 **Condylar.**
5 **Ellipsoid.**
6 **Saddle.**
7 **Ball and socket joints.**

These can be seen in action performing a variety of movements, in combination with muscles which provide the leverage or pulling power through

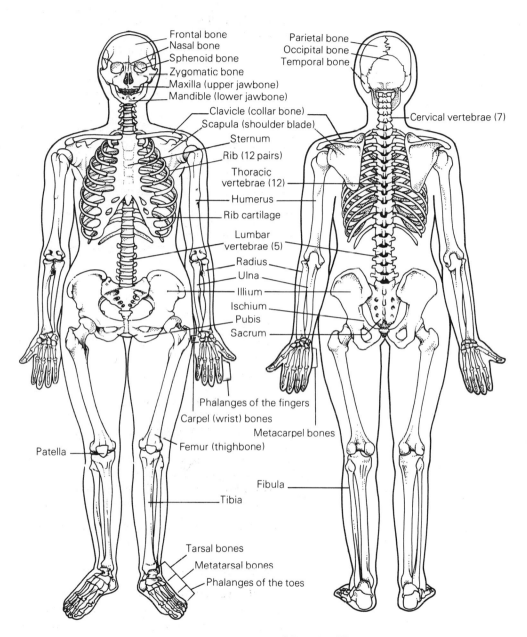

Frontal bone
Nasal bone
Sphenoid bone
Zygomatic bone
Maxilla (upper jawbone)
Mandible (lower jawbone)
Clavicle (collar bone)
Scapula (shoulder blade)
Sternum
Rib (12 pairs)
Thoracic vertebrae (12)
Humerus
Rib cartilage
Lumbar vertebrae (5)
Radius
Ulna
Illium
Ischium
Pubis
Sacrum

Parietal bone
Occipital bone
Temporal bone
Cervical vertebrae (7)

Phalanges of the fingers
Carpel (wrist) bones
Metacarpel bones

Patella
Femur (thighbone)

Fibula

Tibia

Tarsal bones
Metatarsal bones
Phalanges of the toes

The Skeleton – Anterior and Posterior View

their contractability. If the four main types of joint movement are considered, it is evident that a variety of different and special movements come under these general classifications. If these are considered in relation to their muscular connections (attachments) on to the bones, it becomes evident that muscles that move a part are not normally found overlying that part but lie proximal to it (closer to the trunk or body's medial plane).

Gliding Movements – are found between the closely articulating bones of the tarsals and carpals (feet and hands) permitting only very small degrees of movement.

Angular Movement – which include:

Flexion, which brings about a change in the angle between the two articulating bones, normally decreases the size of the angle causing a bending or folding movement.

Extension, being the return from flexion, a straightening movement which, if allowed to progress past the normal anatomical position, becomes hyperextension, commonly seen in the legs.

Abduction, which moves the bone away from the midline of the body (medial plane), an example being arm lifting sideways.

Adduction, being the opposite of abduction, moving towards the midline of the body.

Rotation – is the pivoting or moving of a bone on its own axis, and takes many forms. Some degree of rotation is present in most joint movements throughout the body.

Circumduction – where the bone follows an imaginary cone shaped path as it moves, combining elements of flexion, abduction, and adduction in its muscular action.

Special Movements – which describe unusual actions of parts of the body, and include:

Supination, a movement of the forearm which turns the palm forwards.

Pronation, a forearm turning movement which brings the back of the hand forwards.

Inversion, a movement which turns the sole of the foot inwards (inverts).

Eversion, a movement which turns the sole of the foot outwards (everts).

Skeletal Muscle Movement

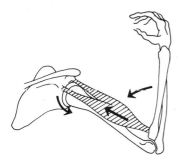

Flexion Movement
Biceps Muscle
Humerus –
Radius – bones (long)
Ulna –
Elbow joint (hinge)
Shoulder joint (ball and socket)

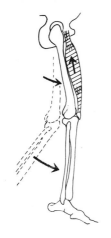

Extension Movement
Rectus femoris muscle
(quadriceps group)
Femur –
Tibia – bones (long)
Fibula –
Knee joint (hinge – diarthrotic-synovial cavity)

Abduction Movement
Deltoid muscle
Scapula bone (flat)
Clavicle bone (long)
Humerus bone (long)
Shoulder joint (ball and socket)

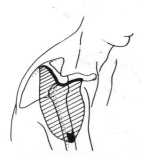
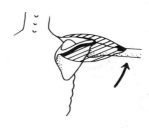

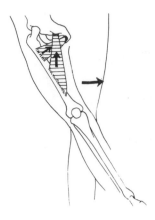

Adduction Movement
Adductor muscles
Femur bone (long)
Pubic bone (part of Pelvic Girdle)
Hip joint (ball and socket diarthrotic)

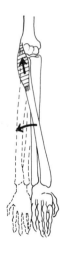

Rotation Movement
Supinator muscle
Humerus –
Ulna – bones (long)
Elbow joint (hinge)

Circumduction Movement
Pectoralis major muscle
Deltoid muscle
Humerus bone (long)
Shoulder joint (ball and socket)

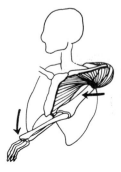
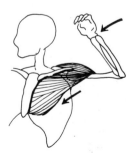

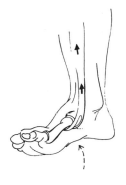

Inversion Movement
Tibialis anterior muscle
Tibia bone (long)
Medial cuneiform bone (short)
Metatarsal bone (short)

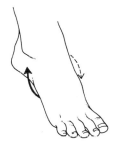

Eversion Movement
Peroneus longus muscle
Fibula bone (long)
Metatarsal bone (short)
Ankle joint (hinge)
Medial cuneiform bone (short)

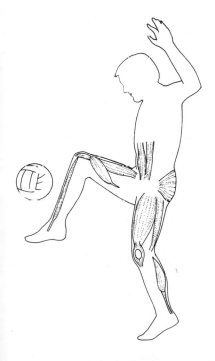

When some of the body's movements are considered, it is possible to see the co-ordinating force of the skeletal and muscular systems in action; for example kicking a ball, where some muscles act to give thrust to the bones of the leg, whilst others add strength to the movement and stability to the body's balance.

The skeletal structure has vital importance when posture is considered. If postural faults are present they will be skeletal in origin, e.g. the pelvis may be tilted incorrectly on the femoral heads, too far forward, causing hollowing of the back, or too far back, resulting in protrusion of the abdomen.

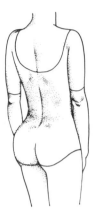

Hollow Back

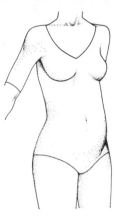

Abdominal Protrusion

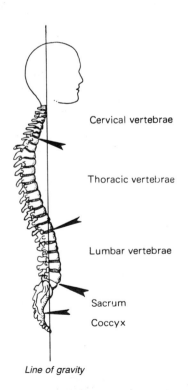

Cervical vertebrae

Thoracic vertebrae

Lumbar vertebrae

Sacrum

Coccyx

Line of gravity

Maintaining an upright posture with the support of anti-gravity muscles is another task of the skeleton. The constant opposition of the effects of gravity would make this a fatiguing task for the muscular system, if it were not for supporting ligaments and fascia which assist and so save energy. The shape of the spinal column, formed into curves, is ideally designed to keep the body upright without strain, if the body's centre of gravity is correctly placed. Incorrect posture throws the body out of balance, and postural faults develop, bringing with them pain, limitations of movement and faulty body alignment.

Recognition of good posture has to be developed both by viewing the standing position (see Chapter 2), and by repeated conscious correction of faulty alignment. An awareness that good posture is being maintained improves the total picture the client presents. If the client can recognize poor posture developing, it can be quickly corrected, and strain and fatigue avoided. This point is of importance to working therapists as well as to their clients.

THE MUSCULAR SYSTEM

Having seen how the structure and attachments of the skeletal system make movement possible, it is necessary to consider how the movement is actually achieved by muscular action. Muscle tissue is able to contract and extend, and has properties of elasticity, all actions being under the influence of the nervous system. The physiological unit for movement is known as the neuromusculoskeletal unit, combining nerve, muscle and joint activities and function. The action is produced by combined effects, and anything that affects one aspect of the unit can cause restricted or abnormal movements, or a loss of movement. Polio and multiple sclerosis affect the neural part of the unit, whilst muscular dystrophy affects the muscle, and arthritis the skeletal part or joint. All can bring about changes in body action, illustrating the integral co-ordination of muscular activity.

Muscular Action

Some basic knowledge of the principles of muscular action is useful in planning exercises, as it shows the varied role the muscular system has to fulfil, both in posture maintenance and free movement. How the muscles are able to work most effectively has to be recognized and used to get effective but not harmful routines established.

The different ways in which muscles can produce movements can be used to the full in exercise choice, to determine the type of exercise needed, and its duration. This also provides guidance as to how fully the muscles can be worked without strain. There are occasions where free exercise is restricted, as in the older or overweight client, and the muscle strength has to be developed. Understanding how muscles work will make this possible.

Skeletal muscles contract only if stimulated by natural or aritificial means, via their motor unit (nerve supply), and can produce either precise or more general movements, this being according to the number of muscle fibres to which the somatic motor neuron is attached at its myoneural junction on the muscle. Some muscles produce actual movements when they contract, these being termed 'prime movers'. Others, termed 'synergists', work to hold a limb or area of the trunk in a fixed position, to make a more stable base for other muscles which produce movements.

Normally when prime movers are contracting, other muscles, termed 'antagonists', are relaxing (extending) to permit the movement. Muscles can sometimes reverse their roles and act in either a prime mover or antagonist capacity, depending on the movement being performed; rather like a see-saw action, with one contracting, the other extending, and vice versa. Flexors and extensors of the forearm can be seen to act in this way.

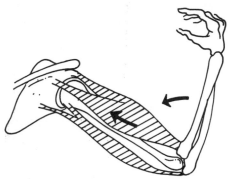

Antagonistic Action of Biceps/Triceps

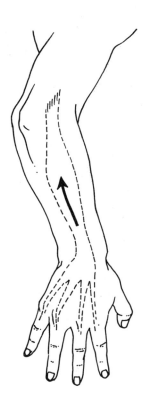

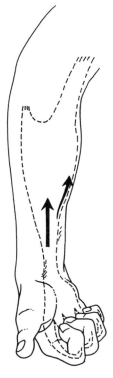

Extension   *Flexion*

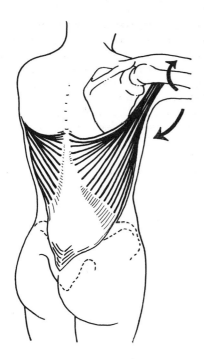

Other muscles, like the pectoralis major (flexor action), with the trapezius and latissimus dorsi (extensor action), have an established range of movement which, although varied, tend to be within certain limits. Here the antagonist action is anterior and posterior to the trunk of the body, and is seen in action in curling up and straightening movements of the trunk, and in abduction and rotation of the arm.

It has been seen that muscles move bones by pulling on them, using them as levers, with the joints acting as fulcrums of these levers. A lever being a rigid bar (the bone) free to turn about a fixed point called its fulcrum. By the muscles shortening, contracting, and becoming thicker, movement is produced and the attachments are brought closer together. The attachment which is most fixed (static) is known as the *origin*, and the more movable attachment the *insertion*. Usually the insertion is pulling back towards the origin and movement occurs: for a muscle is incapable of pushing. It can only shorten or hold against resistance any position between its longest and shortest lengths.

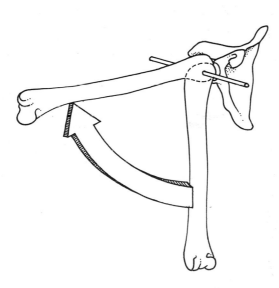

Fulcrum of Joint

There are some muscles where both attachments are fairly movable, or both fixed, and here the origin and insertion is more difficult to define. By noticing which direction the muscle works towards, however, its most static point can be noted, simplifying identification.

It has been noticed also that muscles move the area distal or adjacent to themselves (furthest from the midline or next to them), which provides another means of identification. So the forearm affects the hand, the shoulder the upper arm, and the calf muscles, the foot.

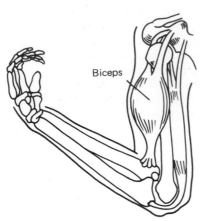

Muscle Shortening onto **Fixed Point**

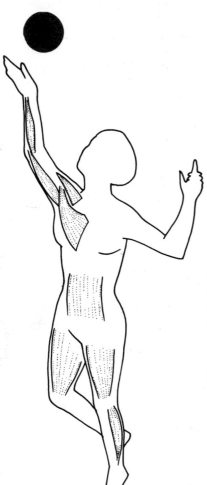

Skeletal muscles almost always act in groups, rather than independently, and when planning exercise routines, it is these groups that will be made to work to improve the figure. Within a muscle group may be prime movers, their antagonists permitting the movement, and synergists steadying the movement: all muscles working under the control of the nervous system, directed by conscious control from the brain. The muscles can reverse their roles occasionally, and are also capable of acting in different ways, matching the demands made upon them. When a new exercise routine is advised muscles have to alter in their action and strength to accomplish the task. Given adequate time to adjust to the new demands, muscles are found to be capable of great variability and mobility, if the exercises are well chosen.

Muscles contract with different degrees of strength at different times. For example, antigravity muscles either maintain static posture, or are involved in general activity.

Muscle Co-ordination

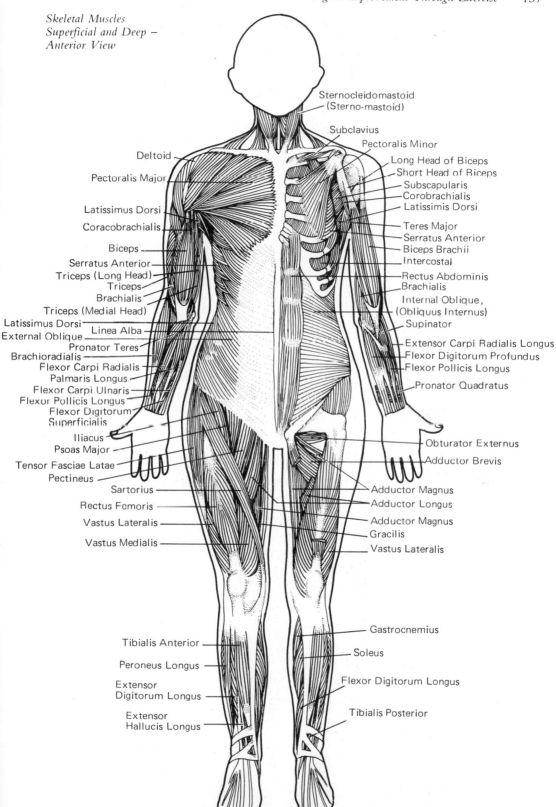

Skeletal Muscles
Superficial and Deep –
Anterior View

Sternocleidomastoid
(Sterno-mastoid)

Subclavius

Pectoralis Minor

Deltoid

Long Head of Biceps

Short Head of Biceps

Pectoralis Major

Subscapularis

Corobrachialis

Latissimis Dorsi

Latissimus Dorsi

Coracobrachialis

Teres Major

Serratus Anterior

Biceps Brachii

Biceps

Intercostal

Serratus Anterior

Triceps (Long Head)

Rectus Abdominis

Triceps

Brachialis

Brachialis

Internal Oblique,

Triceps (Medial Head)

(Obliquus Internus)

Latissimus Dorsi

Supinator

Linea Alba

External Oblique

Pronator Teres

Extensor Carpi Radialis Longus

Brachioradialis

Flexor Digitorum Profundus

Flexor Carpi Radialis

Flexor Pollicis Longus

Palmaris Longus

Pronator Quadratus

Flexor Carpi Ulnaris

Flexor Pollicis Longus

Flexor Digitorum

Superficialis

Iliacus

Obturator Externus

Psoas Major

Adductor Brevis

Tensor Fasciae Latae

Pectineus

Sartorius

Adductor Magnus

Rectus Femoris

Adductor Longus

Vastus Lateralis

Adductor Magnus

Gracilis

Vastus Medialis

Vastus Lateralis

Gastrocnemius

Tibialis Anterior

Soleus

Peroneus Longus

Extensor
Digitorum Longus

Flexor Digitorum Longus

Extensor
Hallucis Longus

Tibialis Posterior

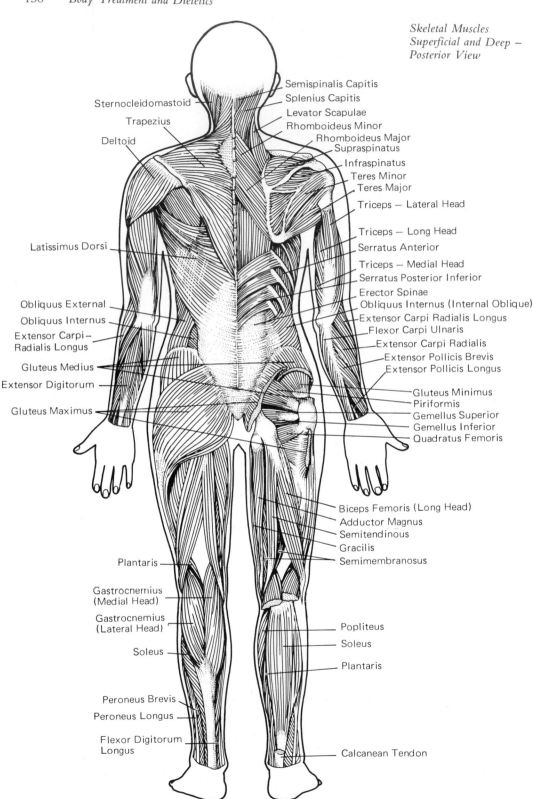

Skeletal Muscles Superficial and Deep – Posterior View

Semispinalis Capitis
Splenius Capitis
Levator Scapulae
Rhomboideus Minor
Rhomboideus Major
Supraspinatus
Infraspinatus
Teres Minor
Teres Major
Triceps — Lateral Head
Triceps — Long Head
Serratus Anterior
Triceps — Medial Head
Serratus Posterior Inferior
Erector Spinae
Obliquus Internus (Internal Oblique)
Extensor Carpi Radialis Longus
Flexor Carpi Ulnaris
Extensor Carpi Radialis
Extensor Pollicis Brevis
Extensor Pollicis Longus
Gluteus Minimus
Piriformis
Gemellus Superior
Gemellus Inferior
Quadratus Femoris

Sternocleidomastoid
Trapezius
Deltoid
Latissimus Dorsi
Obliquus External
Obliquus Internus
Extensor Carpi–
Radialis Longus
Gluteus Medius
Extensor Digitorum
Gluteus Maximus

Biceps Femoris (Long Head)
Adductor Magnus
Semitendinous
Gracilis
Semimembranosus

Plantaris
Gastrocnemius
(Medial Head)
Gastrocnemius
(Lateral Head)
Soleus
Peroneus Brevis
Peroneus Longus
Flexor Digitorum
Longus

Popliteus
Soleus
Plantaris
Calcanean Tendon

Muscle Identification

To build a working knowledge of skeletal muscles as a base for exercise choice, it is useful to consider them from the point of view of their:

Actions – flexors, extensors, abductors, adductors, etc.

Location – bone attachment or proximity, e.g. rectus femoris or tibialis anterior.

Shape – deltoid (triangular) and trapezius, etc.

Number of divisions – biceps, triceps, quadriceps, etc.

Attachments – bone attachments such as the sternocleidomastoid. Considering skeletal musculature in this way should make identification simpler and more interesting.

Muscle Tissue Characteristics

Skeletal muscles have certain characteristics which, when understood, explain the different actions muscles are capable of. All muscles possess properties of irritability, conductivity, contractability, extensibility, and elasticity.

Irritability and Conductivity – the ability to respond to a stimulus and transmit impulses, being necessary for natural exercise and movement, and for electrical muscle contraction.

Contractability – the ability to contract (thicken) and produce movement. This property being the biggest element in body locomotion and survival.

Extensibility and Elasticity – extensibility is the ability to stretch (extend and lengthen), and elasticity is the return from that stretch to the original shape. The rectus abdominis muscle's elasticity is impaired after pregnancy, being too long and needing to be made shorter between its two attachments, the sternum and pubis. So though the muscle's ability to extend is good, it may need help through exercise to improve its elasticity.

Theory of Muscle Action

When voluntary muscles receive a stimulus from the brain via the motor nerve, they develop tenseness and bring about movement. The theory of muscle action is the series of reactions or processes that come about on receipt of the nervous impulse.

Each muscle has its store of food in the form of a carbohydrate called glycogen, (muscle sugar), supplies of which are stored in the liver. On receipt of the nervous impulse, this sugar breaks down and forms a substance called 'lactic acid'; also energy is released and a movement comes about. To ensure continuous movement glycogen must be available to supply the energy, and the lactic acid must be removed, as when this reaches a sufficient concentration it prevents or interferes with the development of tenseness in the muscle. So there exists an ingenious system that prevents this lactic acid piling up in the muscle. A muscle therefore should be able to go on working in-definitely on the receipt of nervous impulses provided that:

(*i*)   Sufficient supplies of glycogen are replaced.

(*ii*)   Sufficient oxygen is available to oxidize the lactic acid.

(*iii*)   Waste products are removed.

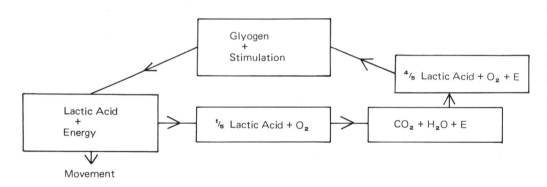

Glycogen Cycle

The Oxygen Debt

During physical activity automatic adjustments occur in the normal working of the body to satisfy these three requirements. However, in actual prac-tice fatigue does set in, with the lactic acid being present in greater quantities, so the process breaks down. This is not due to lack of sugar, but to the fact that the body is unable to supply the muscles with the quantity of oxygen they require. The body has used up more oxygen than it had avail-able, and so rest is required. The oxygen supplied during rest is known as the 'oxygen debt'. Both in extreme activities, such as running, and in daily life this process is seen in action, with people stopping for a breather to refresh themselves, and to enable them to resume former activities.

POSTURE

If body posture is discovered to be poor with faulty alignment during the figure diagnosis (Chapter 2), this should be remedied before progressing to natural exercise for correction of figure faults. If good posture is not attained, exercise programmes will not be completed correctly, and performing the exercises may cause strain, discomfort, and could also discourage the client.

Body posture or position is thought to be good when the maximum efficiency of the body is maintained with the minimum effort. Posture is the attitude assumed either supported during muscular relaxation or during muscular activity, with the muscles co-ordinating to stabilize a base, and constantly adapting it to suit movement around it.

Posture is considered as being *inactive* as in sleep, where muscles work only to maintain respiration, circulation, etc., or *active*, which is used in static and dynamic forms, to hold the body or cause movement. Good posture in the standing position (see Chapter 2) sees anti-gravity muscles working against the downward pull of gravity to maintain an erect figure. The tonicity (tone) of muscles pulls against this force, and by a continual re-adjustment of nervous impulses controlling muscles, and therefore bones, the figure is maintained in an erect state whilst awake (static posture). In sleep the nervous system cannot control skeletal muscles or co-ordinate actions, and so the muscles are at rest (inactive posture).

The Postural Mechanism

There are three main ways in which posture is maintained:

1   **Anti-gravity muscles** – where muscle groups work to overcome gravitational pull, and to maintain an erect position.

2   **Nervous control** – posture being maintained by neuro-muscular co-ordination, with impulses passing in the cycle of muscle, nerve, spinal cord, brain, spinal cord, nerve and muscle.

3   **Postural reflex** – this being the bodily response to gravity. By co-ordinated use of eyes, ears, and skin sensation, the brain causes the correct impulses to pass to muscles which maintain posture.

Good Posture

The importance of good posture can best be judged when it is not in evidence. Apart from its relevance to figure beauty, its importance to the body as a whole should not be underestimated. Posture affects the respiration, digestion, the circulation, and can have far reaching effects on general body health. Poor posture places a strain on muscles which affect the ligaments and bones, altering the body's balance. The body attempts to compensate, and this throws more work on anti-gravity muscles, supporting ligaments and fascia, leading to fatigue and pain.

The value good posture has in avoiding pain and disability arising from postural defects is well known, but its positive benefits seldom get enough publicity to encourage interest in maintaining posture for its own sake. In consequence many working days are lost, and pain suffered through strain and injury to anti-gravity structures, particularly the lower back area. Backache, stiffness, lack of mobility, and overall fatigue are all signs that posture has become faulty. Depression, which may or may not be associated with actual physical ill-health, is another aspect of incorrect body alignment.

Posture is poor when it is inefficient and hinders movement. Balance is affected and alters the performance of many normal activities like walking, running, etc. (dynamic posture). Good health, vigour and confidence are seen when posture is correct, and anxiety, tension, depression and pain may be experienced when it is lacking: for health and posture are inter-related, with environmental factors playing a large part in the maintenance or absence of efficient posture.

Good posture is developed if the following conditions are observed:

1   A stable psychological state, evident in an alert confident manner, and an interest in life.

2   A good environmental situation, with adequate sleep and nutrition, and attention to personal hygiene.

3   Free active movements performed naturally without strain or pain.

Advice may therefore be necessary upon background factors, attitude to hygiene, life style, etc., whilst the client is being guided in posture improvement through exercise. Insufficient sleep or exercise, poorly planned meals, or an unhappy home situation, all reflect in the body posture.

Encouragement and interest from the therapist will also help to improve the client's mental attitude towards her improvement. The positive and negative aspects of posture can be discussed with the client, in order to gain her support for the exercises planned. If the good aspects of posture can be made to relate to the client personally, then co-operation will be established, and the therapist's role will become advisory rather than supervisory. Persuasion is always better than dictating to the client what has to be done.

Correction of Postural Faults

When a fault is observed it is advisable to show the client the necessary correction by using a full length mirror, so that she can see and feel what happens at the same time. Repeated conscious correction of faulty alignment, and maintenance of good posture lead to improved postural habits. If the fault can be corrected by a little effort, then encouragement to feel and hold the position should be given, and if necessary exercises given to mobilize or strengthen muscles around a part.

Developing the client's sense of correct posture is a fundamental part of posture correction. Although at first the corrected position may feel strange (even though it looks correct), this feeling soon passes and the improved posture becomes habitual. Eventually the incorrect position becomes the uncomfortable one, and the advantages of an easy and correct posture become clear.

Generally faults may be helped in correction by:

1 Mobilization of joints.

2 Increase in muscle power.

3 Relaxation therapy.

Any corrective postural work that causes pain, or is beyond the client's capabilities is contra-indicated for therapy practice, or indicates that the exercise needs revision. A progressive approach should avoid strain developing, and uses the principle of building strength and mobility to suit a client's individual needs and abilities. Abnormalities of spinal curvature, chest deformities, knock knees, etc., have to be recognized, because they limit or prohibit (contra-indicate) some postural and active exercises (see Chapter 2).

As the planning of exercises for correction purposes progresses, the need for a sound knowledge of the skeletal and muscular systems becomes evident. The more knowledge of the therapist has of the way the body works, the more effective and yet safe will be the exercise routines advised.

Exercise Starting Positions

Exercises may be undertaken in many ways and can be varied to suit individual circumstances by using different starting positions. Different positions may be required for several reasons:

1   To alter the stability of the base. If an easy exercise is needed the base must be large, such as lying, sitting or a hands and knees position. If a more difficult exercise is indicated, requiring balance, then a position with a small base is more suitable, such as standing.

2   To alter the position of the centre of gravity.

3   To alter the body in relation to gravity. Gravity may be used as an *aid* to the movement, or as a *resistance*, or it may be *eliminated*. For example, using gravity to aid quadriceps contractions: prone lying with knees bent, lower the leg till the knee joint is straight. Using gravity as a resistance, with the starting position being high sitting, lift the lower leg till the knee is straight. To eliminate the gravitational effect, the quadriceps can be exercised from a side lying position, with the knee bent and then straightened.

4   To stabilize a part of the body, so that a movement can be localized to the required area, without other areas compensating or helping the movement unduly. For example, when long sitting, alternate toe touching with the opposite hand to exercise the obliques, and increase mobility in the back and hamstrings.

5   To make the muscle work as easy or difficult as required.

6   To provide the best position for the particular exercise, e.g. back extension is best performed in a prone position (facing downwards), such as prone lying, and prone kneeling.

It is convenient to have titles for these start positions so that the following exercises are quickly understood. The most usual start positions used in therapy are as follows:

Arm Positions

Wing

Bend

Across Bend

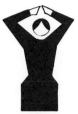

Head Rest

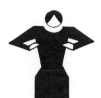

Across Bend

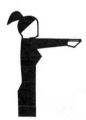

Reach

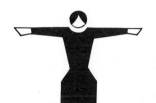

Yard

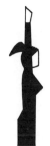

Stretch

Leg Positions

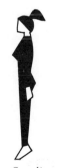

Toe Standing

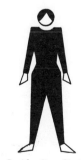

Stride Standing

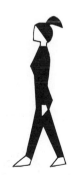

Walk Standing

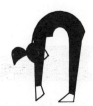

Lax Stoop Standing

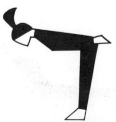

Stoop Standing

Sitting Positions

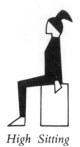

High Sitting

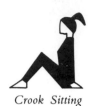

Crook Sitting

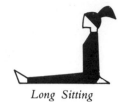

Long Sitting

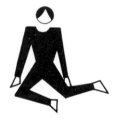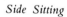

Side Sitting

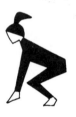

Crouch Sitting

Lying Positions

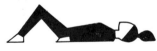

Crook Lying

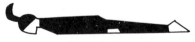

Prone Lying

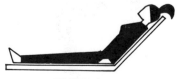

Half Lying

Side Lying

Kneeling Positions

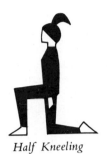

Half Kneeling

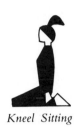

Kneel Sitting

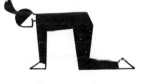

Prone Kneeling

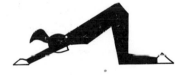

Inclined Prone Kneeling

CORRECTION OF
POSTURAL FAULTS

Any postural faults recognized during the primary diagnosis should be improved as much as is possible before exercises for general or specific figure improvement are undertaken.

Head Tilt – Round Back

In the correction of a rounded back, or **kyphosis**, which often results in an associated forward tilt of the head, certain muscles have to be trained (thoracic sacrospinalis group), and other muscles have to be stretched because they become tight and shortened (anterior intercostals and pectoralis major and minor). These postural corrections also improve round shoulder problems, and improve the the bustline through corrected stance. Simple but correctly performed exercises can slowly bring about an improvement in mobility, and increase capacity for general exercise programmes.

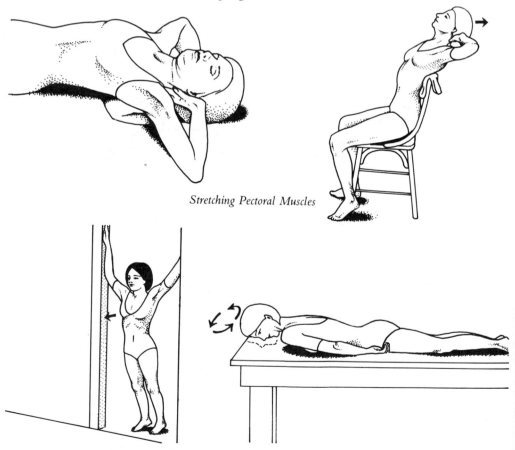

Stretching Pectoral Muscles

Increasing Shoulder Girdle Mobility

Shoulder Girdle Correction – Round Shoulders

Two common faults of the shoulder girdle are round shoulders, and abducted and forward tilted scapulae. The round shoulders may be due to shortened pectoral muscles requiring stretching, or due to overall weakness of the muscles in the area requiring strengthening. Both kinds of round shoulders are associated with weakness of the scapular adductor muscles. The muscles that need to be improved, trained or strengthened are the rhomboids, and the trapezius (middle and lower fibres), whilst the pectoralis major and minor need to be stretched.

In this exercise the scapulae are strongly adducted, then relaxed. The exercise progresses by slowly unclasping the hands, and lettting the arms be lowered to the ground slowly, before relaxing the scapulae adduction.

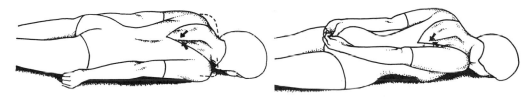

Shoulder Girdle Correction

Trunk: Lumbar Region – Pelvic Tilt Correction

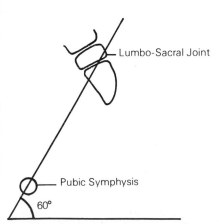

To correct a sway back, hollow back, or abdominal protrusion, certain muscles have to be trained and strengthened. The obliques and hip extensors require training and the hip flexors and lumbar extensors need stretching. Correct postural awareness is a vital factor in correction of pelvic tilt, and the client should be encouraged to recognize the correct stance which achieves pelvic balance.

When judging the degree of pelvic tilt, the therapist should remember that a correct position would find the pubic symphysis and the anterior superior iliac spines in the same plane visually: the pelvis being held on the femoral heads tilted at an angle of 55°—65°. To assess pelvic tilt draw an imaginary line through the lumbo–sacral joint, and the pubic symphysis, then draw a line horizontal to this, and the angle of tilt lies where they meet.

Exercises that work to mobilize and strengthen this area of the lower back include flattening the back, back arching, and stretching the lumbar area and hamstring muscles.

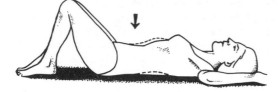

Flattening the Back

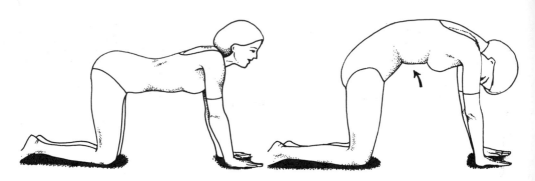

Back Arching

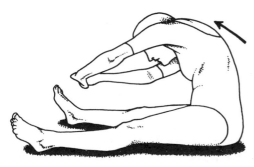

Stretching the Lumbar Region

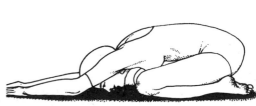

Stretching the Hamstrings

The Abdominal Area

As on many occasions the abdominal muscles act as stabilizers for other movements, rather than prime movers in their own right, it is necessary to exercise them specifically with isotonic (active) routines. The effects of pregnancy and overweight make this possibly the worst body fault for women, and one that relies heavily on postural correction for its remedy. Trunk raising, or sit up exercises in the supine position, works the muscles isotonically and makes them contract and shorten.

Hyperextension of the lumbar spine should be avoided, and if evidence shows that the movement is too difficult, it must be altered and made easier. This can be achieved by *extending* rather than *contracting* the muscles, with an exercise such as lying down from a sitting up position, where the body is working *with* gravity rather than *against* it. If really weak, the area can be exercised isometrically (static contractions) working in a way that is a more normal, therefore easier, action for the abdominal muscles. As the muscles normally contract isometrically (without a change in length) to stabilize or fix the part of origin of other muscles (for movements of the arms, legs and head), this activity can be increased to strengthen the area.

Repetition of isometric abdominal contractions eventually bring about an unconscious control of the abdominal wall, preventing protrusion and improving the digestion process. Strength in the abdominal and pelvic floor muscles also reduces the incidence of prolapse of the womb, after pregnancies or in later life.

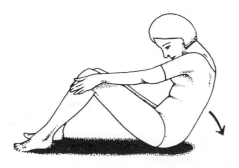

Eccentric Movement of Rectus Abdominus

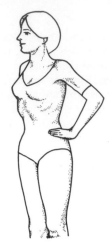

Abdominal Retraction

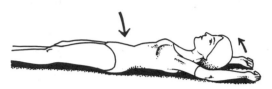

Abdominal Retraction and
Chinning Forward

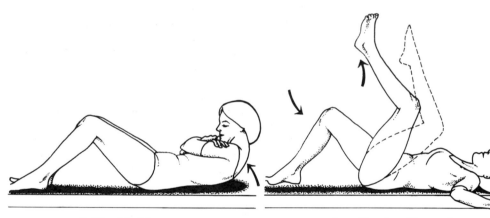

Rolling Up Movement

Legs Flexed to Chest and
Extended

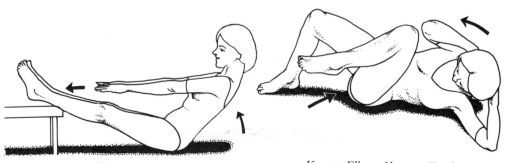

V-sitting

Knee to Elbow Alternate Touching

**Thigh – Leg and Foot
Alignment**

Knock knees, bow legs and back legs when noticed in diagnosis require consideration, as they are an indication that the anti-gravity postural muscles used in standing and walking need strengthening. Excessive internal rotation of the thigh can also be corrected by voluntary contraction of the hip external rotator muscles. Tenseness and shortening of the hamstring muscles can also be a contributory factor to poor posture in this area, and is another very common problem.

Many faults in the legs can be traced back to the feet, and they can in fact cause the total body posture to be poor, if not correctly aligned or weak. Well arched, strong feet give a good basis for correct posture. So flat, or displaced feet may need exercise to improve overall body posture.

Where established faults exist, such as flat feet or knock knees, exercise routines can be adapted to avoid strain or discomfort. If some improvement in the actual faults seems possible, clients should be advised to seek physiotherapy help. The therapist's role is one of recognition in this case, not one of treatment. Normally postural faults of this type are long established, and have become habitual movements of the client, so they have to be considered when planning an exercise programme. Making the client aware of good posture and balance with special reference to the feet, must always be an advantage, and should help prevent faults developing. So here the therapist's preventative role comes to the fore, to help maintain physical health.

MOBILIZING JOINTS

Overall figure posture and dynamic posture can be affected by stiffness or lack of mobility in joints, which alters movement in the surrounding muscles. The mobility of a joint depends on its anatomical structure and the efficiency of muscles working around it.

If pain is experienced on movement of an area, the therapist should advise her client to seek medical guidance to discover the cause of the stiffness. If the lack of mobility is discovered to be due only to muscular weakness, then the exercise plan can be chosen and can take several forms:

Passive (assisted movements) applied and controlled by the therapist, which activate the synovial fluid of the joint, and bring increased blood circulation to the tendons, ligaments and muscles surrounding the joint. Passive movements are used only if the muscles are very weak, and are always followed by the more normally applied active movements.

Active movements are either assisted by the therapist to reach full range movements, or free rhythmical movements performed entirely by the client's own efforts.

Lots of rhythmical swinging types of exercises are the best kind to mobilize a joint, with encouragement to push harder, swing higher, stretching and holding a movement. The client's efforts will be more evident to her if goals are set, such as stretching to achieve a previously difficult movement, e.g. toe touching from a long sitting position, with legs outstretched.

Mobilizing Exercises

As full a range of joint movements as possible should be aimed for within an exercise programme, insuring mobility, suppleness, and preventing restrictions and discomfort from developing in everyday movements. Most normal exercise routines will include mobilizing elements, but the inclusion of a range of specific mobilizing exercises will be particularly worthwhile especially for the older client.

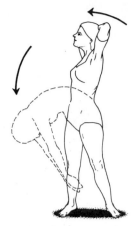

Trunk Rotation

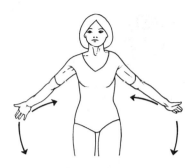

Arm Swinging

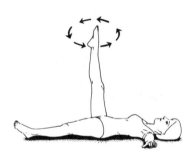

Leg Circling

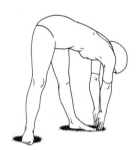

Toe Touching

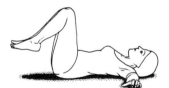

Hip Rolling

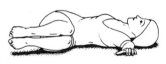

Head Rotation

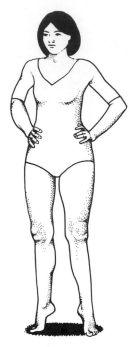

Raising on Toes

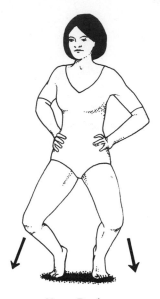

Knees Bend

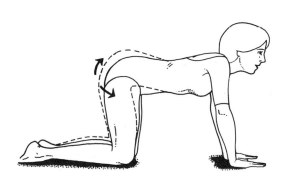

Tail Wagging

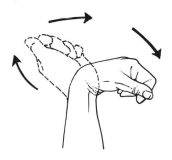

Wrist Rotation

GENERAL EXERCISE

When correct body alignment is established and the client has acquired a postural awareness, then more general exercise can begin to reinforce the correction achieved. In some cases posture correction and mobilizing exercises will not be necessary prior to general movement but can be incorporated into the initial active routines. However, working quickly through the standard checks on alignment, tests for muscle strength, joint mobility, etc., is always worthwhile as general exercise will never be performed well if posture is incorrect.

Furthermore, the risks of strain are increased as the exercises increase in their effectiveness and are made more difficult to perform. The specific correction also prepares the client for more active and strenuous routines, by loosening up muscles, improving respiration and increasing mobility.

Active Movements

Active movements come in two types, *free*, which are performed by the client unaided, and *assisted* or *resisted*, where the operator assists the client or acts to bring resistance into the exercise.

Free active exercise is the kind normally used to improve general body health and vitality, and has several benefits if performed regularly:

1   Active movements strengthen the heart beat and the general circulation is improved.

2   Repeated active movements require an increased supply of oxygen, and so the respiratory organs have to do more work to supply this demand.

3   The nervous system is invigorated and clearer nerve paths are formed, improving co-ordination.

4   Active movements develop and strengthen muscle slowly, especially in the inner range movements (where the muscle works from half contraction to full contraction and vice versa).

5   The vascular supply and nutrition to the muscles is improved, thus improving muscle tone.

Resisted exercises, though still active, are performed under muscular tension in either a *concentric* or *eccentric* manner, with either the operator, gravity, or the client's own weight forming the resistance. Concentric (contraction) and eccentric (extension) muscle work is used in muscle testing procedures (see Chapter 2), and in progressive resistance exercises to build bulk and strength in muscle tissue (body building or figure shaping).

Most general improvement programmes are made up of free or assisted movements, with resistance exercises being more involved in specific correction or reshaping of the figure.

PERFORMANCE OF EXERCISES

Co-ordination

When exercises are performed really well they demand considerable expenditure of nervous energy and thought. It is essential to have perfect co-ordination of mind and body. If strain is experienced on performing the exercise, it must be altered so that it is within the client's capacity and muscular tolerance. Maximum achievement is not the aim of successful exercise routines, but working to personal capacity and progressing whilst still retaining co-ordination.

As muscles become strengthened, the controlling motor nerves bring about a faster response and the tone of the whole body is improved. Each muscle fibre possesses a nerve fibre, and whilst it can be considered an independent unit having the power of contraction, this contraction is only made possible by the muscles through the controlling nervous system. So movements are really represented in the nerve centres and not in the various muscle groups. This is an important point in both natural exercise and electrical contraction of the muscles within the clinic.

The particular nerve cells responsible for movement are situated in the cerebral cortex of the brain. The nerve fibres leaving these cells pass through the medulla oblongata and become part of the spinal cord. The transmission of impulses from the mind to the muscle is a complicated procedure, but when a clear nerve path is discussed, it is this transmission that is being considered. The more that is understood of the nervous system, the greater will be the effectiveness of both natural and artificially induced exercise.

Client Guidance for Exercise Routines

Ensure that the client:

Always performs exercises with regular breathing.

Never exercises on a full stomach or if extremely hungry.

Wears comfortable clothing and normal supporting underwear if large busted or very overweight.

Graduates exercises according to age and abilities.

Checks her general health before embarking on an exercise programme.

Concentrates upon each movement and completes it correctly to gain the maximum amount of joint and muscle movement.

Performs exercises regularly for maximum benefit.

Adopts a progressive approach to exercise, starting with easy exercises and moving through the exercise range to more difficult movements.

Breathing

To get the most out of exercises, the client must be taught to breathe well so that plenty of oxygen is available to the muscles. Respiration is an involuntary action and its depth is dependent upon the mobility of the thorax. The lungs need to be fully expanded and relaxed continually to work most efficiently. A direct result of deep breathing is to increase oxygenation of the blood, and disperse waste products more rapidly, so producing a feeling of well being.

Beauty therapists will find many of their clients do not fully expand their lungs, either because they lack exercise and have not needed to breath deeply, or because of obesity slowing them down, and forming a layer of fat on the chest wall. It is only necessary to guide clients in correct breathing routines, to achieve full expansion of the lungs, in a rhythmical fashion, moving easily from inspiration to expiration without strain. Although therapists are not involved with remedial breathing routines, they should have a sound understanding of the mechanism of respiration, as the trunk acts as a steadying or control force for many other exercises. So if respiration is erratic, the body will not have a firm supporting action in the thoracic and abdominal areas. This control is particularly important in the abdominal area where the muscles act like a natural corset, where there is no bony structures to hold the abdominal contents in.

Areas of breathing are upper costal, mid costal, lower costal and diaphragmatic. So the client can be helped to gain full chest expansion by breathing out against the pressure of her own hands placed first above the breasts, then at the sides of the chest, and lastly on the lower ribs at the sides. Diaphragmatic breathing is the deepest type, where the diaphragm, a sheet of strong muscle between the thorax and abdomen, moves upwards on expiration and downwards on inspiration. As it domes upwards it forces air out, and as it domes and spreads downwards over the abdominal contents, it makes as large a space as possible for the expanding lungs to fill. The lungs are roughly triangular in shape, the apex lying just under the clavicle, and the base at the bottom of the ribs.

The actual process of respiration involves many muscles of the trunk including the sterno-mastoid, the pectorals, and the serratus anterior being connected with inspiration, and the abdominals and latissimus dorsi with expiration. The rib-cage and its intercostal muscles change in shape during inspiration, with the thorax increasing in width, depth and vertical size. The close involvement of respiration to general movement is clearly seen when exercises are attempted. The natural inclination to hold the breath when under strain, or whilst concentrating to perform an exercise shows this close connection in action.

Breathing Exercises

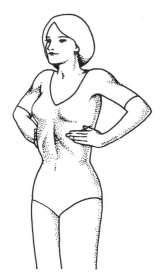

1 Stand the client in a relaxed but correct posture, with the hands on the lower part of the ribs with the fingertips touching on the medial line of the body. She may then breathe in and the ribs will lift up and outwards, pushing the fingers apart. Then exhale slowly and steadily and the ribs close gradually inwards, and the hands come together and can push to expel the maximum air from the lungs. A general feeling of uplift is promoted, with the movements keeping well above the waistline, and being supported in this position by the steadying abdominal muscles which are held drawn in.

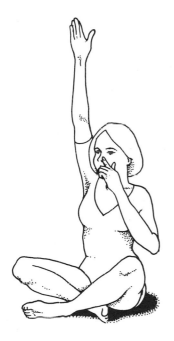

2 Sit the client in a comfortable position and have her lift one arm overhead whilst inhaling, gaining full stretch and rib expansion down the side of the body. The arm may then be dropped, keeping the ribs expanded. The client should then exhale and repeat the movement with the other arm.

   Ideally the breathing exercises should be done in fresh air, and open air walking or sports improve general respiration tremendously. If, however, this is not possible, at least clients can be encouraged to breathe deeply and recognize an improvement in their respiration, which will aid their exercise routines.

ACTIVE EXERCISES FOR
FIGURE IMPROVEMENT

A few examples will illustrate the type of exercise needed for general work, then from knowledge of body musculature and movement, a wide variety of exercises can be developed by the therapist for her clients.

1 Utilise the three walking points of the foot. The heel, the outer side of the foot, and then the inside of the foot.

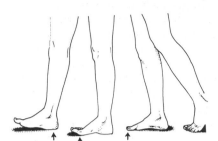

2 Inversion of the foot, ensuring that the foot is held well on its medial arch, not rolling inwards.

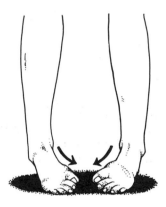

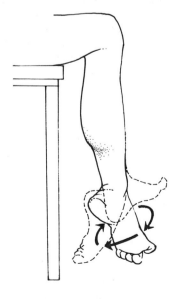

3 Sitting, plantar flex one foot to the limit, invert (turn inwards) and form a circular path attempting full rotation of the ankle, finishing at the start position. Perform the exercise with as much tension in the ankle and foot as possible. Repeat with the other foot.

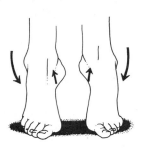

4 Stand with chair or bar support, rise onto the balls of the feet, with tension in the calves and legs, hold for a few seconds, and then lower to the start position, unrolling arched area of feet slowly. Repeat and progress to performing the exercise without the supporting chair when able.

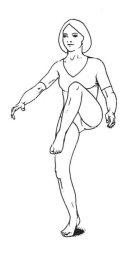

5 Stand erect, arms in wing position (on hips), and bring one knee as high as possible towards the chest, pointing the toe towards the floor (plantar flexed). Perform the movement alternately with each leg and gradually speed up the exercise until it becomes a high prancing movement. Attempt to keep breathing rhythmical and repeat only 20 times initially to avoid strain.

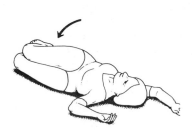

6 Crook lying, arms in yard position (outstretched), swing the hips and legs first to one side then the other, so that the thighs slap the floor sharply on each side. Keeping the shoulders and head as straight as possible, repeat the exercises six times on each side. The strength and mobility of the back should be checked before advising this exercise for clients, as it has a strenuous effect on the lower back. So it should not be attempted by clients with a history of weakness in the back, or slipped disc problems.

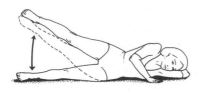

7   Side lying, with the head resting on one arm, and the upper arm supporting the trunk. The upper leg is raised 12 in. off the floor, and the other leg raised to meet it. Both legs are slowly lowered to the start position and the exercise is repeated 5—6 times. The movement is then repeated on the other side of the body. This exercise has particular effect on the muscles of the outer and inner thigh, the tensor fascia lata, the vastus lateralis and the adductors (inside thigh).

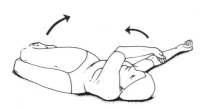

8   Crook lying, with arms stretched to one side, drop the knees to the opposite side, and then rock the legs and arms to alternate sides. The exercise strengthens the internal and external obliques, as well as involving the rectus abdominus, the quadratus lumborum, and the latissimus dorsi of the back.

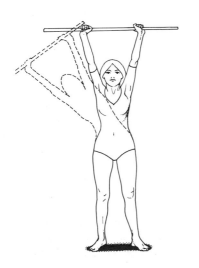

9   Stride standing, arms in yard position (outstretched sideways), bend the trunk as far as possible to the right, sliding the hand down the outside of the leg, then return to the start position. Repeat to the left side and perform the exercise alternately 10 times to each side. Keep the legs straight, and avoid the trunk bending forwards, thus gaining the most effect on the muscles of trunk rotation. This exercise can be made easier by simply rotating the trunk, and flinging the arms as widely as possible. It can also be made more difficult by keeping the outstretched arms position, whilst bending to the side. Holding a bamboo rod or stick helps to maintain the arm position and aids balance. In addition to muscles of the trunk, the quadriceps and hamstring muscle groups of the thighs are stretched and strengthened by these exercises.

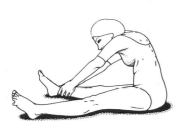

10   Sitting with legs outstretched, grasp the ankles and pull the body as close to the floor as possible. Release the hands and return to the original position. Repeat six times and for younger women follow with alternate toe touching, left hand to right toe, right hand to left toe, repeated 10—12 times. The latter part of the exercise can be made less difficult by guiding the client to reach as far down the leg as possible, rather than straining for the toe. This type of exercise exerts great strain on the lower back area, and so should be progressed gradually.

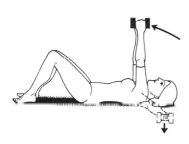

11   Supine lying, arms stretch, with small weights in the hands (books can be used at home), the arms lift to directly above the head, then slowly lower to yard position. The movement reverses to the start position and is repeated 5—6 times. The movement has to be concentrated in the pectoral area if bust improvement is sought. This can be achieved by tension in this area, so preventing the biceps of the arms taking the strain of the movement. Clients can be taught to localize the effects of exercises to achieve the best results. In this way general exercise is a good preparation for more specific muscle building or figure improvement routines.

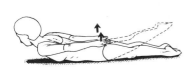

12   Prone lying, arms at sides, then legs and arms lift to form the winging movement, then return to the start position. Repeat the movement 5—6 times, increasing its difficulty and effect by raising the trunk and legs higher off the ground when sufficient strength and stamina is established. The pectoral muscles are stretched, and the lower back, buttocks and back thigh areas are also under considerable tension during the movement. Tension in the neck and upper fibres of the trapezius muscle can be helped by this exercise, and so prevent muscular discomfort developing.

ISOTONIC AND ISOMETRIC EXERCISES

Isotonic Exercise

Isotonic exercises involve active movements where the muscles concerned change in shape to bring about the movement. It has been seen that muscles work as levers, pulling on bones to bring about movement (locomotion). Muscles contract on their long axis (length), and as they become tense, shorten and thicken in shape. In extension the muscle lengthens, stretches out, and as it extends becomes thinner, flatter and loses some of its tone and tension. Most general exercise will be of the isotonic, free, active type, this being beneficial to the whole body, improving respiration, circulation, and using up energy.

However, not all clients like active exercise or are able to perform it easily. Obesity, disability, lack of time or inclination are all reasons why isotonic exercises are not followed regularly. Lack of space is another problem encountered. Rather than viewing these reasons as weak excuses from the unenthusiastic client, it is better to turn to another more convenient, socially acceptable, and still effective method of exercising – isometrics.

Isometric Exercise

Isometric exercises are some of the most useful for beauty therapists, as they can be adapted to suit every kind of person. The word 'isometric' comes from the Greek *iso*, meaning the same, and *metric*, meaning length. Isometric contraction refers therefore to the tensing or tightening of a muscle without changing its length. The tone or tension in the muscle increases, but no movement takes place.

Isometric contractions are similar in activity to static contractions as seen at work in anti-gravity muscles. The degree of tension in the muscle is, however, much greater. The muscle contracts as hard as possible against an immovable resistance such as the floor, a wall, or a heavy table. Anything can be used to provide the resistance, any available object, another person, or even the person themselves. The exercises may be performed anywhere, anytime, and for this reason appear to be followed with enthusiasm.

Convenient and popular as they are, Isometrics still need careful guidance from the therapist to ensure the client gains the most from the exercise. Clients have to be shown how to localize the main effort or contraction of the static exercise into the right area of their body. Correct breathing has to be established, and strain from overexertion prevented. Initially the therapist will need to guide the client to achieve contractions in the correct area, building concentration and control over specific muscle groups.

If general toning effects are needed, a short plan of isometric exercises can be followed which includes an exercise for each part of the body. If toning, reshaping, or muscle building is required, the exercises can be more specific and more regularly performed. The aim is to gradually improve the tension, strength and stamina of the muscles until unconsciously they are held in a state of improved tone. Athletes are an example of the benefits of being well toned, able to avoid fatigue or injury. Some of these benefits can be easily acquired by regular isometric exercise.

The principle of isometrics is to decide which muscles need exercise, consider their action, and then accomplish this action against strong resistance.

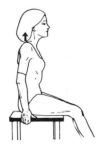

1   The trapezius muscle can be contracted by sitting the client on a chair holding the sides of the seat with the hands, and then attempting to pull up the shoulders.

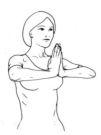

2   The pectorals can be exercised whilst sitting, with the palms pushed hard together to form a strong contraction.

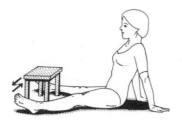

3   The adductors can be worked hard by sitting the client on the floor, with a chair in front, and placing the feet either side of the chair legs. The client then attempts to pull the legs together against the resistance of the chair.

Before each contraction a deep breath should be taken. The breath should be held in whilst a smooth contraction takes place for six seconds, breathing out and relaxing after that time. A few seconds rest between each contraction prevents too much fatigue and provides the extra intake of oxygen for the concentrated effort of isometric work.

The contraction principle of isometrics makes the list of possible exercises endless, but for general toning a programme of 10—15 exercises, taking only a minute or two to complete, is an ideal starting point. If reduction or building effects are required, more concentration and repetition will be required. Building unwanted muscles is not a likelihood, without the additional resistance of weights into a programme (see Exercise Progression page 172).

Short Exercise Programme

Neck and Head   Hands behind the head, press back hard against the hands (extension).

Hands on the forehead, press forward hard against the hands (flexion).

Hand on one side of the head, attempt to bend head sideways.

These neck exercises can also be performed by the client at home, on a bed using a pillow as the resistance.

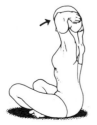
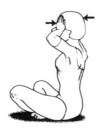
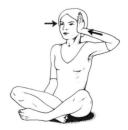

Chest and Bustline   Stand with edge of the door between the hands and pull in opposite directions.

Stand sideways in a doorway, place the hands either side of the door jamb at eye level, and push as hard as possible for six seconds.

Lower the hands to chest level and repeat.

Lower the hands to waist level and repeat.

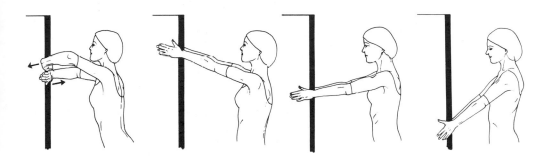

These exercises would need to be repeated for any bust improvement to be accomplished. The exercises develop all fibres of the pectoralis major and minor, and by bringing extra nourishment into the area (increased vascular supply), slowly build muscular bulk underlying the breasts.

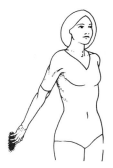

Arms   Standing with the back against a wall, form the hands into claws, with the fingers spread apart and slightly bent. Contract hands and arms strongly, with the pressure being exerted against the wall's resistance. The movement develops strength in the arms, and helps to firm the underside of the upper arm. The movement can also be accomplished sitting, grasping the chair arms behind the back, concentrating the movement in the upper arm (triceps muscle area).

The exercise can also be successfully taught for home use, for the client to do first thing in the morning whilst in bed, pressing the clawed hands hard down into the mattress. This routine needs guidance initially, to get clients to feel the contraction in the correct area of the arm, and localize its effects.

Waist

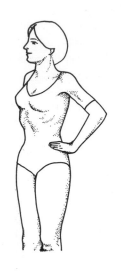

Abdominal retraction is one of the best exercises for waist reduction, and uses the body's own weight and gravity as resistance. Performed standing up, it then tightens the gluteal muscles of the buttocks as well as the rectus abdominus and obliques muscles. The muscles of the abdominal cavity are drawn in and held for a count of six whilst the buttocks are also under tension.

This exercise is excellent preparation for, and reinforcement of, active exercises for the abdominal area, and builds unconscious control of the abdominal wall, preventing forward protrusion of the abdominal contents. It can be used in pre-natal and post-natal routines, and wherever abdominal weakness is present. Overweight or really obese people can also benefit from its action as preparation for isotonic routines, when the excess weight is lost.

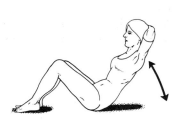

A progression from retraction is to have the client crook lying, holding a book behind the head, then attempting to sit up as far as possible and hold that position for a few seconds. Then release and lower gently to the floor. The exercise can be made more difficult by raising the legs onto a stool, a chair or up a wall. The rectus abdominus muscle is then shortened on its long axis, and a firmer flatter abdominal appearance is gained.

Side and Hips

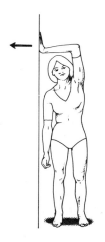

Stand the client with the left side to a wall, with the feet 12—18 in. from the wall. Place the right hand over the head with the palm against the wall. Guide the client to push hard, and feel tension forming in the muscles of the side and hip. Reverse the movement and repeat. The muscles concerned are the latissimus dorsi, the obliques, and the gluteals.

Thighs   With the client sitting with legs outstretched for all the thigh exercises, first place the feet either side of a waste bin and, keeping the legs straight, attempt to bring the feet together.

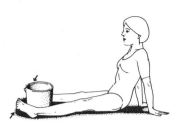

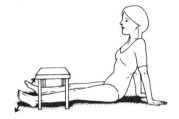

Next place the feet inside the legs of the chair, and guide the client to push out, concentrating the effort on the muscles of the thighs, the vastus lateralis and hamstrings group (posterior).

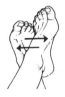

Then cross the ankles and, using the feet as resistance, have the client attempt to pull the feet apart.

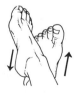

Lastly, place the left foot on top of the right one at the ankle, and have the client try to lift the right leg up straight whilst holding down with the left. Then reverse the movement.

Both active and static movements can be used freely in any exercise plan, and will be effective if followed. Recognizing the client's interest and inclination towards exercising will help the therapist to choose the best exercise plan. For it is better to give a routine that the client will follow, rather than one that she may not, however good its overall benefits can be seen to be.

EXERCISE PROGRESSION

Exercises are normally used to tone and invigorate the body, but they can also be made to build muscle tissue and change the shape of the figure. Many clients wish to improve their figure, whether to improve on nature, or because of weakness, lack of stature, or absence of shapely curves. Whatever the reason, the same principles apply. Muscle bulk can be added slowly by constantly using the muscles, or with isometric contractions, or more quickly by exercising against a steadily increasing resistance such as weights. Muscles do develop from normal usage, but the process is slow, and often more muscles than are desired become involved in the process.

Figure shaping or body building (male clients) is quite a specific art and can be used to develop only those muscles which need additional muscle bulk. Women quite naturally do not want to build large muscular shoulders or arms, but may desire extra inches on the strong breast supporting muscles, the pectorals, so that the bustline is improved. Likewise the shape of the legs may need improvement, the adductor, and vastus lateralis muscles, etc., but the anterior part of the quadriceps muscle would not normally benefit from extra development in women.

Male and female clients look for quite different improvements in their programmes, and their wishes should be considered closely. Men will require development of muscle bulk, wanting a strong, hefty looking body to give the appearance of power and virility. Women will use figure shaping to add inches in certain areas, to round out bony figures, and to give a glamorous image.

For both effects, isotonic free exercise is used in different degrees, with the addition of weights in varying forms to produce the progressive resistance exercises.

PROGRESSIVE RESISTANCE EXERCISES

When clients express a desire to shape their figures by natural exercise means, they have to understand what a long term business it will be before results occur. For this reason they often give up or turn to salon treatments to help them in their search for figure improvement. The improvement can, however, be produced by personal effort, as seen in male body building achievements. Few women seem to have the same dedication to perfecting their figures as do the men who follow this interest.

The resistance for the exercises can take many forms, small bar-bells, weighted bags, standard weights of increasing size, and exercise equipment. A range of equipment in a pleasant exercise room really becomes necessary if full weight training routines are to be interesting and enjoyable for clients. This additional service to clients is often found in conjunction with leisure centres, or alongside sauna rooms in health hydros, hotels or health clinics.

Progressive resistance routines must follow on from normal exercise, so that the client is fit, supple and has correct posture and breathing established. Exercise against resistance improves muscle strength and shape, and develops the narrow fibres in the muscles, so that the muscle bulk increases. The exercise routines can be very strenuous, and so if the client is underweight she should be encouraged to eat a balanced diet with plenty of protein and moderate carbohydrate content. Very active physical exercise always has a problem of creating appetite, which can produce a vicious circle effect for the client trying to improve her figure and lose weight.

For most purposes bar-bells and exercise equipment of the bicycle type will be all that is required for figure improvement in women. Clients will need to use the bar-bells at home if any progress is to be achieved. Exercises are performed in continuous repetitions of 10, or 5 if necessary initially, and should be performed smoothly. These repetitions form a set, and the set can be repeated after an interval to allow the breathing to recover. When the sets become very easy to do, the weights can then be increased. If the movement becomes jerky, the client is attempting more than she can manage and should be dissuaded.

The areas of the female body that may benefit from resistance exercises are: the bustline (pectoralis major and minor), the shoulders and back, if very thin (trapezius), and the legs, if underdeveloped, (gastrocnemius).

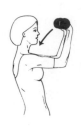

An effective routine for general figure development would be:

(i)   Exercise for the trapezius and deltoid muscles.

(ii)   Trunk raising backwards.

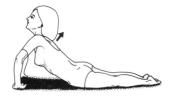

(iii)   Head raising.

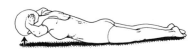

(iv)   Quadriceps development, with sandbags over the feet.

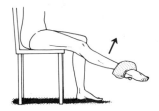

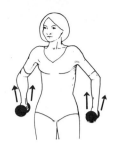

(v)   Arms raising sideways, involving the pectoralis major muscle.

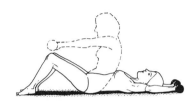

(vi)   Overhead pullover, involving the pectoralis major and rectus abdominus muscles.

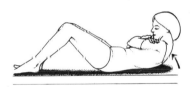

(vii)   Trunk curls, involving the rectus abdominus muscle.

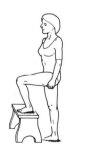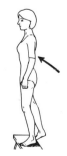

(viii)   Bench stepping, for general strength development.

CONCENTRIC AND ECCENTRIC MUSCLE WORK

It has been seen that muscles are able to work in many ways, and to maintain good condition, tone and range, the fibres must be allowed to contract and relax frequently. In isotonic work the fibres lengthen or shorten, causing movement of a joint to occur. In isometric work the muscle increases in tone, without a change in length. In resistance work the fibres are worked freely, but against an increasing load, so causing fibre development to occur.

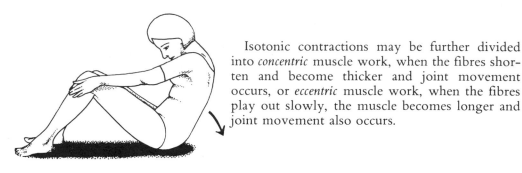

Isotonic contractions may be further divided into *concentric* muscle work, when the fibres shorten and become thicker and joint movement occurs, or *eccentric* muscle work, when the fibres play out slowly, the muscle becomes longer and joint movement also occurs.

Eccentric Movement of Rectus Abdominus

These forms of movement can be used to increase or decrease the effect of an exercise on the muscle groups concerned. Eccentric and concentric movements have already been seen within the tests for muscle strength used in diagnosis, in this case with the therapist adding the resistance to the movement. If a muscle or area is seen as very weak then eccentric muscle work can be used to gradually build strength. Often a weak muscle will be able to play out its fibres slowly, whereas it cannot contract concentrically. When there is some increase in power, concentric exercises can be given as progression. An example of this gradual approach is seen with the rectus abdominus muscle after childbirth, or caused by general weakness. The client may be unable to sit up from a supine position, but can unwind to the supine floor position from a sitting up start. The fibres are extending eccentrically and starting off the strength building and rehabilitation programme.

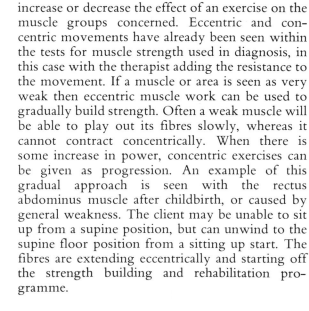

Biceps

Concentric Movement of Biceps

Range of Muscle Movement

Muscles work in a range from full contraction to full stretch and cause a joint to move. This range is called 'full range'. This can be divided into 'inner range' – when the muscle works from half contraction to full contraction or vice versa; 'outer range' – where a muscle works from half contraction to full stretch and vice versa; and 'middle range' – contraction between inner and outer range.

When exercising muscle to increase power it is necessary to work them in full range, with some extra concentration on the outer range to gain additional strength. Middle range movement is the most commonly used, and muscles are in fact most efficient in this range.

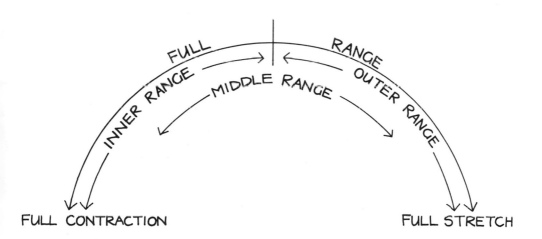

GROUP EXERCISES

A therapist may have to plan exercises specifically for a client or be called upon to run an exercise class for a group of individuals on a more general basis. In a group class there is naturally less scope for correction of specific faults, but there is always the opportunity to include generally beneficial exercises. Some figure faults are very common within any age group, so a plan can include some general and some specific elements.

A general plan of exercise should include:

Mobility exercises – to warm up, and prepare for more specific work.

Strengthening exercises – for specific correction of a fault or weakness.

The form the class could take for a half hour session might be:

1   Assemble the group and assess the individuals – age, mobility, etc., and then establish correct posture.

2   Start with respiratory exercise, deep breathing, or a vigorous exercise to cause deep breathing.

3   Exercises for the extremities; mobilizing, swinging, jumping type of exercises for the arms and legs.

4   Exercises for the head and shoulder girdle areas, to reduce tension.

5   Exercises for the trunk and spine, strengthening exercises for the abdominal muscles, and to increase mobility in the back.

6   Check posture once more, and return to mobilizing elements as a rest from the strenuous routines.

7   Exercises for the arms and legs, stretching, mobilizing elements.

8   Respiratory exercises, deep breathing or relaxation exercises.

9   Postural correction.

This rather general frame can be utilized for classes where mobilization, strengthening or reduction is desired, and has to be kept flexible to maintain client interest. Specific correction can be built into the plan if most members of the group have a similar fault, i.e. overlarge hips and thighs, and have similar ability to perform the exercises.

Group sessions will never seem as satisfactory to the therapist as individually supervised exercise plans, but they do have great value to the individual, and increase awareness of physical health.

Specific Exercise Plans

Correction or improvement of specific faults can be planned into a routine of exercises, at the strengthening stage, after mobilizing elements, and they may also be taught for home use. The schemes suggested form a useful background from which to devise personally tailored plans for clients.

REDUCTION

Exercise Schemes for Obese Clients

(in conjunction with diet control)

Neck Area   With the client in a sitting position.

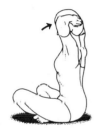

1   Head forward and back pushing.

2   Head sideways bending, aiming the ear to the shoulder.

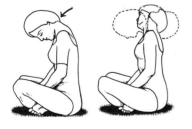

3   Head rotation to alternate sides.

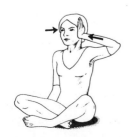

4   Pushing hands against the head, and the head against the hands using isometric principles.

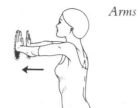

Arms

1 Standing, arms swinging forward and back.

2 Standing, arms swinging sideways and across body.

3 Yard standing, arms backward circling to make small circles, increasing and decreasing in size.

4 As in movement 3 but forwards circling.

5 Standing, hands flat on a wall, elbows bent, straighten and bend elbows.

6 Standing sideways onto the wall, one arm against the wall, push hard against the wall (isometric).

7 Prone kneeling, bend the elbows and stretch on leg out behind, straighten the elbows and lower the leg (adapted press-ups).

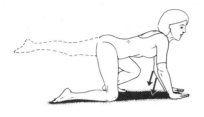

Midriff

1 Standing, hands on the lower chest wall, perform lower costal and diaphragmatic breathing against the hands.

2 Crook lying, perform sit ups.

3 Sitting cross legged, rotate the trunk to alternate sides, flinging arms.

4 Prone lying, head and shoulders raising.

5 Prone kneeling, alternate arm sideways flinging.

6 Standing, trunk circling.

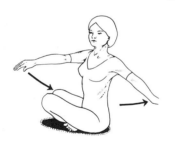

Abdomen

1 Standing, trunk circling to alternate sides.

2 Crook lying, perform sit-ups.

3 Stride lying, side bending, pushing the hand down to the knee on the same side.

4 Standing, alternate arm swinging to touch the opposite foot.

5 Sitting, trunk rotating to alternate sides.

6 Crook lying, both knees lifting to alternate shoulders.

7 Crook lying, with the knees dropping to one side, the arms reaching out to the other side, the movement rocks to alternate sides.

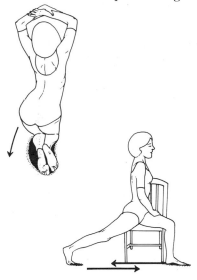

Hips and Thighs

1 Prone lying, alternate straight leg raising.
2 Prone lying, both legs straight raising.
3 Kneeling, lowering to sit on alternate sides of the hip.
4 Side lying, upper leg raising.
5 Standing, stepping on and off a chair.
6 Sitting in front of a chair, the legs inside the chair legs, push out (isometric).
7 Sitting in front of a chair, legs outside chair legs, push in (isometric).
8 Sitting, moving forwards and then backwards on the buttocks.
9 Standing, perform stride jumps.
10 Back against the wall, standing, perform knees bend and straighten.

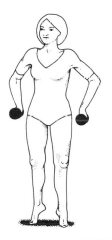

Lower Legs

1 Standing, heels raise, knees straighten, heels lower.
2 Standing, walk on toes.
3 Standing, walk on heels.
4 Standing, step onto a block with one leg, raising that heel, then lower.
5 Standing, walk on the toes, then the heels, carrying a bar-bell weight in each hand.

Each exercise in the previous scheme may be repeated as many times as the therapist considers suitable for the client. For full effect they need to be followed daily at home, so the therapist must ensure that they are performed well in the clinic before suggesting them for home use.

MOBILIZING

Exercise Scheme for Mobilizing the Shoulder Joint

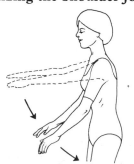

1 Standing, slightly inclined forwards, swing the arm vigorously forwards and backwards.

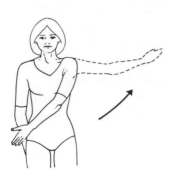

2   Standing as in *1*, swing the arm across the chest and out sideways.

These two exercises can be varied in speed, but all movements should be relaxed. To gain a little more range of movement, when the swing reaches an extremity, i.e. forwards, the client may be told to hold the arm there for a moment and push it a little harder in the forwards direction.

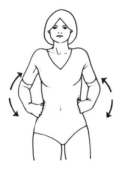

3   Standing, elbows bent, rotate arms in and out.

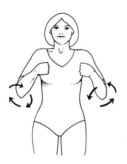

4   Standing, elbows circling, forwards and backwards.

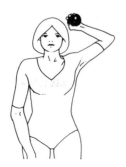

5   Standing, throwing ball or bean bag from behind the head.

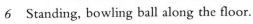

6 Standing, bowling ball along the floor.

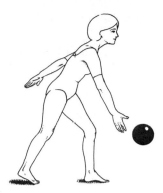

7 Sitting, holding towel over one shoulder with one hand and at waist level with the other, rub up and down the back as if drying it.

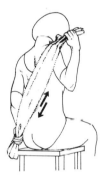

8 Standing, alternate arm circling.

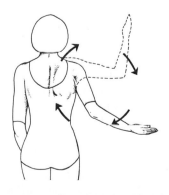

Exercise Scheme for
Mobilizing the Knee Joint

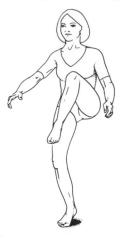

1   Standing, running on the spot, lifting the knees as high as possible.

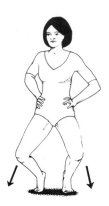

2   Standing, knees bending and straightening.

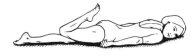

3   Prone lying, alternate leg bending, aiming to touch the buttocks.

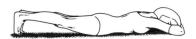

4   Prone lying, feet pushing into the floor, and knee straightening.

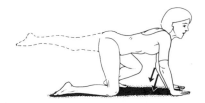

5   Prone kneeling, alternate leg bend to the chest and stretch out behind.

6 Standing, perform crouch jumps.

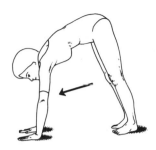
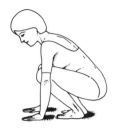

7 Long sitting, tense the legs till the heels are raised from the floor.

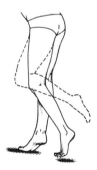

When mobilizing a joint, every possible movement of that joint must be made so that full range is gained. So a full understanding of joint movement is necessary before deciding the exercise plan.

STRENGTHENING

Exercise Scheme for Strengthening the Quadriceps

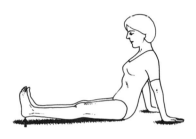

1 Standing, running on the spot.

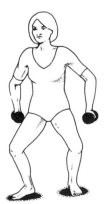

2 Standing, holding bar-bell weights, slowly bending the knees and then straightening.

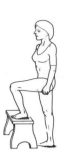
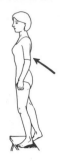

3   Standing in front of a stool, slowly stepping on and off.

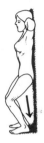

4   Back against wall, standing, slowly bending and straightening knees, keeping the back in contact with the wall.

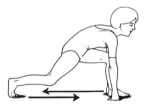

5   Commence exercise in the start position for running, with one leg straight, and one bent, then alternately bend and straighten legs with jumps.

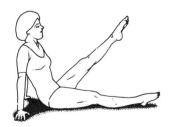

6   Long sitting, straight leg raising, foot turned out, then pointed ahead, then turned in, performing several lifts in each position.

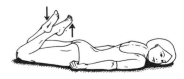

7   Prone lying, knees bent and crossed, push the upper leg down on the lower leg to give self resistance, then slowly straighten the leg.

**Exercise Scheme for
Strengthening the Back
Extensor Muscles**

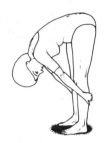

1   Standing, trunk curling and straightening.

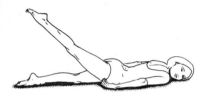

2   Prone lying, alternate legs raising, progress into both legs raising.

3   Prone lying, head and shoulders raising.

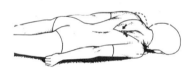

4   Prone lying, legs, head and shoulders raising.

5   Kneeling, trunk curling and stretching back, arms lifting over the head and stretching back.

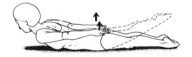

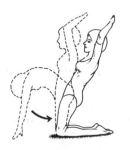

These few suggestions for schemes illustrate how all forms of movement can be incorporated into an exercise scheme. The therapist's role will be to devise interesting, flexible routines, which arc effective, and can be accomplished safely by her clients.

POST-NATAL REHABILITATION

As many of the therapist's clients are of child bearing age, she will frequently find a need for post-natal rehabilitation to help clients regain their figures. Ideally the involvement should be throughout the entire pre- and post-natal period, so that guidance can be given to minimize the effects of the pregnancy on the figure. The therapist can act to reinforce the medical ante-natal care with guidance and encouragement on diet, skin care and postural routines.

Encouragement to keep weight gains down to 9—10 kg (20—24 lb), and practise deep breathing and postural exercises will help the client to stay healthy and aid recovery after the birth. Clients normally receive excellent ante-natal advice, and the therapist simply has to ensure that it is followed. A sympathetic therapist with a keen interest in the well being of her regular clients can be very effective in maintaining morale during the course of the pregnancy.

Treatments can be adapted until well into the pregnancy, and clients advised on home care for their skin, hands and feet. Feet can be cared for professionally with pedicure routines, to minimize the effects of strain on the weight bearing surfaces.

Foot exercises can be suggested as the weight increases and the centre of gravity moves forward.

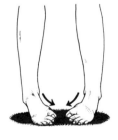

1   Foot arching, to strengthen the arch of the foot.

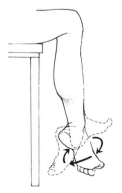

2   Ankle circling, to keep the ankle mobile and prevent oedema (swelling).

Breathing exercises, combined with posture correction are also very beneficial to the whole body's vitality at this time.

Post-natal Guidance

Immediately after the birth, medical post-natal exercises will be given, and the therapist can ensure that these are religiously followed for the first six to eight weeks. After the post-natal examination (six weeks after the birth), the client can commence clinic exercise routines to reinforce progress already achieved. The strength of the muscles should be carefully tested before deciding exercises, to ascertain the effectiveness of the post-natal work accomplished.

Mothers need a lot of encouragement to undertake exercise regularly, having a lot of other responsibilities with new babies. The importance of regaining a trim figure should be explained to the client to gain her support for the routines advised. The womb has to return to its original size and position in the abdominal cavity, to make further successful pregnancies possible. This also helps to prevent a condition which may occur in later life, that of prolapse of the womb.

Post-natal Exercises

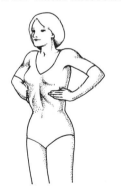

1 Diaphragmatic breathing.

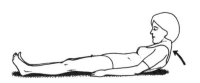

2 Supine lying, raising the head and shoulders to look at the feet, progressing slowly to sit ups.

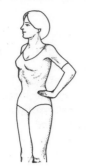

3 Abdominal retraction, initially performed lying supine, gravity assisting, progressing to standing up retraction.

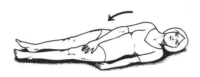

4 Lying supine, touch right hand to left knee, return to lying position, and repeat with left hand to right knee.

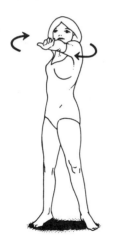

5 Trunk rotation, arms swinging.

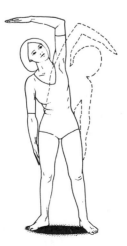

6 Side bending, sliding the right arm as far as possible down the right leg, whilst stretching the left arm, stand up and repeat to left side stretching the right arm.

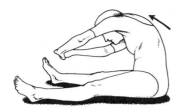

7   Toe touching, stride sitting.

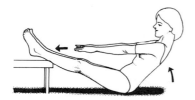

8   Lying, feet on a stool, touch the hands to the stool, return to the lying position. Slowly raise height of the foot support to chair height. Gradually this exercise shortens the rectus abdominus muscle, which has been overstretched by pregnancy.

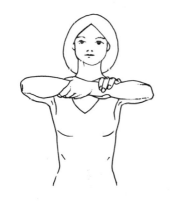

9   Isometric exercises for the pectoral muscles (see isometric exercise).

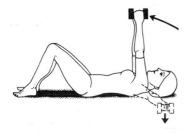

10   Lying supine, arms raising from stretch position, with weights or books in the hands, lift to an upright position over the head, lower to yard position and reverse back to the start.

The therapist is able from a wide range of exercises to devise routines to answer all the client's figure needs. If the action of muscles is understood, and the purpose of the exercise decided, then the therapist can plan individual routines, using her own skill and knowledge.

RELAXATION TECHNIQUES

Therapists will find many instances where it is beneficial to teach clients relaxation techniques to relieve mental and physical tension. Teaching relaxation reinforces the effects of manual massage, and can be supervised before the massage begins. Its main aim is to help the client to recognize tension building, and has the means through relaxation work to prevent its formation.

Relaxation is a reduction of muscle tension, and the degree of relaxation varies. The degree of tension in the muscles gives an indication of overall nervous tension in the body, and this can be determined by palpation of the muscles. Tension evident during massage will point to a need for relaxation instruction.

A therapist who is able to relax the client so thoroughly during massage that sleep is induced, has mastered the art of teaching relaxation. In order to maximize the effects of relaxation certain points should be followed.

The client should be warm whilst in the clinic, and be dealt with sympathetically. The atmosphere should be restful, and the decor conducive to relaxation. The client should be placed in a lying position, with pillow supports to maintain the relaxation posture. The most comfortable position may be side lying, or the client's normal sleeping position which can be adopted after the relaxation exercises are completed.

The relaxation routine commences with the client supine, and undertaking deep breathing in a rhythmical manner. The client should be encouraged to pause slightly at the end of each expiration, and consciously 'let go' of her whole body. If the client is able to concentrate deeply and absorb herself completely in the deep rhythmical breathing, absolute relaxation may be achieved without further treatment.

If the client needs further instruction, progressive contraction and relaxation of muscle groups is the next stage towards full relaxation. Beginning with the legs, each group of muscles is tensed and relaxed several times. The arms, trunk, neck and face muscle groups are progressively contracted and relaxed.

The client may fall asleep at any time during the routine, and will naturally assume the most comfortable position. If the therapist feels the client is close to sleep, she can gently guide her to assume a side lying position, which can then be supported with pillows if necessary.

At the conclusion of the relaxation treatment the client's whole body should be totally relaxed, and this effect should be maintained as long as possible, with the client being allowed to wake naturally. Relaxation therapy is easiest to apply in a residential situation like a health hydro, where the client can be left to rest and unwind in peace. In a normal clinic situation the therapist's role will be mainly to teach the principles of relaxation, for clients to apply in their normal daily life.

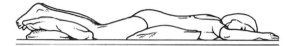

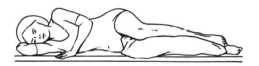

Chapter 5

Manual Massage

GENERAL EFFECTS AND BENEFITS OF MASSAGE

Among the skills of the beauty therapist, ability to perform a relaxing massage must rate as an essential ingredient for commercial success. Many treatments produce more visible effects, with recorded results, but nothing can match the relaxing or invigorating power of skilful manual techniques on the body. Because the results are less obvious, there is a temptation to underrate the value of manual massage.

When the effects of massage are fully understood, its value in modern life becomes clear. Skilfully applied by a thoughtful and caring masseuse, it can take on a three dimensional quality, producing effects of relaxing, maintaining, or stimulating the body's systems to greater efficiency. Whilst nothing can replace the role of exercise in maintaining physical health, manual massage has a valuable contribution to make through circulation improvement. The effects on the muscular system of the body bring about increased interchange of tissue fluids, relieving fatigue and preventing a build up of tension.

Recognition of muscular tension may show that stress, anxiety, or depression are present, and may indicate that the calming, soothing elements of massage are needed. Tight, hard muscles, with fibrous thickenings and discomfort on movement, all point to a need for muscular relaxation. This allows the muscles to co-ordinate to their fullest efficiency. Where discomfort is felt, muscles will attempt to compensate to relieve the strain and so stiff muscles are formed. All these minor problems could be avoided if massage was used as a preventative treatment to keep the body in peak condition.

Care of the body, and relaxation of the mind through massage is an ancient art, with its value proven over centuries for dispelling the cares and tensions of daily life. Its presence is recorded at different times in history, but it is best known from Roman times, where it was an integral part of their social culture. In association with steam heat, dry heat, and cold baths, massage formed part of the cleansing and relaxation ritual, and great importance was placed on anointing the body with scented oils.

In recent times the study of massage has become more scientific, with the differing movements studied for their effects on vascular, lymphatic, and muscular systems of the body. In 1813 the Royal Central Institute was established in Stockholm, Sweden, and from this Institute came most of the systems of general massage known as 'Swedish'. There are many schools of thought on the effects of different movements, and combinations of movements, to create special effects on the body. Medical opinion is divided over its value in restoring the function of muscular tissue, and its role in physiotherapy has diminished over the years, due to the pressures of time and convenience of application.

However, as therapists are not concerned with restoring the function of muscles, but with simply maintaining and promoting healthy bodies, massage is a valuable tool in their range of treatment. The relaxation and enjoyment that is gained from massage is fully appreciated by the general public and the medical profession, and this provides a tremendous opportunity for the therapist to use her skills. Having the time and ability to offer a massage personally tailored to the client's physiological and psychological needs, she is in a unique position, and should use it to the full.

General Massage

The therapist is primarily concerned with general massage, where all areas of the body are manipulated to different degrees, to bring about relaxation which eases physical and mental tension. By altering the combination of movements a more stimulating effect can be created, which leaves the client feeling toned and invigorated, rather than relaxed and sleepy.

However, manual massage is normally considered for its relaxation powers, for which it cannot be equalled. No other treatment provides the degree of personal contact found in the manual skills, and for this reason they remain the pivot point for all the other skills the therapist must acquire.

Whilst developing manual skills, the therapist can learn a great deal about the body; how it feels in tension, and the changes occurring as relaxation develops; the difference between young and old muscular tissue, and skin texture; and the problems which life itself brings to the body. Also, client handling and conversation abilities develop at the same time as the manual techniques are improving. The therapist certainly learns more about her client and how she can help her from a one hour body massage than from any other form of treatment. Skilled hands and a thoughtful mind are still the best diagnostic tools in existence.

Before a truly effective massage routine can be applied, certain background information is required of the general circulatory and muscular systems of the body. It is known that muscles co-ordinate into groups to perform essential movements, and this knowledge is vital to the therapist for planning exercise work. It also reinforces the information gained of the superficial musculature, which more closely affects the masseuse. It has to be remembered that the muscular bulk of the body is three dimensional, and in conjunction with bones, joints, and tendons, is responsible for the erect and moving body.

The stimulus for the movements is naturally through the nervous system, but for massage purposes the primary concern is the muscular system and the position of individual muscles. Also important is a sound knowledge of the vascular system of the body, as correctly applied massage can aid the venous and lymphatic circulation. On its own massage has a local effect, but in conjunction with heat treatments the entire body circulation is increased temporarily. The pulse quickens, the heart beat is increased and the stimulation to the whole physical system is considerable.

Although this effect is only temporary, it does appear to have long term benefits in improved vitality and feelings of well being. Insufficient medical research has been completed to fully prove the value of massage in improving circulation, but for therapy purposes proof is not necessary. Clients understand the value of massage by the way they feel, and judge its worth on a personal level. Improved vigour, supple joints and flexible muscles, plus feelings of regeneration, are all benefits clients derive from massage. Improved skin texture, a reduction in circulation problems, (swelling, varicosity, and chilblains in the legs) and freedom from fibrous accumulations, are all additional bonuses. Most important, however, is the effect prized above all others – that of total relaxation – which frees the mind and body from anxiety and tension.

This effect has real benefits in health terms, and maintains the body functions naturally, avoiding the need for drugs to produce calming or anti-depressant effects. The use of medically prescribed drugs for anxiety, depression, or stress, is vast, and shows that a tremendous need exists for relaxation techniques. Massage, skilfully and sympathetically applied, must be seen as a better way to cope with the stresses of life, dealing as it does with the client's physical and psychological need for relaxation.

THE VASCULAR CIRCULATION

The circulatory system of the body is extremely complex and must be studied in depth. Although this is beyond the scope of this book, a few points to demonstrate the relationship of massage to the circulatory system may prove useful.

Transportation is the primary function of the circulatory system, with food and oxygen being carried to all the body's cells. It also plays a large part in maintaining the body's hydric balance and metabolism. Its role as a defence against infection is also vital to survival. All these functions occur through the system's transportation network of arteries, veins, and the connecting smaller blood vessels, the capillaries. All arteries except the pulmonary artery and its branches carry oxygenated blood from the heart, or serve as distributors, carrying the blood to the capillaries. Veins function simply as collectors, returning de-oxygenated blood from the capillaries to the heart. The heart acts as a pump, keeping the blood moving through the system of vessels, to meet physical demands. The entire circulatory system works to keep the capillaries supplied with an adequate amount of blood for its needs. Increased demand on the capillary network of the body, perhaps through massage stimulation, is answered by an increased response of blood circulation, either locally or generally; for functionally the capillaries are the most important blood vessels, permitting the interchange of tissue fluids to take place, and allowing essential nutrients to reach the cells of the body.

Principal Arteries of the Body

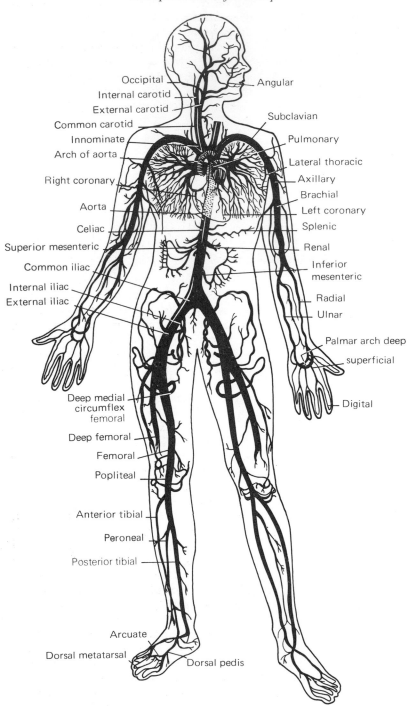

Occipital

Internal carotid

External carotid

Common carotid

Innominate

Arch of aorta

Right coronary

Aorta

Celiac

Superior mesenteric

Common iliac

Internal iliac

External iliac

Deep medial
circumflex
femoral

Deep femoral

Femoral

Popliteal

Anterior tibial

Peroneal

Posterior tibial

Arcuate

Dorsal metatarsal

Angular

Subclavian

Pulmonary

Lateral thoracic

Axillary

Brachial

Left coronary

Splenic

Renal

Inferior
mesenteric

Radial

Ulnar

Palmar arch deep

superficial

Digital

Dorsal pedis

Principal Veins of the Body

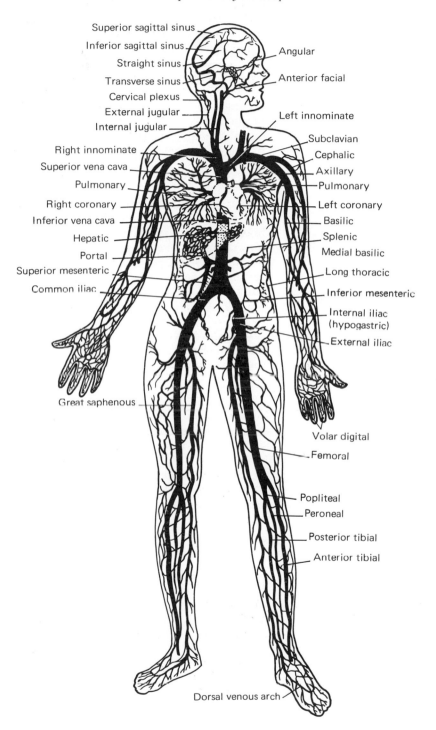

Superior sagittal sinus
Inferior sagittal sinus
Straight sinus
Transverse sinus
Cervical plexus
External jugular
Internal jugular
Right innominate
Superior vena cava
Pulmonary
Right coronary
Inferior vena cava
Hepatic
Portal
Superior mesenteric
Common iliac
Great saphenous

Angular
Anterior facial
Left innominate
Subclavian
Cephalic
Axillary
Pulmonary
Left coronary
Basilic
Splenic
Medial basilic
Long thoracic
Inferior mesenteric
Internal iliac (hypogastric)
External iliac
Volar digital
Femoral
Popliteal
Peroneal
Posterior tibial
Anterior tibial

Dorsal venous arch

EFFECTS OF MASSAGE

It has been seen that in therapy work it is unnecessary to 'prove' the effects of massage, simply to understand its benefits and apply them to the best advantage: unlike medical practice, where physical changes have to be measured, and research proved, before a treatment can be prescribed. Where restoration of function is needed in medical work, the need for proven results becomes evident to justify its use within the physiotherapy field. A great difference of opinion exists regarding the physical therapeutic effects of massage on patients, and its use has declined in the hospital service.

This approach to analysing the effects of massage clinically has been useful to beauty therapists, however, as it prevents false claims or misunderstanding over the effects massage can create within the body. For the therapist applies massage for maintenance of physical health and well being and to induce relaxation, and not to restore function. The remedial aspects of massage for correction of physical conditions, muscular, respiratory, etc., are within the medical province of the physiotherapist and play no part in the beauty therapist's work.

The range of effects available to a skilled masseuse/therapist within manual massage is vast, and worthy of appreciation in their own right. Therapists who understand and believe in the effects of massage will be able to accomplish extremely beneficial treatments for their clients. They may also be suprised by the effectiveness of their routines, with clients seeming restored in mind and body simply by application of an age-old technique.

There exists a view that massage may indeed have a healing influence, which comes from the process of 'the laying on of hands' seen since biblical times. There are many clients who would support this view, and there is no doubt that a sympathetically, skilfully applied massage does bring about a restfulness of mind and body that is hard to define.

EFFECTS OF MASSAGE ON THE SKIN, MUSCLES AND ADIPOSE TISSUE

Effects on the Skin

Application of general massage with a suitable medium for the skin type, has several benefits. Talc or no medium is used for greasy skins, or one prone to perspiration. Fine oils or cream are used for the normal or dry skin to feed the skin whilst helping the movements.

Massage – improves skin texture by helping the skin to function more efficiently.

By improving the skin circulation through vaso-dilation of surface capillaries, skin colour is improved.

Through increased removal of waste products via the lymphatic system, skin imperfections become less evident.

Improved circulation delays the formation of fibrous imperfections, skin tags, epidermal warts, cysts, etc.

Small fibrous skin growths and milia can disperse naturally.

On dry skin the sebaceous secretions are increased. This effect is enhanced by use of fine penetrating oils or cream within the massage.

The skin becomes soft and smooth, and rough skin is gradually desquamated (shed).

The skin remains supple, intact, and so at less risk from bacterial invasion.

Wrinkles appear to be delayed, or appear less obvious. The skin's elasticity is increased by regular massage; an important point for the older or post-natal client.

Effects on Muscles

Massage – will not increase the strength of normal muscles, but keeps them in good tone.

It relieves fatigue in muscular tissue, by removing the accumulation of lactic acid in the tissues.

Regular massage will prevent the formation of fibrosis in muscular tissue, or reduce its development.

Massage acts to help the muscle function at its maximum efficiency.

Tense, contracted muscles can be relaxed by suitable massage routines.

Effects on Adipose Tissue

Massage – has no direct effect on adipose tissue deposits, which may only be removed by reduced food intake.

In conjunction with a reduction diet massage can be useful to help firm the contours, and improve the circulation of the body.

Locally applied massage and specific exercise can help ensure stubborn, long established fat deposits are reduced as well as the subcutaneous fatty tissue, within a diet plan.

Soft fat deposits, connected with ineffective circulation, can be improved by locally applied massage. Here the massage is working to improve the circulation and remove intercellular infiltrations, and must be part of a treatment programme for success.

THE DEFINITION OF MASSAGE

Massage is classically defined as manipulation of the soft tissues of the body, performed by the hands, for the purpose of producing effects on the vascular, muscular and nervous systems of the body.

For therapy purposes general massage can be seen as a means of either inducing relaxation, or invigorating the system, depending on the choice and combination of massage movements. Whatever the effect desired, the basic components for massage remain constant, being based on a range of varied massage movements.

Classification of Massage Movements

Massage movements are described or classified in many different ways, and it is convenient to know into which category or group each type of movement falls, so that its purpose is understood. It does not matter what a movement is called, as long as its purpose and effect is understood, so that it can be applied safely to good effect. Massage movements come under three main headings:

(*i*)   *Effleurage* or *Stroking* movements.

(*ii*)   *Pétrissage* or *Compression* movements.

(*iii*)   *Tapotement* or *Percussion* movements,

with most movements being able to be placed by effect into one of these groups. There are also:

Vibratory movements, which are a group on their own, not fitting into any of the above classifications.

These main groups can be further divided, and it becomes apparent that most well known movements fall into one of these main groups. All movements may be varied by altering pressure, direction, and the area of the hand used in the application. A uniform speed of seven inches per second, and an even rhythm has to be maintained during the massage wherever possible.

Effleurage or *Stroking Movements* include:

Superficial effleurage.

Deep effleurage.

Superficial stroking.

Deep stroking.

Pétrissage or *Compression Movements* include:

>>> Kneading – Palmar kneading.
>>> Double handed kneading.
>>> Thumb kneading.
>>> Digital kneading.
>>> Wringing (double handed).
>>> Rolling.
>>> Pinchment.
>> Frictions – Finger or thumb frictions.

Tapotement or *Percussion Movements* include:

>>> Beating.
>>> Pounding.
>>> Clapping.
>>> Hacking.

Vibratory Movements include:

>>> Digital vibrations, static or running.
>>> Thumb vibrations.
>>> Palmar vibrations.

DESCRIPTION OF MASSAGE MOVEMENTS

Effleurage or Stroking Movements

These movements commence, link and complete the massage routine, and are applied with the entire palmar (palm) surface of the hand, or as large a part of the palm as will fit the area available. The movement commences with superficial strokes, moving over an extended area of the body, and may be applied in a centrifugal direction to follow the normal direction of bodily vellus hair. As the pressure used is so light the direction may be towards the heart (centripetal), or away from the heart (centrifugal). The stroke may return to the start position with constant pressure, or can be free from the client. The making and breaking of contact with the client's skin at the start and finish of a stroke should be so gradual as to be imperceptible. The hand contours to the area under treatment, and exerts equal pressure over the entire contact area. The thumbs are abducted, and the fingers held close together in a flexible manner. When sufficient relaxation has been achieved the pressure of the strokes can increase to become deep effleurage or stroking.

Deep strokes are applied towards the heart, and bring about a physical response from the surface capillary network. The movement maintains constant but increased pressure, and pays special attention to rhythm and the speed of the application. The upward deep strokes are returned with superficial strokes, and contact is then maintained throughout to develop relaxation.

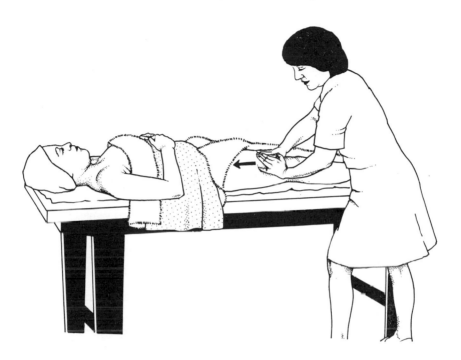

Benefits of Effleurage/Stroking

Superficial

1   Stimulation of sensory nerve endings brings about a reflex response in the skin's circulatory network.

2   The venous and lymphatic flow is increased locally.

3   Relaxation of contracted, tense muscle fibres may be obtained through the reflex response to stroking.

4   Generally a feeling of relaxation is accomplished which can be very sedative in effect.

Deep

1   Aids venous circulation by a mechanical response to the pressure used.

2   Arterial circulation is aided by removal of congestion in the veins.

3 Lymphatic circulation is improved and absorption of waste products is hastened.

4 Aids desquamation (skin shedding process).

5 Aids relaxation in preparation for further massage.

6 Re-establishes relaxation during the massage routine when used to link more active movements.

7 Brings about relaxation of contracted muscles.

Pétrissage or Compression Movements

Kneading Movements

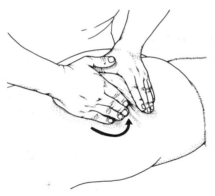

A compression movement is performed with intermittent pressure, either with one or both hands, or parts of the hands. The pressure is smoothly and firmly applied, then relaxed, and the movement progresses to an adjacent area and is repeated. The movement normally follows the shape of the muscles working from the insertion to the origin, usually distal to proximal towards the heart. The pétrissage or compression movement, termed kneading, may be performed in many ways and is described by the part of the hand used to accomplish the massage, i.e. palmar or thumb kneading.

The pressure used must vary according to the purpose of the massage and the bulk of tissues under treatment. The degree of pressure has to be reduced as the muscle bulk decreases, and this can be aided by reducing the area of the hand used to achieve the movement. Whatever the routine and combination of kneading movements, the heavy pressure must always be applied towards the heart (centripetal) to aid the venous and lymphatic flow.

The rhythm and rate of movement (established rate seven inches per second) are equally important in the pétrissage/compression movements, particularly as the pressure is applied intermittently. Care must be taken to avoid pinching the skin at the end of strokes, and effleurage used freely to link the movements in a purposeful manner.

Frictions

Frictions are compression movements but as they have a different purpose from the kneading type of pétrissage/compression massage, they may be considered separately. Frictions are concentrated movements exerting controlled pressure on a small area of the surface tissues, moving them over the underlying structures. The movements are applied in a circular manner with the thumb

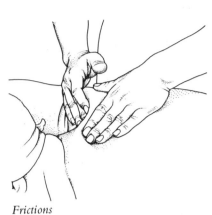

Frictions

pad of the palm, the fingers, or the distal phalanx of the thumb. The movement completes several small circles over a limited area, placing a degree of stretch on the underlying structures. The pressure is then relaxed and the hand moves on to an adjacent area without losing contact.

The movement may be applied along a muscle, or be more generally applied, for as its purpose is to produce a stretching releasing effect on tissues, it need not follow a centripetal path. It is useful, however, if the linking deep effleurage movements which follow do move firmly towards the heart, to aid the venous and lymphatic return.

Effects and Benefits of Pétrissage or Compression Movements

The *immediate effects* and *long term benefits* of all compression movements are:

Kneading

1 Compression and relaxation of muscle tissue causes the vascular and lymphatic vessels to be emptied and filled, thus increasing the circulation and hastening the removal of waste products.

2 This in turn eliminates fatigue, by removing lactic acid from the muscular tissues.

3 Hard contracted muscles are relaxed, so preventing the formation of *fibrositis* in the tissues.

4 Correctly applied compression movements produce a toning effect on muscular tissue, and can act as a reinforcement to natural exercise.

Frictions

1 Prevent the formation of skin adhesions.

2 Free adhesions or prevent their formation in deeper structures.

3 Prevent the formation of fibrositis in muscular tissue if applied regularly, particularly in the trapezius muscle of the upper back.

4 Aids absorption of fluid around the joints, particularly swelling (oedema) in the ankle area. This may only be applied if the condition is medically checked, and attributed to poor circulation, tiredness, etc., and is not connected to any systemic condition.

Tapotement or Percussion Movements

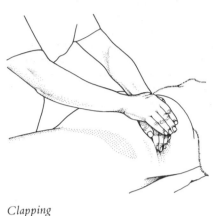

Clapping

All percussion movements are stimulating and should only be used if a general toning effect is required from the massage, rather than relaxation. Percussion movements come in many different forms, the best known are clapping (also known as cupping), beating, pounding and hacking. Sufficient muscular and adipose tissue must be present for these movements to be applied to any part of the body.

Clapping is performed with the hands formed into loose cups, which rhythmically strike the body, producing a distinctive clapping sound. The hands form a vacuum like effect on their palmar surfaces, appearing to draw up the bulky tissues, creating an immediate erythema reaction (skin reddening).

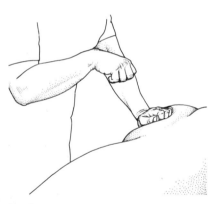

Beating

Beating, where the hands form into loose fists, and the movement is performed with the assistance of gravity, with the arms dropping from shoulder level to strike the client's body. The strokes are repeated rhythmically, slowly or quickly depending on the degree of stimulation required. A change in skin colour and temperature should be instantaneous if the movement is correctly applied.

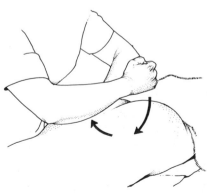

Pounding

Pounding, where the outer borders of the hands are used to accomplish the movement, with the hands loosely closed, and the impetus coming from the therapist's elbows and forearms. The hands quickly strike and turn inwards, back towards the therapist in a glancing fashion. The hands circle each other, and the movement is fairly rapid in application, although equally as stimulating as beating.

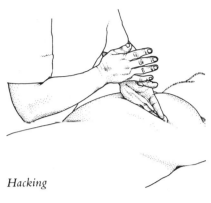

Hacking

Hacking, which is a much lighter, faster movement than the others, is performed with the hands at right angles to the wrists, the palms facing but not touching. The elbows are held well away from the body, the shoulders should be relaxed and the hands slightly flexed. The hands twist and the fingers flick against the skin in rapid succession, to produce light glancing movements. The fingers touch and leave the skin's surface very rapidly, with the outer three fingers of each hand being most involved. Hacking is always performed across the muscle fibres, and is also very stimulating both to the circulation and to the sensory nerve endings.

Effects and Benefits of Tapotement or Percussion

Clapping, Beating, and Pounding

1   A very stimulating effect is produced on the circulatory system.

2   Erythema is produced locally.

3   There is a local rise in skin temperature.

4   Sensory nerve endings are irritated, so bringing about vaso-dilation of blood vessels.

5   Reflex contraction of muscle tissue is produced.

Hacking

1   Causes muscle fibres to contract momentarily as a response to stimuli. Nerve paths become clearer, and muscles improve in tone and muscular response.

2   Blanches the skin if given for a short period, due to contraction of the superficial blood vessels.

3   Causes dilation of blood vessels, erythema, and a change in skin temperature, etc., if given heavily for a longer period.

It can be seen that percussion movements can be very effective in stimulating the circulatory and nervous systems of the body. If these effects are desired they may be incorporated into the general massage. Sufficient bulk of tissues must be available for the movements, and pain should never be experienced. Contra-indications must be checked carefully (reasons why the treatment may not be given), to avoid unwanted effects occurring.

When skill and control of percussion/tapotement movements is developed, they may be applied to less protected areas of the body, such as the back, shoulders, upper arms. Initially these vigorous movements should be restricted to the buttocks, and possibly the thighs if sufficient bulk is present.

Vibrations

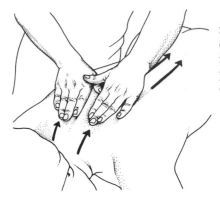

Vibrations are fine trembling movements performed on or along a nerve path, by the fingers or distal phalanx of the thumb. The muscles of the forearm are continually contracted and relaxed to produce this fine trembling or vibration, which can be applied either in a static or a running form.

Effects of Vibrations

1 Stimulates and clears nerve paths.
2 Brings about relaxation and relieves tension.

REQUIREMENTS FOR GENERAL MASSAGE

The most important requirement for massage is a skilful application, based on thoughtful concentration and understanding of the purpose of the massage chosen.

Technique

Correct technique forms the basis of requirements for massage, and is even more important than the routine of movements chosen.

The therapist should have a correct and easy posture, to permit free movement without fatigue.

Massage should be applied in a rhythmical, calm manner.

The correct rate of movement should be used wherever possible, to increase the client's relaxation effects (established rate seven inches per second).

Pressure should be altered to meet changes in the amount of muscle bulk available, and the tension present in the muscle.

Massage movements should be altered in duration, intensity, and sequence if this appears to be necessary or more beneficial.

Flexible, strong hands which can contour to the area under treatment should be developed.

A caring attitude, and restful personality will increase the effectiveness of all forms of massage for the client.

Equipment For Massage

Unlike many other aspects of beauty therapy, manual massage requires very little equipment for successful treatment to be possible; the most important elements being the skilled and sympathetic masseuse, and her client. Other equipment needed would include:

A firm plinth or massage couch of a suitable working height.

A warm, light, washable blanket or bath sheet to keep the client comfortable.

Towels, sheets or disposable tissues to protect the bed and the client.

Pillows, large and small, for head and limb support during massage.

Massage medium – talc, oil, or cream according to skin type.

The treatment area should be restful, with natural or indirect lighting if possible. Overhead lights which glare down directly into the client's eyes should be avoided. Co-ordinating colours in towels, blankets, gowns, etc., create a harmonious and luxurious effect which adds to the client's enjoyment.

There should be adequate space for the therapist to move freely around the massage plinth, to accomplish the massage. The plinth should be wide enough to support the client, but not so wide that she has to be moved in order that a movement can be completed. Tall or very small therapists should alter their working position by either raising the plinth, or raising themselves. This can be accomplished by blocks on each leg of the plinth, or by working on stable duckboards all around the massage position. Permanent positions of work would justify the purchase of a couch made to the exact height required. The therapist will never be able to complete a really satisfactory massage until her working stance is correct.

Working Stance

The therapist works in a relaxed and easy posture, which gives freedom to the arms and control to the hands. Body weight should be supported between both feet, and the general posture should be upright, not bent over or with the back hollowed and buttocks protruding. The strain of heavier movements will be less fatiguing if the load is spread, using body weight to relieve strain in the shoulders and upper spine. The therapist can sway gently back and forwards when completing sweeping movements, to help body rhythm. The posture when working should appear to lift from the hips, with the back straight and the shoulders relaxed to avoid back strain developing.

Body weight can be used to regulate pressure in massage movements, and it will always be needed by the more slightly built therapist. Unnecessary use of the body and swaying movements should be avoided however, and as strength and skill develops, the movements become localized to the therapist's arms and hands. Unnecessary movement is wasteful of the therapist's energy and distracting to the client's relaxation.

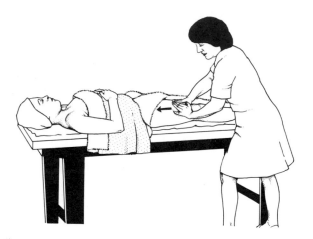

Correct Working Posture

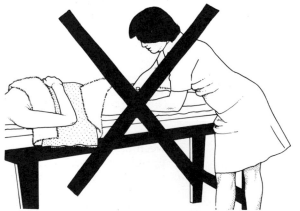

Incorrect Posture

Hand Contact and Flexibility

All massage is applied directly to the skin, using a suitable medium or no medium if it seems unnecessary. The therapist's sense of touch develops gradually as the understanding of underlying structures and musculature grows. An awareness of tension, discomfort, or pain in an area can be detected by touch alone, if sufficient thoughtful concentration is being used to guide the hands.

Differences in skin and muscular tone and texture, requiring different methods of treatment, can also be decided by touch. It has been seen how manual massage acts as a part of the figure diagnosis process if improvement is needed, and this effect can be extended in massage to gain maximum benefit for the client.

Flexible hands can be developed by practise of massage procedures and also by simple hand exercises. Strength in massage tends to come with experience, and naturally is linked to the therapist's size and stamina. The hands must contour to the area of treatment like a second skin, flowing over the surface with gentle but firm movements. The maximum amount of palmar surface should be in contact during stroking movements, so this requires a mobile and relaxed hand. The joints of the hands should be freely movable, and the fingers and thumbs capable of hyper-extension, to bring their pads into skin contact, so avoiding nails scratching. The nails should be short, and the cuticles smooth, to avoid catching the skin. The hands should be soft, warm and dry for maximum comfort.

Simple hand exercises can be performed to speed the hand mobility process, and can be linked with mobilizing exercises for the arms and shoulder girdle. This ensures that the breathing is correct and that strain does not develop on performing the massage, which initially is found quite strenuous.

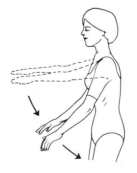

1   Arm swinging backwards and forwards.

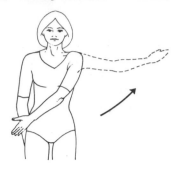

2   Arm flinging outwards.

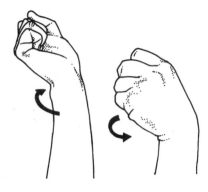

3   Rotation of wrists, inwards and outwards.

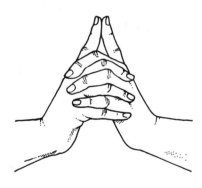

4   Pushing the fingers back, one by one.

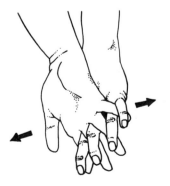

5   Locking the hands and pulling apart.

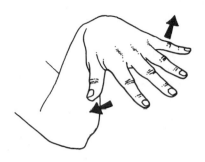

6 Shaking the hands vigorously.

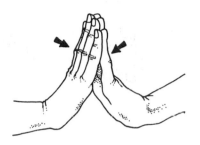

7 Pushing one hand back against the other, to tip the fingers back.

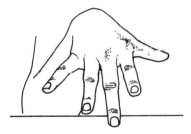

8 Piano movements on a hard surface.

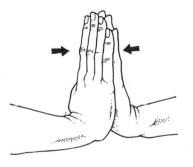

9 Pushing the palms together to gain total contact of the palmar surface.

MEDICAL LIAISON AND CONTRA-INDICATIONS TO MASSAGE

Before commencing massage treatment on a client it is necessary to ascertain the state of her health, to avoid harmful routines being applied. If the client is a regular customer her clinic card will contain details of her general history, and these can be considered (see Chapter 1: Clients' Record Cards). If the client does not know the state of her health she should be advised to check with her own doctor, particularly if the massage is to form only part of an overall treatment plan.

Manual massage does not have many *total* contra-indications, but may need to be adapted to suit the client's physical condition. If the therapist has any anxiety over the client's health, she must ask her to obtain medical approval prior to treatment, explaining the reasons why this is necessary to the client. Few clients will take exception to this point, if it is presented as being for the client's own welfare, and will see it as an example of a professional approach to the work.

Most clients are normal healthy individuals, and have few problems. However, the more difficult clients need not be excluded, as they will gain the most benefit from massage; but their problems *must* be known to the therapist before a routine can be devised. The medical profession is seldom reluctant to co-operate on this point, but is increasingly judging it as a more responsible attitude on the part of the therapy industry, who for so long declined to have its work scrutinized or judged on its merits.

CONTRA-INDICATIONS TO MASSAGE

General Conditions

Massage should not be performed if the client suffers from any systemic illness which affects the circulation, or if she has recently had an operation or suffered a fracture. Conditions such as diabetes, asthma, heart conditions, nervous disorders, or blood pressure problems would not normally be suitable for treatment. The decision, however, rests with the physician, who alone knows the degree of the problem, and whether any benefit could be derived from massage. There are many conditions which would not be altered by massage, but if it makes the client feel better within themselves, it might be considered to be of value for that reason.

Local Conditions

Massage should not be performed over recent scar tissue, which can simply be avoided for 6—9 months, until internal healing is complete or medical permission is gained.

Evidence of a spastic condition, or postural deformity, such as curvature of the spine, requires medical approval and guidance.

Skin disorders that are infectious or carried by cross infection to other clients. Many skin disorders of nervous origin benefit from massage, and if approached in a professional way can be very beneficial. Psoriasis is an example of a skin disorder that can benefit from massage, but of course only the doctor can decide.

Varicose veins or varicose ulcers are contra-indicated to massage. Where the varicosity is established, and the veins are bulbous, dark and bulging on the legs, massage would be painful and harmful. To prevent the formation of varicose veins however, massage is invaluable in aiding the venous return in the legs, particularly within an exercise and general guidance plan.

Acute joint conditions, swelling, bruising, or inflammation of the veins (phlebitis), would be contra-indicated.

Extremely thin or very elderly clients should not be treated with Tapotement/Percussion movements, as bruising and discomfort would result.

Tapotement/Percussion should never be applied over the abdominal cavity due to its lack of bony support.

Temporary Conditions

If the client has a high temperature, or is feverish, perhaps sickening for something, massage should not be applied.

Sunburnt clients who have overexposed their skins, and have taut, painful areas, should not be massaged.

Bites, stings, heavy bruising or cuts should be avoided in the routine.

Abdominal massage should be avoided during the menstrual flow, or at any time it is uncomfortable for the client. Constipated clients may find the massage initially uncomfortable but as muscle spasm relaxes, may find it very beneficial as part of the process, with corrected diet, of re-establishing regular bowel movements. Severe constipation problems must be checked with the doctor.

The later stages of pregnancy are not suitable for massage generally, but local applications can be given to the limbs well into the pregnancy.

In an area where extreme pain or tension seems to be muscular in origin it must be checked with the doctor. Massage and heat may be advised, but it is not the therapist's decision. Apart from courtesy to the doctor, it is primarily for the client's safety that medical advice be sought. Pain in any area may be due to inflammation, for which manipulation and heat could be very dangerous. Inflammation of the ovaries, kidney infections, slipped disc problems, etc., can all produce feelings similar to acute muscular pain, so the dangers are apparent, and the therapist must act in a responsible manner.

It would appear that the reasons for *not* performing massage are many, and that constant adaptation is necessary. In practice the therapist finds most clients able to benefit from some form of massage, possibly adapted slightly to individual needs. This makes massage interesting and a challenge, which gives variety to the work. The therapist has got to be alert to the rare occasion when all is not well with the client, as she works in isolation and does not complete her work under the protection of medical direction.

PREPARATION FOR MASSAGE

Whatever the purpose of the massage, the preparation should always be efficiently carried out so that a well organized appearance is presented to the client. The working position, treatment area, and the therapist should appear ready for the client, who should be welcomed in a pleasant manner. A few words of conversation places the client at ease, starts off the relaxation process and avoids embarrassment or anxiety over the treatment. It also helps the therapist in her choice of massage routine, revealing areas of tension or anxiety to the client, which can be given special attention in the treatment.

Client modesty is important to consider, as this is an area which can cause considerable embarrassment to both client and therapist. The client should be allowed the degree of modesty that feels right to her at that time. Ideally the massage should be completed with the client naked under the protective towels, so that the massage can proceed smoothly without interruptions or restriction of the massage strokes. But if the client feels more comfortable retaining her pants or bikini briefs, this is quite acceptable practice. The manner of the therapist and her ability to put her client at ease will tend to determine the degree of undress. It is a measure of this ability and professionalism, when the client feels completely at ease in her presence, free from embarrassment, that the client is able to benefit fully from the massage. Most of the embarrassment felt is projected by the *inexperienced* therapist, and picked up and reflected by the client. But as skill and confidence grow so do client handling abilities and a more professional approach is achieved.

For most purposes a general massage is used in therapy, and this is the routine learnt initially to develop smoothness, rhythm, strength and control of the hands. Skill in general massage develops the sense of touch needed when more advanced skills of massage are required, such as for localized effects.

The purpose of the routine has to be considered, whether for relaxation, or toning effects. The duration and area of application also must be known, whether general or a locally applied massage. Relaxation general massage may be of 40 minutes to one hour's duration. Sports massage may concentrate on larger muscle groups, and combined with electrical work take 30—40 minutes. Treatment of specific areas, such as the back, may take up to 30 minutes, concentrating on this area exclusively.

The therapist has to be capable of adapting her work to fit the client's and clinic's requirements, without its losing its effectiveness and benefit to the client. A general plan of massage can be used as a frame within which movements can be added, removed, or altered to fit all circumstances. Working on knowledge of the effects of the massage movements, individual routines can then be developed to keep the work varied and individual, but always retaining a consistently high standard of technique.

Client Preparation for Massage

Clients' robing for massage should be chosen to maintain client modesty, whilst permitting the therapist to complete her work efficiently. Unnecessary interruptions in the massage routine to rearrange towels should be reduced by sensible robing in the first instance.

The couch may be prepared with protective towels or tissue sheeting and a pillow placed at the head of the bed. A small towel may be placed in readiness which can act as a modesty towel. The client can then be settled under a covering blanket or bath towel, after removing the robe. A small towel can then be slipped across the breasts on a female client, under the blanket in readiness for massage of the abdomen, to avoid interruptions later in the routine.

At the start of the massage the blanket can be folded back to reveal the length of the leg, hip to foot, and the modesty towel lifted through and folded back to protect the blanket from soiling. This position is reversed for the second leg, and then the blanket is used to cover the body, from the chest downwards. The breast towel protects the blanket during massage of the arms and chest, and when these are completed acts to cover the breasts when the blanket is turned down to permit abdominal massage.

The modesty towel can then be turned over the edge of the blanket to protect it, whilst the abdominal massage is in process. On conclusion of the front of the body, the blanket is drawn up to the chest level once more, and the breast and modesty towels deftly removed. The client may then be asked to turn away from the therapist who holds the blanket firmly to avoid total exposure of her client.

In the prone position the blanket can be quickly re-arranged and protected to expose the back, utilizing the original towels. The pillow may be removed from beneath the head, or a smaller one substituted, and a towel or flat pillow placed under the abdomen if desired. The back may then be completed, and the blanket re-arranged to expose the buttocks. The upper back can be kept warm with another of the original towels till the massage is concluded, if the client is cold.

On completion of the massage the client returns to the supine position, assisted if necessary by the therapist, and is moved into a semi-reclining position to regain balance. Assistance is given to replace the gown, the blankets are removed, and the client is helped from the plinth.

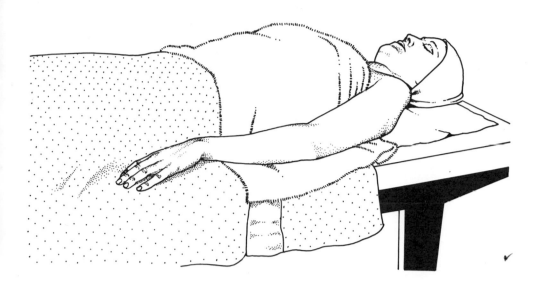

Relaxed Client

GENERAL MASSAGE

Organization and Adaptation

With the client comfortably settled in a supine position, head supported by a pillow and body adequately covered with towels or blankets, the massage commences on the client's right leg. Effleurage movements start the massage, followed by pétrissage movements, both kneading and frictions if indicated, linked and concluded with effleurage. When tapotement movements are used they follow pétrissage within the massage routine.

If strong circulatory effects are desired, the proximal parts of the arms and legs are completed with pressure movements first, rather than distal portions, to create the effect of freeing the vascular and lymphatic vessels in these areas. Then subsequent massage can bring about faster circulatory responses as the blockage or restraint is removed, like the cork being released from a bottle.

The normal routine of work is right leg, right thigh, right lower leg and foot, left leg, left thigh, left lower leg and foot, left arm, chest, right arm, abdomen, shoulders and back, buttocks and finally the back-again.

The posterior aspect of the thigh is not treated separately, unless the client is extremely large and it is impossible to complete the massage working from the front of the body.

This routine can be altered in many ways – all of them correct and successful – as long as the client is not moved or turned unnecessarily, and the work is completed with the greatest efficiency. The therapist endeavours to maintain contact with the client as much as possible, avoiding unnecessary making and breaking of hand contact which can spoil relaxation.

The following routine of strokes should provide a good base for massage work in the beauty therapy field, as it works generally on muscle groups, with a few localized movements. If more concentrated effects are desired, more repetitions of specific movements can be included, and general work deleted. If relaxation only is desired, the tapotement can be replaced by further pétrissage aspects and vibrations. If toning effects are needed primarily, the movements will be of the more active stimulating type, concentrating on the larger muscle groups with a wide range of pétrissage and tapotement movements.

If the time allowed for massage has to be reduced, then areas requiring less attention can be deleted. For example, hands, feet, arms, lower legs, abdomen (if very slight in build), and the chest. Naturally this reduction is bound to have an effect on the benefits derived from the massage, but if circumstances make time reduction necessary, it is helpful if this can be achieved with the least loss to the routine. Therapists have to be realistic in their approach to massage, and if they find themselves having to work to restricted times for massage, must attempt to make the most of the time retained.

MASSAGE SEQUENCE

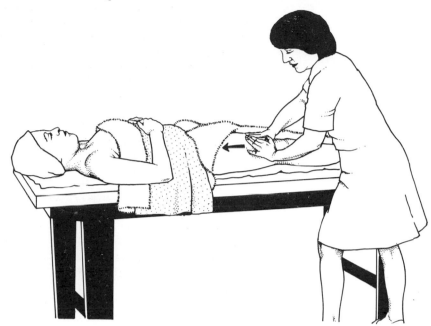

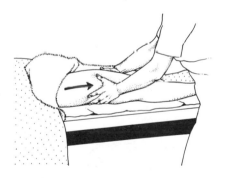

Superficial Effleurage

1   With the client comfortably settled and warm, massage can commence on the right leg with long sweeping effleurage movements superficially given, from the anterior superior spine of the ilium to the foot. On a very long limb the movement will need to be divided, groin to knee, knee to foot, with the therapist changing position slightly. The massage medium can be applied within these strokes, via the therapist's hands. The minimum amount of oil or talc should be used, and it should never be applied directly onto the client.

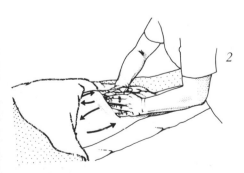

Deep Effleurage

2   Massage strokes continue until a degree of relaxation is felt in the muscles, and the movement then changes to deep effleurage on the thigh, with the pressure being applied towards the heart, with the return stroke being superficial.

3   Palmar kneading on the quadriceps muscle of the thigh follows, with the muscle being picked up above the patella, and worked upon from its insertion to its origin. Alternate lifting pressure movements are used till the muscle bulk diminishes at its origin. The movement concludes with a squeezing, smoothing-out stroke, applied with the right hand, whilst the left hand is free. The right hand returns to the patella with a superficial stroke and the movement is repeated 3—6 times. The movement is fairly active, with a degree of pull and push motion in between the hands. The muscle remains lifted away from its underlying attachments throughout most of the movement, so control, rhythm, and regulation of pressure and speed are very important. The effect on the cirulation is immediate, with the vascular response bringing about warmth, erythema, and a reduction in muscular tension. Small knee supports can be used if this appears to reduce tension in the leg, or if more general support seems desirable. The size and shape of the client determines this point, also the degree of tension present. At no stage should the limbs be loose, floppy or unsupported, so the therapist should have prepared small pillows, or extra towels to use, rolled as bolsters.

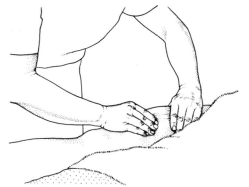 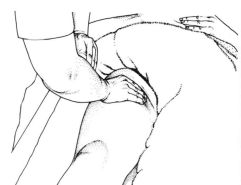

Palmar Kneading on the Quadriceps

4   Single handed palmar kneading on the vastus medialis, rectus femoris, and vastus lateralis of the quadriceps muscle, applied following the paths of the muscles from insertion to origin. The working hand exerting intermittent pressure in a controlled circular movement, with the other hand supporting the muscle and acting as a stabilizing force.

The whole anterior surface of the thigh is covered, with the working hand being reversed on the lateral aspect of the thigh. The movement links with superficial and deep effleurage.

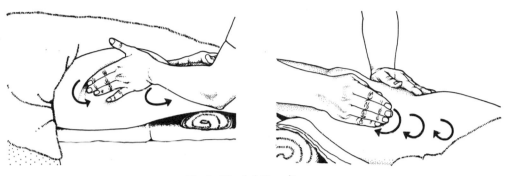

Single Handed Kneading

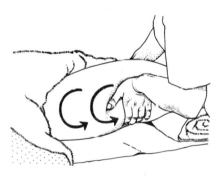

Double Handed Kneading

5   Double handed kneading on the thigh involving the quadriceps, and hamstrings muscles (anterior and posterior to the thigh). The movement commences at the fullest area of the thigh and works back to the knee, exerting forward pressure within circular compression movements. The bulk of the thigh is pushed upwards by the power of the movement. To ensure smoothness the therapist must be attentive to correct breathing, posture and working stance when applying this strenuous movement, otherwise the movement becomes jerky as the hands shake with the effort. The movement may be varied by alternately rolling the muscle bulk between the hands medially and laterally, in a slow, controlled manner. All versions of double handed kneading are linked and concluded by effleurage.

6   Wringing movement (alternate palmar kneading) to the medial and posterior surface of the thigh. The leg is rotated laterally to bring it into the correct position for wringing, and may need a knee support to ensure comfort. The movement picks up the vastus medialis at the knee and applies opposing pressure movements of a 'wringing' type along its length. The hands are placed across the muscle fibres, but the movement works along the muscle's length. The opposition effect is created by the movement of the therapist's elbow joints and forearm muscles, and is transmitted through to the hands. The fingers and thumbs on opposing hands exert pressure

against each other, and create the wringing effect. The movement is continuous, with the right hand squeezing out the tissues at the end of the stroke, whilst the left hand returns to start the movement again at the knee. After six repeats the hands link with effleurage, and repeat the movement on the hamstrings muscles if the client's size allows. The movement concludes with effleurage, and the leg is returned to its normal position.

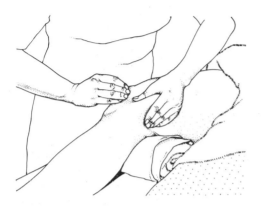
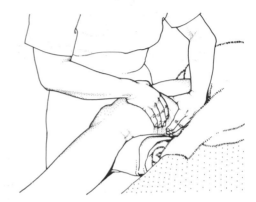

Wringing

7   Deep kneading and stroking around the knee joint follows, with first the fingers, then the palmar surface of the hand applying the movement. The patella must remain in its normal position, and only controlled pressure is used within the movement. The hands adopt a cupped position to apply the circular kneading movement, holding and supporting the knee joint. The movement links with deep stroking over the patella area and is repeated 2—3 times.

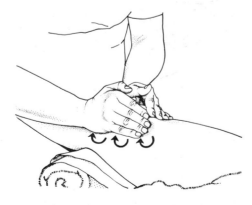
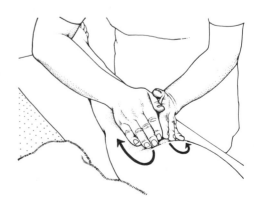

Deep Kneading and Stroking around the Patella

8   Deep effleurage precedes palmar kneading on the calf muscles, with the slightly flexed knee supported by the right hand, and the left hand working on the lateral aspect of the leg. The pressure is applied between the thumb and fingers, with the maximum amount of palmar surface in contact with the muscles. The pressure of the circular movements is upwards, towards the heart, but the movement works down from the knee to the ankle, returning with a deep upward stroke. The hands are reversed and the movement repeated.

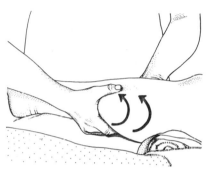

Palmar Kneading on Calf

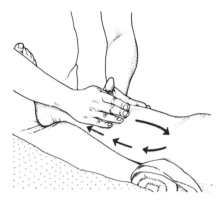

Deep Effleurage

9   Thumb kneading on the tibialis anterior muscle is then firmly applied, with the thumbs working closely together and the hands supporting and steadying the leg. The surface tissues are moved smoothly over the underlying structures by the circular movements of the thumbs. Depending on the intensity and manner in which the movement is performed it may be classed as either a kneading or a friction movement. Both movements come within the pétrissage/compression group, but their purpose and effect are different. The choice will depend on the therapist's assessment of her client's needs. The movement is normally performed from the origin to the insertion of the muscle, concluding at the ankle, with deep effleurage being used to link the 2—3 repeats necessary.

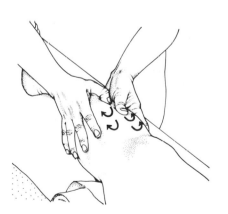

Thumb Kneading on the Tibialis Anterior

10   The massage then moves to the toes, linked by the last effleurage stroke, which brings the therapist to a position at the end of the plinth. Digital stroking commences at the toes, with the fingers in contact and the thumbs abducted. The fingers perform deep stroking

over the surface of the foot, keeping close contact, till the hands divide to stroke over the lateral and medial aspects of the malleolus bone of the ankle. The palmar surface of the hands contours closely over the foot, as the movement returns with a superficial stroke to the toes. Correct rhythm, hand contouring, and speed are necessary for successful application of this popular and restful movement. The movement may be repeated 3—4 times.

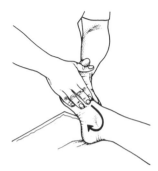
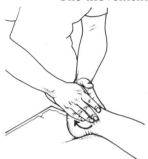
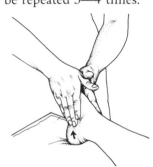

Digital Stroking

11   Frictions around the ankle follow naturally on from the previous movement, and are applied around the ankle with first the fingers, and then the thumbs exerting the pressure. When the fingers work the thumbs support and vice versa. Small circular movements are used until the desired circulation response is achieved; these movements being interlinked with deep stroking effleurage to aid the circulation and increase lymphatic drainage, so helping to remove or prevent swelling (oedema).

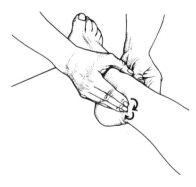
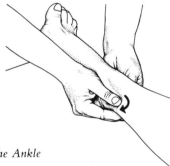

Friction around the Ankle

12   Thumb stroking to the plantar surface of the foot is applied with the hands resting lightly on the dorsal (upper) surface of the foot, with the thumbs on the plantar surface (sole). The thumbs work deeply with circular kneading movements down to the heel, and return with

an upward pulling movement, exerting pressure between the fingers and thumbs. The foot appears spread by the movement, which helps relieve aching tired feet, or postural strain imposed by modern foot wear. Firm movements are necessary when dealing with the soles of the feet, as light movements can be very ticklish and break relaxation.

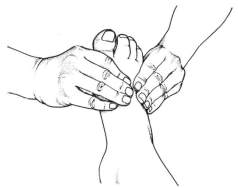 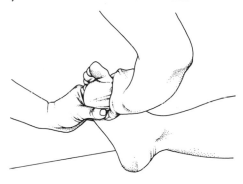

Thumb Stroking of the Foot

13   Palmar stroking to the plantar surface of the foot is applied, with the therapist moving to face across the foot of the plinth, sideways on to the client. The left hand holds and supports the foot, and the right hand works from the toes to the heel of the foot with firm pressure, using the ulnar (outer) border of the hand to produce the movement. The working hand starts supinated, and as it progresses pronates until the palmar surface is in total contact with the plantar surface of the foot. The movement presses firmly downwards, concluding on the underlying massage plinth. The strokes are repeated 2—3 times, and with the supporting hand remaining in the same position, the massage progresses to the next movement.

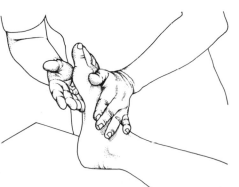 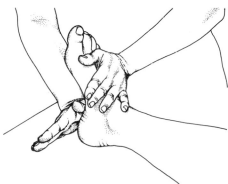

Palmar Stroking of the Sole

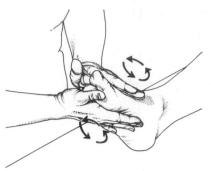

Palmar Kneading

14   The foot is held loosely between the palmar surfaces of the hands, and pressure is gradually applied till the movement becomes a controlled deep kneading of the whole distal part of the foot. Pressure is released slowly, and the hands re-position for the next movement.

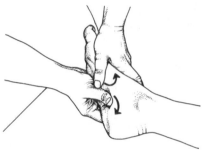

Kneading of the Medial Arch

15   The foot is supported by the left hand over its dorsal surface, and the right loosely in contact with the plantar surface. The thumbs of both hands work deeply along the medial arch of the foot with circular kneading movements, from the toes to the heel. The movement returns with deep stroking of the thumbs, and is repeated 2—3 times. The movements on the foot conclude the massage of the leg if tapotement/percussion movements are not to be included, and the massage is for relaxation only. The addition of more stimulating movements can conclude the routine for the legs, returning to the thighs and lower legs if bulk permits, with beating, pounding, clapping and hacking. The tapotement may also be built into the routine, such as in sports massage, following the pétrissage movements in each area, to achieve a more stimulating effect.

Hacking and clapping can be applied with the leg in lateral rotation after 'wringing' (Movement 6), and with the leg returned to its normal position all forms of tapotement can be applied to the heavy muscle groups and adipose deposits. As tapotement works across muscle fibres, and is generally applied, not following specific muscle paths, its application is similar in any part of the body. Only the pressure alters for the differing bulk of the tissues, and naturally, sufficient bulk must be available for these active movements to be used at all.

Optional Tapotement Movements

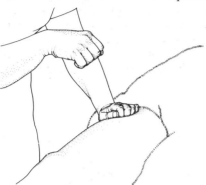

Beating

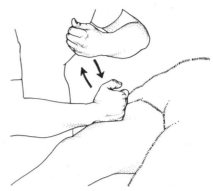

Pounding

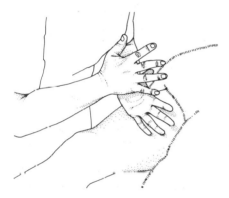

Hacking

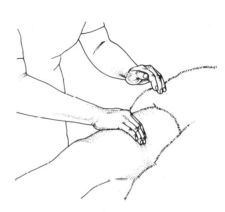

Clapping

The therapist moves to the left side of the plinth and movements *1—15* are then repeated on the other leg, reversing the hands used where necessary. The first leg is covered whilst the second is treated, and then both are warmly tucked under the blanket. The therapist then moves up the plinth to treat the left arm.

16 Superficial effleurage over the entire arm from shoulder to hand commences the massage, with both hands in contact. The stroke is repeated 4—6 times or until relaxation is present.

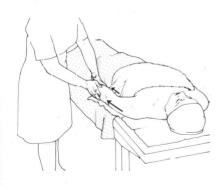

Superficial Effleurage over the Arm

17 Deep effleurage over the biceps and deltoid muscles follows in a centripetal direction, with the hands working alternately and contouring closely to the muscles. The arm is supported on the plinth or on a pillow placed on a small table adjacent to the plinth, if the client is large.

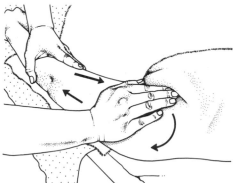
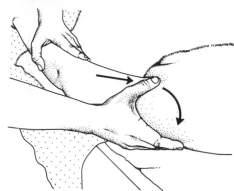

Deep Effleurage over Biceps and Deltoid

18 Alternate palmar kneading to the arm and forearm is then applied, with first the left hand supporting the arm and the right hand working. As the movement progresses from the shoulders to the elbow, the hand support alters, and the arm rests on the plinth, whilst the supporting hand moves to the wrist. The deep kneading movement is repeated on the lateral aspect of the arm 2—3 times, with the supporting hand moving between the elbow and the wrist to maintain the arm in relaxation. The hands then reverse, the arm is placed in slight outward rotation, and the movement is applied to the inner surface of the arm, the triceps muscle, by the left hand. At the conclusion of this movement both hands return to the shoulder with deep effleurage.

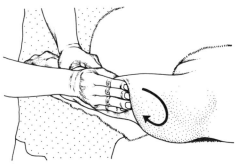
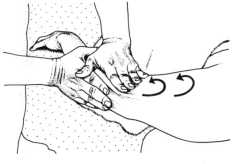

Alternate Kneading

19   With the arm supported in the same position, deep kneading and rolling of the upper arm muscles may be applied. The arm is lifted free of the plinth with its weight supported by the therapist, and deep rolling movements applied. The muscles are grasped firmly, moved towards the body, and then lifted upwards and outwards to form the rolling movement. The movement progresses from the elbow to the shoulder, and returns with deep stroking to repeat 2—3 times. The hands reverse and the movement is repeated, with the direction of the kneading being first outward, then upward and inward. This movement is very stimulating to the triceps muscle and covers it fully, so helping to prevent the loss of tone which occurs so frequently in this area.

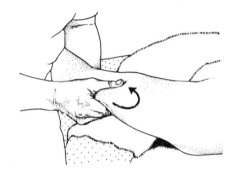
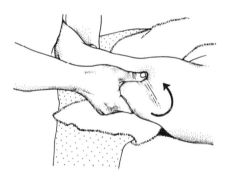

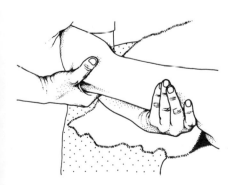
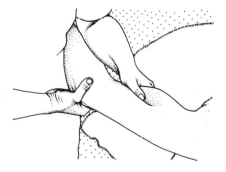

Kneading and Rolling of the Upper Arm

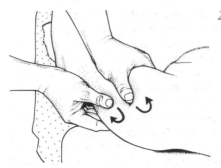

*Thumb Kneading/Frictions
on the Upper Arm*

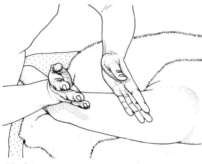

Hacking

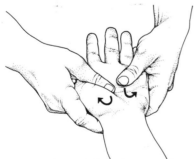

Deep Stroking of the Palm

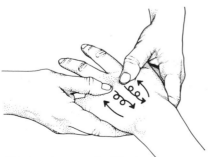

Frictions between the Tendons

20   Thumb kneading/frictions on the upper arm may then be applied, with the entire area being covered, first anterior, lateral and then posterior surfaces. The movement is similar to kneading/frictions on the leg, and the pressure used is chosen for the same reasons. Accumulation of adipose tissue, fibrositis in the muscle, etc., may warrant the use of frictions, otherwise the more general kneading movements may be applied. Effleurage is used to link the movement, and concludes it.

Tapotement movements, if desired, may be added at this stage of the arm massage, or at its conclusion after the hands have been treated. Movements can include pinchment, light hacking, skin rolling and clapping if sufficient tissues are present.

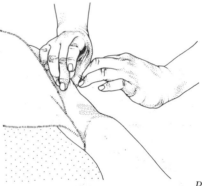

Pinchment

21   Massage of the hands commences with stroking, and then with the client's hand in supination (palm uppermost) supported by the therapist's hands, deep thumb stroking of the area is applied. Smooth deep movements of the thumbs progress towards the wrist, and the movement is linked with effleurage and repeated 2—3 times.

22   The hand is then placed in pronation (palm downwards) and circular frictions applied between the tendons by the thumbs working in an upward direction. The movement links and concludes with effleurage. The thumbs work on alternate metacarpal spaces till the entire surface is covered.

23 The movement progresses to thumb kneading on the client's thumb and finger joints.
With the left hand supporting, the right hand
performs deep kneading movements to the
joints of the outer three fingers, working
proximal to distal. The hand support then
reverses, and the medial aspect of the hand is
completed with the left hand. The kneading
movements must be smoothly applied, and
exert a degree of pull on each joint. Performed well, the movement can be very
relaxing to the client. Deep effleurage completes the massage of the left arm, working
from shoulder to hand with long sweeping
movements. The therapist then positions herself to work on the chest area.

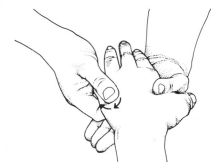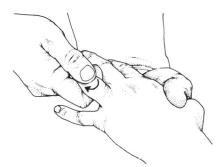

Joint Kneading

24 Superficial stroking is applied from the
shoulders to the sternum, with alternate
hands working so that contact is not broken.
As the right hand concludes its stroke, the left
hand commences, until 6—8 repeats are
accomplished.

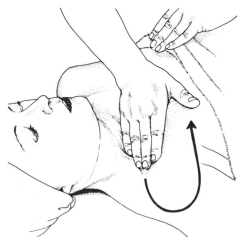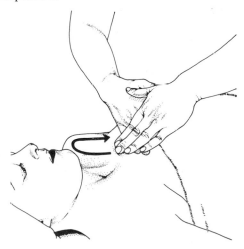

Superficial Stroking

25 With both hands at the sternum, a broad sweeping effleurage movement is applied around the shoulder joints, up the trapezius muscles (upper fibres), and gently back to the sternum. As the client's muscles relax in the shoulder girdle, more forward pressure can be applied in the return stroke, lifting the neck forwards. The movement may be repeated 4—6 times, or until tension in the trapezius muscle starts to lessen.

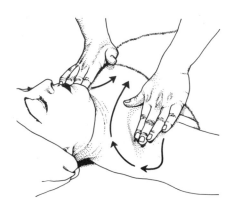
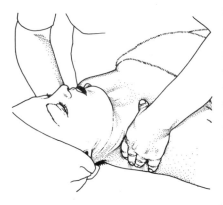
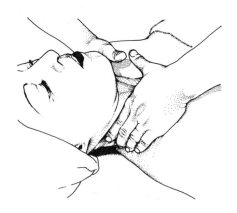
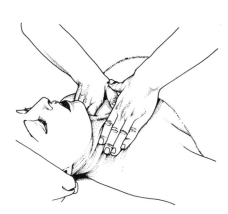

*Sweeping Effleurage and Kneading over
the Trapezius*

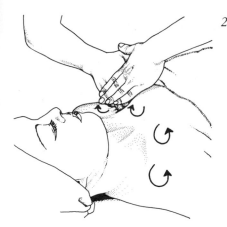

Reinforced Kneading

26 Reinforced kneading over the chest area is then applied, with the right hand working from the sternum to the shoulder, reinforced in its action by the left hand. 4—6 large circles are performed on first the left then the right sides of the chest. The movement links and concludes with effleurage.

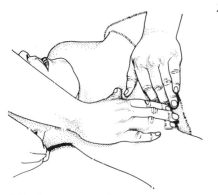

Wringing on Pectoralis Major

27 A picking up and wringing movement of the pétrissage type may then be applied to the pectoralis major muscle, concentrating on its insertion into the humerus bone of the arm. On women the breast itself limits the movement, but it should be applied as fully as possible, to help support the breasts. The movement should be applied to the left then the right side of the chest, being linked with effleurage. The therapist then moves to stand directly behind the client's head to apply the next movement.

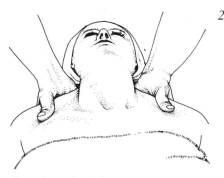

Deep Sweeping Effleurage

28 Deep sweeping effleurage commences the movement, with the hands progressing down to the sternum, outwards and round the shoulder joints, returning to the mastoid process with deep circular kneading movements over the trapezius muscle. The movement exerts smooth forward lifting pressure on the upper fibres of the trapezius, so preventing the formation of fibrositis and aiding relaxation of tense muscle fibres. Deep sweeping effleurage links and concludes the massage of the chest. The therapist then moves to complete the client's right arm, reversing hand positions where necessary.

29   The abdominal area can then be revealed, and massage commenced with deep stroking over the abdominal area. The movement commences at the symphysis pubis, then the hands divide to pass inside the anterior superior iliac spines of the pelvic girdle, progressing to follow the iliac crests until the hands touch in the upper lumbar region of the back. The hands return with firm pressure around the waistline, and conclude with gentle pressure over the abdomen back to the symphysis pubis. The movement is repeated 2—3 times, at a slow speed.

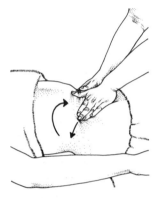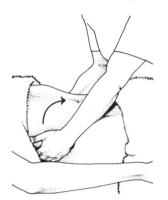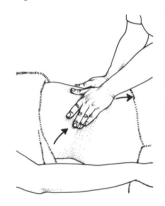

Stroking over the Abdominal Area

30   The therapist stands sideways on to the plinth, weight evenly balanced and back upright to perform the next movement. The right hand is placed with its palm at the base of the sternum, and is reinforced by the left hand. The right hand strokes lightly in a lateral (outwards) direction over the ribs, and then returns to its start position with firm pulling pressure over the upper abdomen. The movement is then applied with the tips of the fingers at the base of the sternum, and the wrists in full extension, to the other side of the body. The movement progresses lightly downwards over the ribs, and then the hands are pushed upwards back to the start position. This movement of 'pulling' and 'pushing' will only be accomplished correctly if body posture is correct. The therapist has to drop her height by bending with the body weight evenly distributed, and must also have flexibility and strength in the wrists. The movement may be repeated 3—4 times on each side.

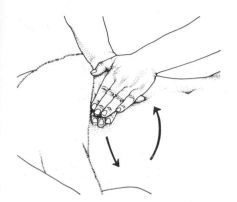

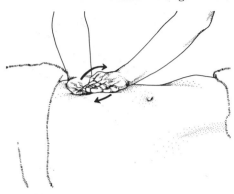

Kneading over the Midriff

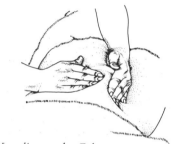

Kneading on the Colon

31 Deep kneading over the colon is accomplished with the hand cupped and pressure being applied along its ulnar border. The movement follows the path of the ascending, transverse, and descending colon, with deep kneading movements. The movement is completed by stroking over the lower part of the descending colon, and this links the movement back to repeated kneading of the ascending portion. The movement is repeated 2—3 times.

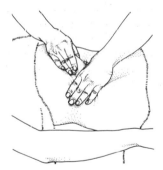

32 If adequate subcutaneous tissues are available, double handed wringing may be applied to the entire abdominal area. The tissues are lifted and kneaded, with the movement progressing upwards and downwards over the entire area, if the client's size permits.

Double Handed Wringing

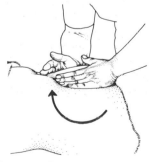

33 Deep stroking over the colon follows, with the right hand working and the left hand reinforcing and steadying the action. The movement is repeated 4—6 times, then superficial effleurage concludes the abdominal massage, applied from the lower ribs to the symphysis pubis. The client is then helped to turn over, her towels, etc. are rearranged, and with the therapist in the same position, massage of the back commences.

Stroking over the Colon

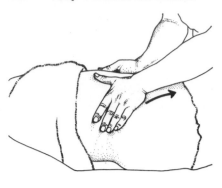

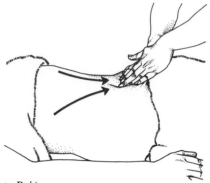

Stroking from Lower Ribs to Pubis

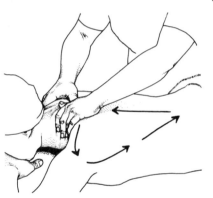

Deep Stroking of the Back

34   Massage commences with superficial and deep stroking over the back, using the entire palmar surface of the hands. Starting at the sacrum, the hands pass either side of the spinous processes of the spine, thumbs abducted, and separate at the neck to work deeply over the shoulders, the hands then drawing the muscles back with the fingers, whilst the thumbs stroke down both sides of the cervical vertebrae. The hands relax and return to the sacrum with deep strokes down the sides of the body. The movement is full and strong, but still rhythmically and calmly applied, and it acts as a preparation for following back movements.

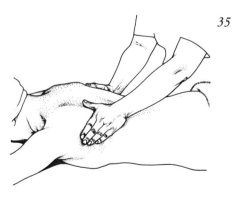

35   The deep stroking may also be applied in an upwards, outwards manner, with the hands starting at the sacrum, and progressing first to waist level and returning to the sacrum. Then the hands repeat the movement to the axilla level (arm pit), and lastly outwards over and around the shoulders contouring closely, to return with a superficial stroke to the sacrum. Firm upward pressure is used in all aspects of the movement.

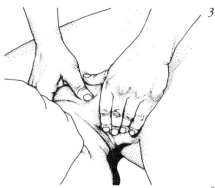

Deep Kneading of the Trapezius

36   Deep effleurage is used to bring the hands to the trapezius muscle area, where deep kneading is applied, the hands working in unison on the upper fibres of the muscle, from its attachment to its insertion in the occipital cavity of the skull. The movement works deeply, fingers supporting and aiding the movement, with the thumbs exerting intermittent but smoothly applied pressure. Effleurage links and concludes the movement, which is repeated 4—6 times.

37   If sufficient relaxation has been achieved in the muscle, double handed wringing may then be applied to the same area, with the movement reducing in pressure as the muscle bulk diminishes. The movement may be 'squeezed out' to end the strokes at the occipital cavity at the base of the skull. It may be necessary to turn the head to accomplish this movement on both sides of the trapezius, or a small pillow can be placed under the head to permit greater access to the muscles. The movement uses effleurage to link the movements and re-establish relaxation, in between the more penetrating strokes.

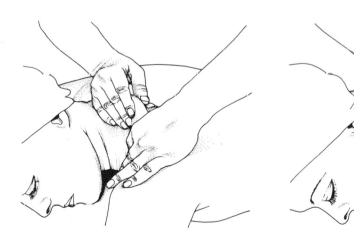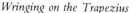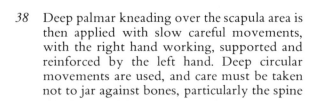

Wringing on the Trapezius

38   Deep palmar kneading over the scapula area is then applied with slow careful movements, with the right hand working, supported and reinforced by the left hand. Deep circular movements are used, and care must be taken not to jar against bones, particularly the spine

of the scapula. The movement is linked with effleurage and is repeated on the other side of the back. Deep kneading may be applied over the entire surface of the back if indicated, working up and down the area, avoiding the spine, and concluding at the sacrum.

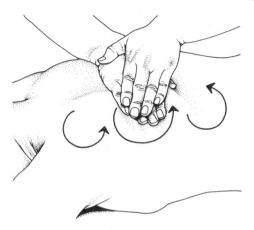

Reinforced Kneading of the Scapula

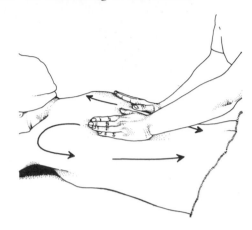

Sweeping Effleurage

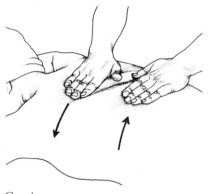

Crossing

39 Sweeping effleurage brings the hands back to the shoulder area, where they move easily into alternate palmar kneading, 'crossing' over the back. The hands move firmly across and back, exerting pressure on both the forward and backward strokes, so that the kneading effect is created between the hands. The movement progresses from the shoulders down to the lumbar area, in an even rhythmical manner.

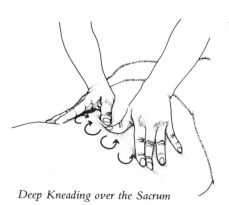

Deep Kneading over the Sacrum

40 Deep kneading over the sacrum follows, applied with the thumbs, the fingers supporting the movement. The thumbs work alternately, and the entire palmar surface of the hand is used to apply linking and concluding effleurage.

41   Effleurage is used to bring the hands to either side of the cervical vertebrae, and the thumbs stroke down firmly either side of the spinous processes. The movement changes from thumbs to a palmar surface contact as the movement is drawn backwards and downwards to the sacrum. The movement may be converted into running vibrations over the same erector spinae muscles, as the therapist's skill and strength grows. The movement is then concentrated into the finger tips, and applied with gentle consistent pressure.

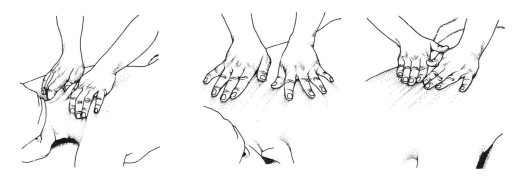

Vibrations down the Erector Spinae

42   Slow, deep, and carefully applied effleurage is then used over the entire back, working up to the occipital cavity, and drawing the trapezius muscle firmly back with pressure applied through the fingers. As the muscles should by this stage of the massage be more relaxed, a greater depth of lifting stroke may be achieved. The movement may be repeated over the deltoid muscles, and the latissimus dorsi area.

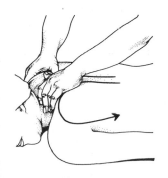
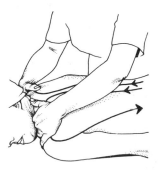
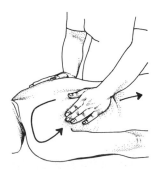

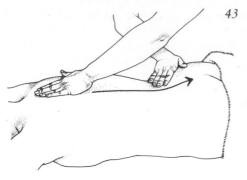

43 Alternate palmar stroking along the spine normally concludes the back massage, with the movement applied slowly and lightly to aid relaxation. The entire palmar surface of the hand is used, from the cervical region to the sacrum. As the first hand concludes its stroke, the second hand commences, with the movement being slowly repeated 6—8 times. The client's towelling is then rearranged to allow treatment of the buttocks, and the back covered if necessary for warmth.

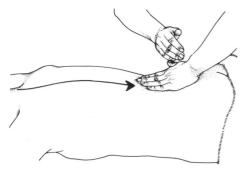
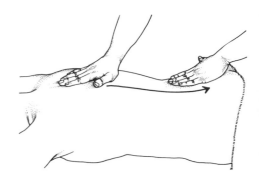

Palmar Stroking of the Spine

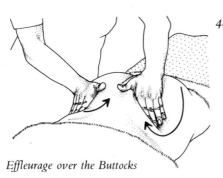

44 The buttocks are first treated with deep effleurage movements, working inwards from the sides to the sacrum to avoid separation of the gluteal fold. The movement works firmly inwards and upwards, and returns with superficial strokes.

Effleurage over the Buttocks

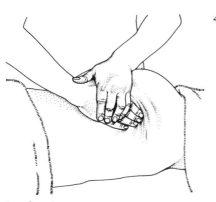

45 Deep reinforced kneading movements may then be applied to the gluteal muscles, first on the right, then the left sides. Firm pressure must be applied to overcome the natural resilience of the adipose deposits in this area. Deep effleurage links and concludes the movement.

Reinforced Kneading over the Buttocks

46 Deep wringing (alternate palmar kneading) may then be applied, with the hand being spread widely to obtain a good grasp of the tissues. The movement may be applied over the buttocks and iliac crest areas, where subcutaneous fat develops, to discourage its formation.

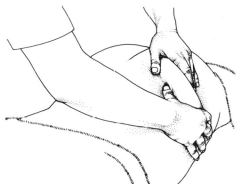

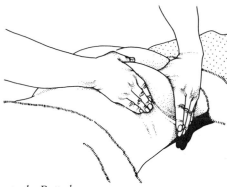

Double Handed Wringing to the Buttocks

Tapotement/percussion of all types may then be applied to the buttocks if desired, with clapping, beating, pounding, and hacking being used in sequence. Effleurage can be used to calm the muscles, and provides natural breaks for both the client and therapist whilst performing these strenuous and stimulating movements.

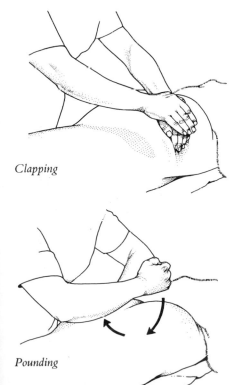

Clapping

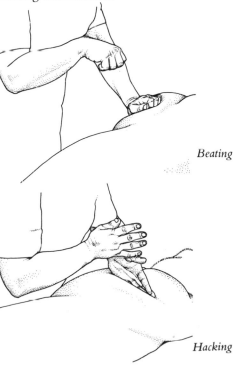

Beating

Pounding

Hacking

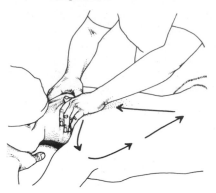

After massage of the buttocks is completed, the entire massage may be concluded with superficial effleurage to the back area, to relax the client. If tapotement has not been included, this is less necessary, but when it has been used extensively within the massage, effleurage is needed to re-establish relaxation. If oil has been used as the massage medium, any remaining on the skin may be carefully removed by towels placed around the therapist's hand.

Superficial Effleurage to the Back

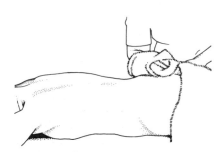

Removing the Massage Medium

STIMULATING TAPOTEMENT AND PÉTRISSAGE MOVEMENTS

More active movements of the pétrissage and tapotement type may be included in the general massage if preferred by the client. They may replace the more soothing elements, or be added to the overall routine. To keep within the normal one hour timing for general massage, fewer repetitions of movements, or deletion of some areas, would be necessary if a full range of both relaxing and stimulating movements were desired.

Many of the stimulatory effects of massage are achieved electrically with heavy duty apparatus, and the need for extended periods of tapotement has diminished. However, the need will always exist for its correct and skilled application, particularly on clients contra-indicated to electrical therapy.

Pétrissage Stimulating movements

Skin Rolling   Skin rolling may be applied wherever sufficient surface tissues are available to accomplish the movement. The back and the abdomen are the normal areas for its application. The movement is performed by the hands pulling the surface tissues away from the midline of the body, to the sides, where the thumbs and fingers apply a rolling pressure movement back to the midline. The movement can also be performed pushing away from the therapist, using the thumbs to push the tissues outwards, with the fingers and thumbs again producing the rolling effect. Great care must be taken to avoid pinching the skin, by applying the pressure slowly, smoothly, and with consideration for the amount of subcutaneous tissue present.

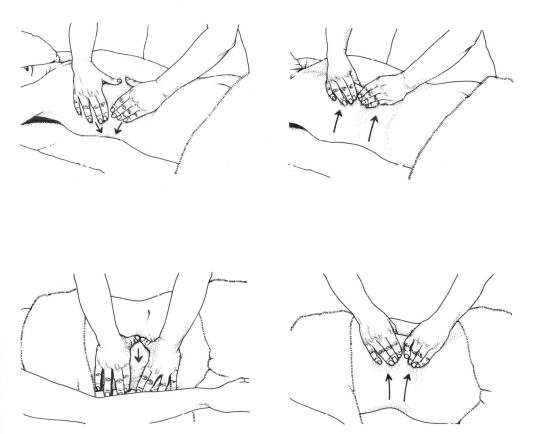

Skin Rolling

Pinchment

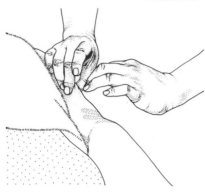

Pinchment is another useful movement where particular stimulatory effects are needed. The movement is a picking up, pinching type of movement, performed with the thumb and index fingers of both hands. The movement is applied generally as it affects the surface tissues, rather than deeper structures. Its immediate effect is erythema, local heat production, and an increased vascular interchange in the area. It is normally applied on the upper arms, back, and abdominal areas for its stimulating and skin toning effects.

Tapotement Movements

Tapotement movements are normally restricted to the larger muscle groups, on the buttocks, thighs, etc., but can be applied to the back, across the shoulders and to the upper arm, if used skillfully, and chosen with care.

Hacking

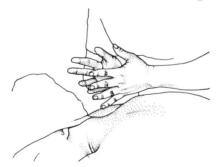

May be used on the upper arm, back and shoulders, as well as the buttocks and thighs. The movements must be very lightly applied, with attention to the changing underlying structures. The movement contours to the shape of the body, by changes in the working position of the therapist. Great control is needed over the speed and pressure of the movements, and the more difficult areas of the body should not be attempted, until proficiency has been gained in general hacking applications on more protected areas.

Clapping

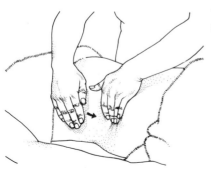

Clapping may also be applied to the sides of the waist, and the back, in addition to its normal application on the buttocks and thighs.

Chapter 6

Heat Therapy and Lamp Treatments

Forms of Heat Therapy

There are many forms of heat therapy for the therapist to include in her treatment range, some elaborate, some very simple. All will produce beneficial effects in differing degrees when combined into treatment routines with massage, exercise, or electrical equipment. Heat produces relaxation of tense muscles, relieves discomfort, and is very sedative in effect. It also improves vascular circulation, increases the heart beat, and raises body temperature so that perspiration is induced. The effects required, and the client's physical condition, will determine the level and duration of heat therapy that may be applied.

The forms of heat therapy used in beauty treatments include:

(i)   Sauna baths.

(ii)   Steam baths, cabinets, or steam rooms.

(iii) Foam baths, hydro/oxygen baths.

(iv)   Radiant heat/infra red lamps.

(v)   Wax baths.

(vi)   Impulse or ordinary showers.

Safety in the Clinic

The forms of treatment vary considerably in their application, but are similar in their need for safe, careful handling and control by the therapist. With total responsibility being carried by the therapist for the well being of her clients, attention must be paid to safety within the treatment situation. Choice, location, and maintenance of the apparatus is important, but even more vital is the therapist's correct choice and application of the treatment for the client.

The correct and safe method of use must be known for all the equipment applied, to avoid accidents occurring. Most mishaps stem from unfamiliarity with machines, and lack of understanding of their possible hazards. Wherever water and electrical power are used to produce heating effects, there exists a potential hazard. Correctly used, with attention to safety procedures, heat therapy is one of the therapist's most valuable tools. It should never be used carelessly, or the client left unattended whilst undergoing treatment, unless all sources of heat are fully protected.

It is in the therapist's interest to be sensible and knowledgeable about heating treatments, so that she can assess the possible dangers, and so protect her client from them. The client will then feel secure, and reassured by the calm efficiency of the therapist guiding her through the treatment. No feelings of panic or anxiety will then be present to spoil the enjoyment of the treatment.

A lack of confidence, in both attitude and application of treatment on the part of the therapist, soon induces anxiety in the client, and may prevent her continuing with a course of heat therapy. Careless handling, lack of guidance from the therapist, or a wrongly applied treatment are all reasons why clients decide against heating treatments. It has to be remembered that sauna, steam baths, etc., are a new experience to the client, one that she will happily enjoy if helped throughout its duration by the therapist.

Initially the client requires guidance at every stage of a treatment, with the therapist being in close attendance to direct her actions, and assess the reaction to the treatment. In some cases, such as sauna baths, the client soon becomes familiar with the routine, and the therapist only needs to intervene if she feels the treatment should be concluded or altered. For it is always the therapist's greater knowledge of the client's limitations, and the physical effects of the treatment that determine the length and level of heat used in the treatment. This is an important point, as clients enjoy the effects of heating the body, and will often overestimate their capacity to take the heat.

Heating the body affects people in different ways, and the therapist should be alert to changes in the client's appearance. Any feelings of faintness, giddiness, or over-exertion, can normally be spotted before they become a real problem. It is necessary to be able to deal with these and any other minor problems which might occur in the clinic, however carefully safety routines have been followed. The element of human error makes it necessary for the therapist to hold a first-aid certificate, so that she can deal with burns, shock, etc., resulting from treatment. If careful precautions are taken to guard against hazards it is extremely unlikely that accidents will happen, but if they do, the therapist must be prepared and offer assistance until medical help arrives.

SAFETY POINTS IN ELECTRICAL THERAPY

1   Choose well made, sturdy equipment that is suited to the task it will have to perform, and is easy to clean and operate.

2   Have electrical equipment professionally installed or checked to prevent overloading of the circuits. Also, avoid the use of adaptors for connecting apparatus to the power supply, as this can cause faults during the treatment, and is not as safe as a direct connection.

3   If a fault develops, turn off the power supply, check the plug and fuses, and if this does not cure it, call in an electrician. If a fuse blows several times, it indicates the fault lies within the equipment, and the unit should be checked by the manufacturer or an electrician who deals with therapy equipment.

4   Have the equipment maintained and serviced at regular intervals, according to the use it receives.

5   Ensure the equipment is correctly wired, and either has an earthing attachment, or is in the form of double insulation symbolized by ▣ on the rating plate.

6   Locate the equipment so that attachment leads are not overstretched or likely to become disconnected from the sockets. Leads should not be allowed to trail over the floor, where they could be tripped over.

7   Lamps, wax baths, etc., must be placed safely, when hot, out of harm's way, and should have a warning notice to indicate they are in use, or still hot.

8   Follow the correct application routine for each piece of equipment, according to the manufacturer's instructions, and become familiar with the application before applying the treatment to clients. Leave the equipment turned off after use, or, if in continuous operation, turned down for economy and safety between clients. At the end of the day plugs should be pulled out from the sockets.

9   Wherever possible, purchase thermostatically controlled apparatus with pilot lights to indicate that the power is connected.

10   Avoid moving mobile heating equipment more than is necessary. Position the unit safely and bring the client to the unit for treatment, i.e. for paraffin wax baths.

11   Don't leave lamps positioned over reflective surfaces or plinths when in use, because of the risks of burns or fire.

12   Apparatus should be checked before use, to see that the performance is constant, and to ensure the unit is clean and ready for use. Any faults or intermittent current will then show up prior to the treatment, and not during it.

13   The preparation of apparatus should be completed before the client's arrival, so that everything is ready and well organized for the treatment. Hurried preparation can lead to oversights, confusion, and accidents.

14   The client should be checked for contra-indications, and if suitable should be gradually introduced to heat and lamp treatments, building tolerance slowly with low heat and short-duration routines.

15   Use the client's comfort as the primary guide to temperature control.

16   Ideally, all the wet treatments, saunas, steam baths, showers, etc., should be separate from the main treatment area, to isolate them for convenience and safety.

17   In the unlikely event of an accident occurring, the therapist must administer first aid, and call for medical assistance. The client may only need to be advised to consult her own doctor, i.e. after recovery from fainting, to ascertain that she is still suitable for steam or sauna baths. The therapist must take responsibility for the client's welfare during treatment, and must not shirk her duty towards the client's safety.

EFFECTS OF HEAT ON THE BODY

If the effects of heat are considered more closely their value in beauty therapy becomes evident. The need to modify these effects on some individuals also becomes clear. When the body is heated the body temperature slowly rises, and the heart beat quickens, in the same way as if active exercise had been undertaken. Surface capillaries dilate in order to lose heat, and the sweat glands are activated to produce perspiration to help in this process. The surface expansion of blood vessels causes the skin to redden and become hot (erythema), whilst the internal blood pressure is lowered slightly. Waste products are lost from the skin's surface and lactic acid, the product of muscular work and fatigue, is dispersed through the vascular circulation. Tense muscle fibres relax, the client feels cared for and comforted by the warmth, and tensions are reduced.

The increase in pulse rate, and vascular interchange brings fresh arterial blood supply to the tissues, producing a feeling of well being and regeneration. If the body is then allowed to return to its normal temperature slowly, the effects are beneficial to pure relaxation, being close to natural exertion and rest. At least half to one hour should be allowed for the body's return to normal pulse and temperature, and this provides the obvious opportunity for massage routines.

If a more stimulating effect is required and the client is fit, the body temperature can be alternately raised and lowered rapidly, with high temperature saunas, cold showers, plunge pools, etc. This places a much greater strain on the heart, and really does not have any merit over moderately hot saunas, warm showers, and a slower return to normal body temperature. The normal sauna routines alternates heating with cold rinses, but it need not be followed slavishly, and can be adapted to meet the physical needs of the client.

Clients may feel totally relaxed after either the toning and invigorating routine, or the sustained heat and resting routine, and it is important to match the treatment to the client's preference. If the client is physically and psychologically at rest at the conclusion of the treatment, then it has been successful.

PRE-HEATING TREATMENTS

Heat therapy may be used to pre-heat the body prior to massage or electrical treatment, improving the effectiveness of the application, and the client's acceptance of it. The body is warm, muscles are relaxed, and the client is free from tension. Surface tissues are moist and amenable to muscle contraction treatment, making its application more comfortable. Hard contracted muscles are relaxed so that deep manual and vacuum massage routines can be applied with less risk of discomfort or bruising. The body is in an ideal condition for further treatment, with heat therapy maximizing the effects of whatever treatment is applied.

Therapists should encourage clients to undertake some form of pre-heating prior to treatment, even if it has to be adapted, or is only of a moderate temperature. Even warm showers, of the ordinary or impulse type, relax the body and help prepare it for further applications. Local applications of heat, with wax or lamps, are also useful if time is restricted or the client is contra-indicated to more general forms of heating.

CONTRA-INDICATIONS TO GENERAL HEAT THERAPY

There are many physical conditions which would require medical approval prior to genera-lized heat applications, including abnormalities of the cardio-vascular or respiratory systems. The therapist should obtain medical approval and guidance for any clients who do not know the state of their health, or who are undergoing med-ical treatment.

Contra-indications include:

1   Any evidence of high or low blood pressure, history of thrombosis, or heat abnormalities such as angina pectoris.

2   History of coronary thrombosis (heart attack), particularly in male clients.

3   Bronchitis, asthma, hay fever or heavy colds.

4   Migraine sufferers, where the heat may trigger an attack. It may not have any effect, but only careful application will reveal this fact.

5   Skin disorders. Certain disorders, like acne vulgaris, can benefit from the drying effects of sauna. Psoriasis also can be helped by the wet heat of the steam bath, in combination with massage. Both conditions require medi-cal approval prior to treatment with heat.

6   Diabetes.

7   Epileptics.

8   Clients should not have just had a heavy meal, or be under the influence of drink or drugs. In large leisure centres or health clubs this pre-sents quite a problem with male sauna users, but in clinic practice the problem seldom exists. The dangers of passing out, being sick, or even having a heart attack are very real when the sauna use is unsupervised.

9   Clients suffering from severe exhaustion, or who are on a very restricted food intake (crash diet), may pass out or become giddy with the effects of heat. A short rest and light refreshments may solve the problem, fol-lowed by a short-duration treatment.

10 During the first 2—3 days of the menstrual flow (monthly periods).

11 If the client suffers from fluid retention, medical approval must be sought.

12 During the later stages of pregnancy.

13 Clients with athletes foot (tinea pedis), verrucaes, or plantar warts, must wear slippers or slip-on sandals throughout the sauna and steam bath treatment.

STEAM BATH TREATMENT

The steam bath treatment is one of the most popular forms of pre-heating the body, and originates from the steam rooms or turkish baths of earlier times. The principle of vapour heat is similar but the application differs considerably. The modern steam cabinet allows the client's head to be free from the steam, and so avoids totally spoiling the client's hair style. The old turkish bath principle is still found in use in the larger health hydros, leisure centres, etc., and is enjoying a revival in many areas. Its relaxation effects are undisputed, but the facilities required make it unsuitable for all but the larger health units.

The system was based on steam rooms of different temperatures, where people could progress according to personal tolerance, through the interlinking rooms, starting with the moderately hot rooms, and progressing through extremely high levels of heat, according to personal capacity. The individual could conclude the ritual with plunge pools into cold water if desired, or simply reverse through the different temperature rooms back to the cooler levels. The whole body was involved in the steam treatment, and the process was a leisurely form of enjoyment, with each individual progressing at her own pace until fully relaxed. This form of deep cleansing and relaxation was very popular in Roman times, and examples of steam rooms, plunge pools, and resting, relaxing areas are still evident in Roman ruins around Britain to this day.

So the therapist is applying an ancient and well proven treatment with steam or vapour routines, although nowadays in a more modern and convenient form for the individual – the Steam Bath. These cabinets are constructed in metal or fibreglass, and permit one person to sit comfortably without restriction, with her head placed through the opening at the top. The height of the seat can

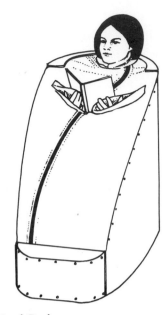

Metal Bath

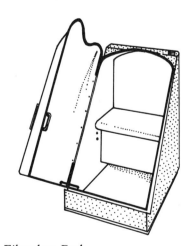

Fibreglass Bath

be altered for clients, so that the head is free from the cabinet. The steam is produced by electrical elements heating water in a bath under the seat, controlled by a thermostat set to the desired temperature.

The size of the water bath, and its position in the cabinet, should be carefully considered by the therapist when choosing a steam bath. For clinic application where continuous use is required, a water tank capable of providing 6—10 baths without being refilled, is necessary. For less frequent use a smaller capacity tank for 4—6 baths will be sufficient. The tank should be rust proof, and contain two elements for water heating. Its position should allow the steam to circulate freely around the client when in the bath, and not funnel up to cause accumulations of steam which could scald the skin.

The shape of the seat in the bath should also be designed to guard against this problem, and modern baths do have improved protection for the client's legs, as they direct the steam away from the sensitive calf area.

If choosing a steam cabinet the different features of the baths available may be helpful in deciding which unit best fits personal circumstances and finances.

Metal baths are durable, can be used continually, offer good value, and have a long working life. However, they get very hot during treatment, so all parts touching the client have to be protected by towels. They are also less easy to keep clean, and have not got such a modern appearance.

Fibreglass baths are very attractive in appearance, need very little maintenance and require less towelling protection, as the cabinet does not become so hot to the touch. Their durability is not so proven as the metal baths, as they have not got such a long working record, and their cost is considerably higher.

So the choice depends on convenience and the general application, with the costs of a cheaper bath perhaps being cancelled out by increased laundry and staff costs incurred in preparation between clients. The tried and tested metal bath performs a very adequate job if correctly towelled up and, if well maintained, will last for years. The more recent innovation of the plastic or fibreglass bath does save time in preparation, needing only paper towels for hygiene, and also being very simple to clean.

Whatever the bath found to be available, the routine of application is similar, and the therapist has to learn to deal deftly with whatever is in clinic use.

Routine of Application

The steam bath is prepared prior to the client's arrival, with the water checked to see that the elements are well covered, and the seat prepared with towels and/or paper tissues according to type. A free-standing seat must have the towels arranged so that they protect the client's legs or back from direct steam. A towel is placed over the top opening of the bath, and heat controls turned to maximum initially, and then set to the desired temperature, when the water starts to heat. The bath will take 15—20 minutes to heat from cold, depending on the size of the water tank. The pilot light should be watched to see that the bath is heating, as often therapists are waiting in vain, only to find that they have neglected to turn on from the wall mains socket. This is a common error, but very annoying if a client is waiting.

When the bath is at the correct temperature as shown on the temperature gauge, or when tested by the therapist's hand inside the opening, the client can be helped into the bath. Her gown is then deftly removed and, as she is seated, her head is guided into the correct position by the therapist. The towel may then be firmly tucked round the client's neck to prevent steam escaping. The temperature of the bath, if comfortable, may then be kept at a steady level for the duration of the routine by setting the thermostat. If no control mechanism is built into the bath, the therapist must manually control the heat by turning off the elements if the heat level becomes too high. Each element can be alternatively turned off and on to keep the heat spread throughout the bath. Again, the more modern the design, the more convenient the application.

The steam bath treatment provides a valuable time to discuss the client's diet progress, exercise plans, or problems arising from the overall treatment plan. The therapist cannot leave the client unless some other skilled supervision is available, just in case the effects of the heat prove too strenuous for the client, so the time should be put to good use. The normal temperature of the bath should be 50—55° Centigrade, although some clients prefer a higher temperature than this. The duration of the treatment should be 10—25 minutes, with 15—20 minutes being the average.

Clients should not be allowed to exceed sensible durations in the belief that the hotter it is, the better.

Any feelings of being restricted, or worries about becoming trapped, should be dispelled initially by demonstrating to the client how easily they can leave the bath, by simply pushing the door open. This also serves to illustrate how the heat can be instantly reduced if it becomes too hot, so they have no worries of being scalded. Clients suffer many minor anxieties over electrical treatment, and large apparatus in particular, most of which are dispelled by the continuing presence of the therapist. The client's anxiety level rises if the therapist disappears, even if only for an instant, and it is then that in panic accidents may occur.

As the steam settles on the skin, it softens the stratum corneum, or horny layer, and dead skin is released. The heat of the body rises and perspiration commences, adding to the cleansing process. Many clients find this form of heating far more comfortable than dry heat, as the body is already moist with vapour and perspiration seems to come more easily. The head is free from the cabinet, and although affected by the change in body temperature is less directly involved, which some clients find more acceptable. Clients with very sensitive skin on their face also find it less damaging to surface capillaries than the dry baking of the sauna.

The treatment may be made more luxurious by wiping the brow to remove excess moisture, with a scented cool tissue. The extra attention involved in steam bath therapy, with its need for close personal client contact, makes it a more expensive treatment than sauna baths, in the normal clinic situation. In a hydro many clients can be supervised at a time, in the steam bath or sauna rooms, by one qualified member of staff.

Steam baths should not be taken more than twice a week, unless under medical supervision as in a residential hydro. The fluid lost during treatment is small and can only *help* to maintain a correct weight; it cannot without diet *reduce* body weight. The body naturally replaces the lost fluid within the next 24 hours by its hydric equilibrium mechanism, retaining more fluid from its intake, and passing less out in urine.

The steam bath treatment concludes with a warm shower and friction rub to remove dead surface skin; then the client must rest for 15—30 minutes. Massage naturally follows the steam bath routine, and is very complementary to it in effect.

SAUNA BATHS

Sauna baths are based on the Finnish principle of log cabins, heated by wood stoves, to produce dry heat effects. The principle of dry heat for therapeutic effects is much more ancient, however, and can be traced throughout history. The log cabin, which has become so popular, does originate in Finland, and it is a version of this sauna that is in use in modern therapy practice. The sauna cabin comes in either a log or panel version and can be built in or be free-standing. The air must be allowed to circulate around the sauna to permit an interchange of air within it of at least seven times an hour. The saunas are made of solid pine logs or panels of wood packed with insulated material to contain more of the heat within the bath. The material the bath is made of must be capable of removing all the moisture from within the bath, otherwise the air would be stale and it would become unhygienic and smell unpleasant.

The heat is produced by large electric stoves which heat special stones placed in a recessed tray, piled on top of the stove. The smaller 3 kilowatt stoves can operate off the normal 13 ampere electricity supply socket, but the larger units (4—9 kilowatts) require a special electricity supply and must be installed professionally. Current similar to that required for a cooker is needed, and the control box must be isolated for safety, well away from the treatment area. It is useful if the temperature control is also placed in this area, rather than outside the sauna entrance, so preventing interference by clients with the sauna temperature.

The temperature inside the bath is indicated by a thermometer placed near the ceiling of the cabin. Light comes from specially insulated light fittings, and the sauna fittings also include resting benches, a guard rail for the stove, duckboards on the floor and sauna bucket, ladle and birch twigs.

Sauna cabins take 20—30 minutes to heat up completely, if of average size; the larger 10—12 seater units take much longer to reach full capacity; up to one hour. When the bath has reached the temperature set, it turns itself off, but the heat continues to increase within the sauna as the temperature of the wood increases. When the walls, etc., have absorbed as much heat as they are able to, it is radiated back into the cabin, creating a build up effect. For this reason clients must be supervised when in the sauna, as the effect of the heat seems to creep up on them and they can suddenly be overcome by it. Because of the build up effect, the initial temperature should not be set too high, but the bath permitted to develop heat which will be thrown back from the walls and ceiling. This, then, is closer to the true effect of a log sauna, with the natural essence of pine resin exuding from the wood all adding to the authenticity.

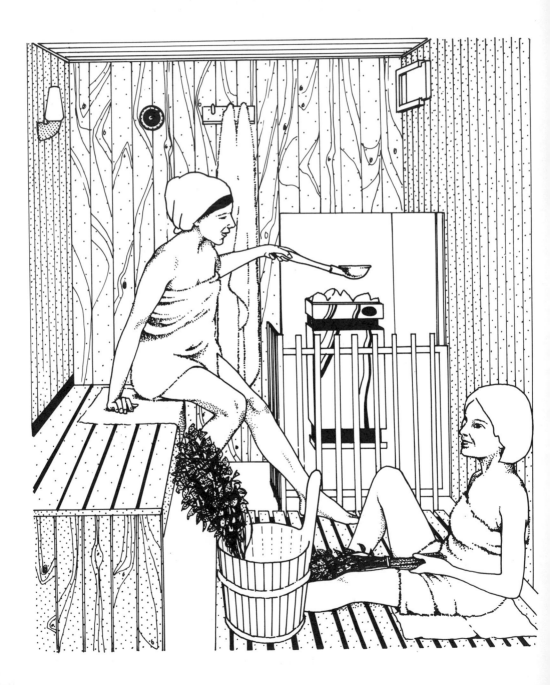

Routine of Application

Having ascertained that the client is fit, the procedure of the sauna treatment can be explained briefly if it is a first visit. On entering the bath, the gown is removed and a towel wrapped loosely around the body. The client should be advised to stay on the lower benches until becoming accustomed to the heat. The head may be wrapped with a towel or left free; if hair lacquer has been used it is better covered. All the body and head will perspire, so the hair style really has to be renewed after the routine. The client can retain the towel or lie naked, relaxed on the benches, according to personal choice. Smaller clinic saunas will have the benches and floors protected by paper roll tissues for hygiene, whilst larger units may not, so clients would be better advised to retain some towelling protection. The temperature in a sauna may range from 60—80° Centigrade, with female clients starting at the lower range. A multiple use sauna may be set at 70° Centigrade, and the only reduction of heat that the client can obtain is to sit on the lower benches, away from the stove.

Some clients do not perspire immediately, but take up to 10 minutes before body heat starts to be released. This can be aided by having the client shower prior to the sauna and enter it whilst still wet. When the client is relaxed and accustomed to the heat, she may be shown how to sprinkle a few drops of water from the bucket on to the stones, using the long-handled ladle for safety. This brings vapour into the routine and alters the feeling of the bath, making the client more aware of the heat present. Clouds of steam should be discouraged, as the air circulation of the bath cannot cope with its removal, and the dry baking effect is then lost.

The routine of the sauna can be alternated with warm or cold showers, or simply periods of rest outside the sauna cabin. Depending on the organization of the clinic and its sauna facilities, the routine can be either a pre-heating routine prior to treatment, or a leisure relaxation treatment in its own right. It is naturally more profitable if it is self-supporting, and tends to build linked business, light diet facilities, exercise participation and instruction, as well as increasing the treatment aspects of the clinic.

At the conclusion of the routine, the client showers, has a brisk rub with a towel or friction rub, and then rests for half to one hour, depending on the body temperature reached

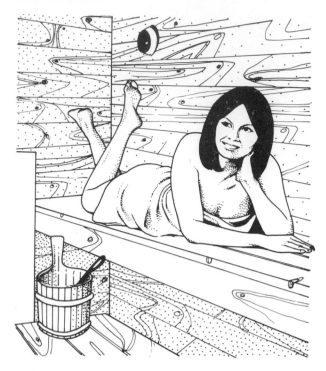

within the sauna. The rest period may encompass massage, electrical treatment, or more minor treatments, or the client may simply sleep. The clinic facilities dictate to a large extent the way the sauna treatment is promoted, but to be profitable the bath needs to have a regular flow-through of clients to justify its heating costs. A medium size bath will comfortably hold 3—5 people, depending on whether they lie stretched out or sit up. Friends can be encouraged to try the sauna together, as it is a very communal treatment, and this can lead to further business for the clinic. Sauna is a very convenient treatment to operate, requiring only supervision rather than close personal attendance. The ideal way to organize linked sauna and treatment is to book the therapist's time for the treatment and allow the client to come in for the sauna ahead of this time. So that if clients like long, lingering saunas, they may come in an hour ahead, or more normally complete the routine in 20—25 minutes, and still be ready when the therapist is free to treat them.

COMPARISONS BETWEEN THE STEAM AND SAUNA TREATMENT

It may be useful, when deciding which heating routine is most suitable for the client, to compare the advantages and disadvantages of each routine.

The steam bath may be personally adjusted to the client's heat tolerance and offers privacy, which older clients may prefer. The client's head is free, so she may feel less enclosed or claustrophobic than in a sauna. The wet heat is found more acceptable and comfortable to clients with sensitive skin. But it does require personal supervision, has greater maintenance and preparation needs, and can only treat one client at a time so, although less expensive to run, it is also less profitable than sauna. It tends to be used mainly as a pre-heating treatment rather than as a treatment in its own right.

The sauna is normally a communal treatment and is enjoying popularity at this moment. It provides relaxation, social elements, and is undertaken as a leisure routine or as pre-heating prior to treatment. It is low on preparation and maintenance and only requires supervision. Many clients can use the sauna, showers, and rest area at any one time, so potentially it is much more profitable.

Some clients find it claustrophobic and regret the lack of privacy it affords. The temperature set may not suit all the clients undertaking treatments as it is set for general purposes, not according to individual needs. The dry, baking heat is found less comfortable by some clients, particularly older people. As the head is involved in the treatment, the hair really requires washing after the routine.

Clients will normally like one routine or the other, depending to a large extent how it is presented to them. Clients with a low heat tolerance may be safer in a steam bath, or in a small individual model sauna, which then can be set for the personal temperature chosen. Small saunas are popular in salons where a more personal service is offered, but where both sauna and steam bath effects are desired.

Many different physiological and psychological effects are attributed to steam baths and sauna baths, but the important thing to remember is that both have heat as their main force. The overall aim is relaxation, without over-exertion or strain placed upon the heart and circulation to achieve this. The client should feel free from tension, but not exhausted by the routine; just gently sedated with a desire to rest.

The overall benefits should be improved vigour and vitality, plus freedom from muscular and nervous tension. A renewed capacity to deal with the stresses and strains of everyday life is also felt, sometimes described by clients as being recharged for the week ahead.

CARE AND MAINTENANCE OF STEAM AND SAUNA BATHS

Where heat and moisture are involved in treatment, there exists an ideal situation for bacterial growth, which will decompose, smell unpleasant and damage equipment if not removed. Valuable equipment deserves regular care and maintenance to keep it in good condition and prolong its life.

Steam baths need to be wiped out after use, using the towels initially to remove excess moisture. The inside can then be thoroughly cleaned with an antibacterial disinfectant solution, which is non-irritant in action. The bath may then be prepared for further use with paper tissue on the floor and towels and paper sheets on the seat. If treatments are concluded for the day, the bath should be left open, free from towels, to dry thoroughly. If the steam bath has a zip opening, this must be kept oiled, as it is often the first area on a bath to become faulty, through rust. If the steam bath rests in a drip tray, this must be cleared regularly and cleaned to prevent debris accumulating.

Sauna baths need to be really scrubbed at regular intervals, depending on their usage, to free the wood from accumulated secretions from the clients. Clients leaning against walls and other surfaces, leave body oils and dead skin which build up unpleasantly. Soap and water is used to thoroughly scrub the benches, walls, duckboards, etc., and permit the natural air interchange to take place efficiently. It is sometimes thought that the high level of heat acts to kill all bacteria in a sauna, but a visit to a large municipal sauna at the end of a busy day dispels this illusion.

During operation the sauna can be kept fresh with a disinfectant wipe over the surfaces, and adequate use of disposable materials on the resting and floor surfaces. For a sauna to be sweet smelling, it must have adequate circulation, and fans will need to be installed in the vicinity if the sauna is rather enclosed or is positioned in a basement. The wood has to breathe and the bath should be left open to air at the end of the day's treatments.

To avoid the risk of cross infection, disposable materials should be used to protect the floors and seats of baths, and nearby areas where the clients may walk with bare feet. Larger establishments may have marble type floors than can be rinsed down. If the heat and shower areas are isolated from the main treatment area, the floor surface can be chosen for its easy cleaning advantages. The situation can be kept clean without appearing cold and clinical. Clients particularly appreciate a high standard of hygiene and, if not evident, will decline to use the facilities available.

PARAFFIN WAXING TREATMENT

Wax baths provide a convenient means of heating areas of the body, normally the limbs – although the wax can be used to accomplish a complete body treatment. In residential clinics, hydros, etc., total immersion baths of large capacity are installed, into which the client relaxes in a sitting position. The body is able to tolerate a very high level of heat within the paraffin wax treatment, as the heat is evenly spread throughout the wax. If full body treatments are applied within the salon, the wax is applied sectionally with a brush, and the client wrapped to retain the heat. Although not as simple in its application, the effects are very similar to immersing the body. All waxing treatment is based on paraffin wax, with several different varieties available for specific effects.

Paraffin Wax

Paraffin wax is used for treatment of stiffness in the joints and improvement of skin texture, colour and general appearance. It provides a means of generating a steady, high level of heat throughout the tissues, so relieving pain. Paraffin wax is solid and cloudy-white in colour when cold, and has a low melting point. When heated to its working temperature of 120°F/49°C, it becomes clear, completely fluid and capable of forming a second skin of wax over the treated area on exposure to the air. When sufficient wax encloses the limb, heat is built up, perspiration is induced and relaxation of the tissues results.

Parafango Wax

A mineral-based wax, similar in action to paraffin, but reputed to have additional cleansing, toning, relaxing and invigorating actions on the tissues. Muscular pain is eased, joints are relaxed and sweating can be induced if a sufficient area is treated. Parafango wax is dark greeny-brown in colour and requires the same method of application and maintenance as paraffin wax. Its additional effects are credited to the mud-based mineral content of the wax, which is obtainable only from volcanic areas of the world.

WAX TREATMENT OF THE LIMBS

Equipment

Paraffin Waxing

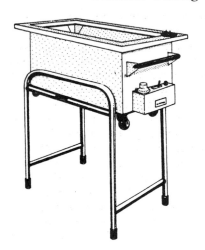

Small quantities of paraffin wax may be prepared in a single unit waxer, but for immersion of limbs, a larger bath, with a built-in water jacket and thermostatic controls, is desirable. The wax is pre-heated and maintained at the correct temperature (49° C) automatically, so minimizing the risks of overheating or burns. Sufficient time should be allowed for pre-heating the wax prior to treatment, particularly in the case of the larger baths, where one hour should be allowed prior to the client's arrival.

Preparation for Wax Therapy

The working area should be protected with heavy grade polythene sheeting to prevent fragments of wax adhering to the floor coverings, or couch surfaces. Both vinyl and carpet-type floor coverings require protection. The couch should be covered first with polythene, followed by rough paper sheeting, to prevent damage and speed the clearing procedures after treatment is concluded. Towels, if used, must be protected by disposable paper, as a paraffin wax cannot be removed easily from fabric but forms a fast bond. Clients' clothing must be adequately covered and, if a large area is being treated, it is preferable for the client to replace her clothing with a salon gown to avoid mishaps. Careful application of technique with the wax at the correct temperature and consistency should avoid unnecessary mess caused by liquid wax dripping during the application.

PARAFFIN WAX THERAPY

Preparation

Paraffin wax may be applied by (1) painting the wax over the area with a large brush, or (2) dipping the limb into the wax bath. Preparation for both methods involves pre-heating the wax, protecting the working area and ensuring the necessary commodities are ready for use.

Items required include:

(*i*) **2 sufficiently large foil sheets to enclose the limbs.**

(*ii*) **2 medium sized towels.**

(*iii*) **Nourishing cream and spatula.**

(*iv*) **Large brush for application (if used).**

The working position should permit safe and efficient wax application, whilst maintaining client comfort. The limb should be washed, or wiped over with a soapy, antiseptic solution and, in the case of hand treatment, all jewellery removed if possible.

Application

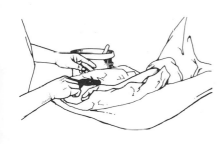

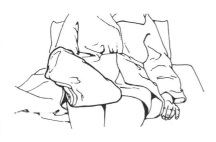

With the client adequately protected and in a comfortable position, the limbs are covered in a thin film of nourishing cream and then dipped into the warm wax to form a thin coating. The fingers or toes remain together, and the process is repeated (5—6 times) until a fairly thick layer of wax is formed. The limb is then wrapped in foil and towels to maintain the heat. The second limb is treated in a similar manner, and then the client should be allowed a few minutes' rest to permit maximum heat build up to produce a satisfactory circulation improvement.

If a small wax container is employed, the wax may be brushed on to the prepared limb, which rests on a foil sheet, placed over a towel protecting the operator's lap. When sufficient layers of wax have been applied, the foil is wrapped firmly around the limb, enclosing the wax, and towels bind the package to retain the heat. Due to the fluid nature of the heated wax, care must be taken to protect the garments, towels, etc. and the surrounding area from drops of wax spilt during the application.

Removal

Removal is easily accomplished due to the nourishing cream application. The wax peels off in one piece, if it has been evenly applied, requiring the minimum of additional cleaning. The limb will be found to be relaxed, warm, with increased circulation, improved skin colour and appearance. The tissues are in an ideal relaxed condition for manual massage treatment to reinforce the circulation improvement action commenced by the hot wax.

If applied, a full 10 minutes massage is desirable to release dead skin, ease stiffness and tension in the joints and muscles, and reinforce the improvement in appearance. Senile skin, dehydrated and dry flaky conditions benefit particularly from paraffin wax applications, as the action is two-fold, promoting internal circulation, whilst achieving a cosmetic improvement in epidermal cells and skin tissue.

FULL BODY WAX TREATMENT

Good organization and preparation are required to accomplish a total wax treatment successfully. A larger quantity of wax is set to heat, ideally a 22 kg (50 lb) approximate capacity bath, which will require 40 minutes to one hour to reach the correct working temperature. The wax can be set to 50—55° Centigrade as it will lose its heat rapidly on the larger body expanses. An infra-red/radiant heat lamp should be placed in readiness and the bed and floor areas protected. The plinth has first blankets, then thick polythene sheeting, placed upon it, which will be used to wrap the client.

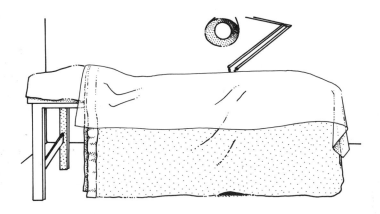

Routine of Treatment

The client removes her gown and, naked, is settled on the plinth, lying on her side. The therapist checks the temperature of the wax and applies it rapidly with broad sweeping strokes down the back with a 10 cm (4 in.) paint brush. The gluteal fold is protected from the wax by a tissue.

When the back and back of the legs are entirely covered with several layers of wax, the client turns supine. The therapist then turns the heat lamp on and continues to apply wax to the lower and upper legs. When these are complete, the polythene sheeting is wrapped round the legs and blankets tucked round to maintain the heat. The heat lamp is then placed 60—90 cm (2—3 ft) away from the legs to keep the heating effect in action as long as possible. The application continues up the body, with the pubic area again being covered with disposable tissues and excluded from the application. When the trunk is completed, it is wrapped and, finally, the arms are painted and the client is then totally enclosed with only the head free. The neck area is firmly tucked with towels for comfort and to retain the heat, and the client is left to rest for approximately 20 minutes. The heat lamp may be placed more centrally over the body or, if available, a second lamp placed to heat the client. An overhead multiple lamp is very useful in this instance, if it can be used for heat alone rather than ultra-violet and infra-red combined.

After 20 minutes the lamps may be removed, the client unwrapped and the wax removed, first from the legs, trunk and arms and, with the client sitting up, lastly from the back. A warm shower concludes the routine, followed by massage if desired. The wax treatment frees dead skin from the surface, and perspiration is also lost during treatment. Waxing has a very skin-softening effect and brings about great improvements in skin texture in addition to the normal effects of heating. The skin is very warm and pink after waxing, and appears plumped out by the treatment.

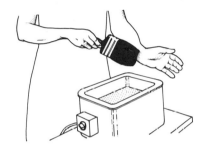

Testing the Temperature of the Wax

1

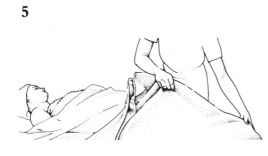

2

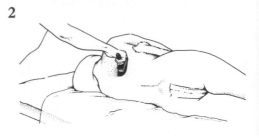

3

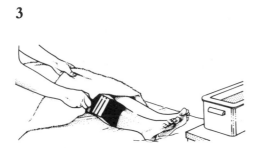

4

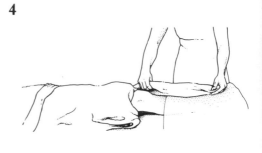

5

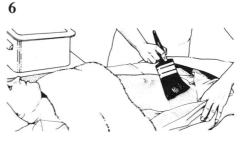

6

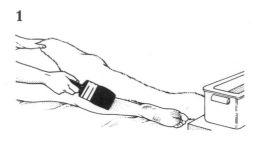

7

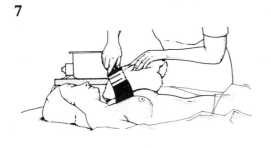

8

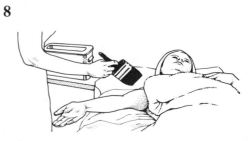

9

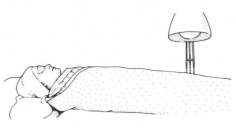

Waxing completed

10

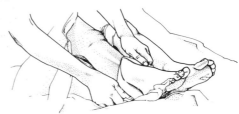

Removal

11

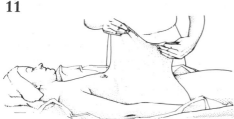

12

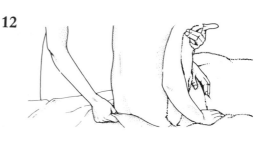

CONTRA-INDICATIONS TO WAXING

Treatment of the limbs has few contra-indications, apart from:

(*i*) **Skin diseases, particularly athletes foot.**

(*ii*) **Varicose veins, or any varicose ulcers.**

(*iii*) **Sunburn, or windburn.**

Total body treatment has the normal contra-indications to general heat therapy, as the heat effects created by the build up of warmth in the body are physically similar to steam and sauna baths.

SAFETY PRECAUTIONS AND MAINTENANCE OF WAXING EQUIPMENT

Safety Precautions

Well made waxing apparatus which complies with the B.S.I. standard of safety should be employed. The equipment must be earthed or double insulated, correctly wired, and should have enclosed heating elements to prevent over-heating of the outer casing. The heater should be sited for use on a metal- or wood-topped mobile trolley, protected with rough paper tissues. Glass trolleys must not be used as the risks of shattering are high, and could result in serious damage to anyone in the vicinity.

The wax should not be left to heat and melt close to any inflammable materials, plastic goods, curtains, etc., due to the risk of fire. Covered containers reduce both the pungent odour of the melting wax and reduce the fire risk. The wax pans should be free from adhering wax on the rims and bottoms, otherwise they may ignite and cause a serious fire hazard. Regular supervision should be given to the wax, to check its progress, even with thermostatically controlled units, and as modern apparatus is designed with client presentation in mind, it may be prepared within the treatment situation, close to the operator and the client.

The best form of safety precaution in waxing is knowing the best wax for the application, and then becoming proficient in its use and maintenance, thus avoiding areas of danger.

The following faults reduce the safety level and proficiency of waxing, and so must be avoided at all times:

1 **Overheating the wax.**
2 **Inadequate protection of the client and working area.**
3 **Incorrect working consistency, too hot or cool.**
4 **Neglect in testing the wax temperature, in relation to the client's tolerance.**
5 **Careless application, producing untidy removal and unsatisfactory results.**
6 **Moving the wax whilst hot.**

Paraffin Wax Maintenance

Small quantities of used wax may be filtered through a very fine gauge mesh sieve to remove waste particles before being replaced for future use. Larger waxing units incorporate an efficient cleansing system, which functions on the principle of drawing off the waste elements upon the addition of water into the wax container. As the wax cools, it rises to the surface and, when solid, the water debris may be drawn off from a release tap at the side, leaving the wax clean and ready for use.

Paraffin waxing units based on the principle of a container surrounded by a water jacket and heated by an enclosed element are the safest in use, as at no time can the limbs come into contact with an open source of heat during the treatment. The water level must be maintained, by checking before use and by the addition of fluid if necessary, through an opening at the side of the tank.

FOAM AND HYDRO-OXYGEN BATHS

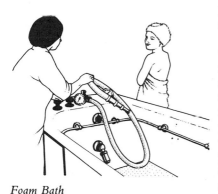

Foam Bath

These more specialized baths are only likely to be found in larger establishments, where fairly continual use would justify their considerable expense. The simpler foam baths work on the principle of aerating the water of a bath, to create stimulating and heating effects. The power is obtained from an air-compressor which forces air through tiny holes in duckboards placed on the floor of the bath. The bath may be filled with a small amount of hot water 10—13 cm (4—5 in.) sufficient to cover the boards, and concentrated foam essence 13—15 g ($\frac{1}{2}$—1 oz) added. The air pressure creates foam which fills the bath, into which the client steps and relaxes in a sitting position. Heat is built up within the body and the client is virtually surrounded by foam which acts as an insulator and holds the heat. Seaweed or natural flower essences may be used, and clients find the treatment very luxurious and bracing.

The air pressure may also be used with the normal quantity of water in the bath, and with the addition of essences or extracts, and the whole of the bath becomes aerated. The client remains in either type of bath for 10—15 minutes, and then showers or simply is dried normally.

The same principle in a more elaborate form is used in the hydro-oxygen bath, in which the client reclines to be stimulated with warm to hot water jets, whilst the whole cabinet is diffused with oxygen. Heat is created and the client feels refreshed and invigorated by the treatment.

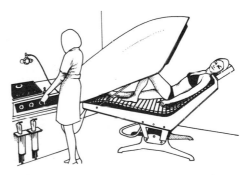

Hydro-oxygen Bath

LAMP TREATMENTS

The therapist will use several different forms of ray treatment within her clinic applications; some to provide localized forms of heating to relieve tension, others for cosmetic purposes to produce sun tanning effects. The treatments may be applied via single lamps, with or without reflectors, or by multiple lamp units for more general body applications.

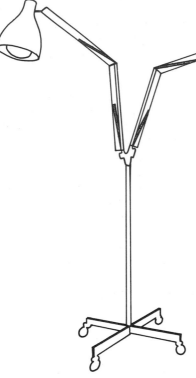

The equipment available is very varied, and a sound knowledge of the underlying principles of ray treatments makes safe and effective adaptation possible, whatever the lamp unit used. Even the modern multiple lamps, although more convenient in application, are based on identical principles and ray sources. Their advantage is in easier, faster applications and increased safety rather than in any change in effect.

All lamp treatments require careful attention to safety, as the risk of overtreatment, scorching the skin or burns is ever present. Some lamp treatments, like infra-red/radiant heat, produce an instant reaction to guide the therapist, whilst others, like ultra-violet, do not produce this immediate built-in safety precaution, and require much more careful timing. The skin reaction created is erythema, sometimes termed hyperaemia when referring to heat reactions produced by ray treatments. This is the normal skin response to heat; increased colour, warmth, rise in local temperature, etc., that has already been considered in general treatments. In lamp treatments the degree of erythema is measured to ensure the treatment does not produce excessive reactions which could result in skin damage or burns.

Twin Headed Treatment Lamp (Ultra-violet and Infra-red)

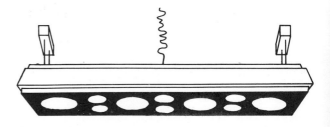

Solarium (Ultra-violet and Infra-red) Ceiling Fitting

The rays used by the therapist in the clinic are ultra-violet, visible light and infra-red rays which are electro-magnetic radiations. Since the sun produces the same radiations they can be called ACTINIC.

Visible light can occur as any one of a whole range or spectrum of different colours, each colour having a different wavelength, and the order red, orange, yellow, green, blue (indigo and violet) of the well known colours in the rainbow is due to this, being the order of decreasing wavelength. These visible wavelengths ranging from 7000 (red) down to 4000 Angstrom units (1 Angstrom unit being one ten thousand millionth of a metre). All the other electro-magnetic radiations are invisible and the diagram shows the complete spectrum of radiations in order of decreasing wavelength.

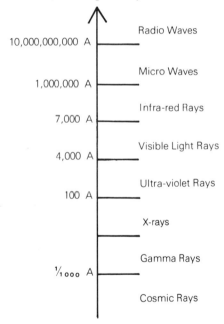

Electro-magnetic Spectrum

	Radio Waves
10,000,000,000 A	
	Micro Waves
1,000,000 A	
	Infra-red Rays
7,000 A	
	Visible Light Rays
4,000 A	
	Ultra-violet Rays
100 A	
	X-rays
	Gamma Rays
$\frac{1}{1000}$ A	
	Cosmic Rays

Solarium (Floor Standing Model)

Ultra-violet rays have shorter wavelengths and infra-red rays have longer wavelengths than visible light. It is the different wavelengths which account for the different properties of the various rays. Radiations of long wavelengths, for example radio waves, do not easily cast sharp shadows and for this reason they tend not to be called rays but are called waves because they travel rather like water waves.

Often ultra-violet radiation is produced mixed in with visible light and seeing where the visible light goes gives a good guide to where the invisible ultra-violet is going. Similarly infra-red radiation is often accompanied by visible light.

The advantage of this mixing of rays in beauty therapy is the increased safety which it provides. The timing of treatments, although still needing care, is not as critical as in medical applications. By providing warmth, largely by the visible and infra-red rays mixed in with the ultra-violet rays, the feeling of warmth acts as a warning to indicate that the treatment should be concluded. Also this heating produces an immediate erythema reaction while the effects of the ultra-violet rays are not produced until six to twelve hours after the treatment. The warmth produced also makes the treatment luxurious and a feeling close to natural sun bathing is achieved, where heat and tanning elements are normally combined.

Lamps for heat-ray treatment are of two main kinds, one known usually as *radiant*, sometimes as mixed or duo-ray lamp, and the other as *infra-red*. In both kinds infra-red radiation is the main source of heat, and since this radiation is invisible it is often described as black heat, like that received from an ordinary room-heating radiator. The difference between the two types of lamp is that the radiant lamp emits red light in addition to infra-red and that the infra-red is mostly of short wavelength, while the infra-red lamp, as its name suggests, produces infra-red rays only (no visible rays) and this infra-red radiation is of longer wavelength. The presence of the visible light coming from the radiant lamp makes it obvious that the lamp is in use and therefore makes this lamp safer. It is only when special effects are needed and when the irritation caused by short wavelength infra-red rays is to be avoided that infra-red lamps are used.

For measuring the small wavelengths of the above mentioned rays the Angstrom unit is often used, as mentioned earlier. However it is becoming more usual to employ the nanometre (nm) which is equal to 10 Å (or a thousand millionth of a metre).

ULTRA-VIOLET TREATMENT (RAY LAMP)

Ultra-violet rays are electromagnetic waves with wavelengths of between 4000 and 136 Å, those within the range 4000 and 1849 Å being available for treatment purposes. Ultra-violet rays are absorbed in the skin, and it is there that the reactions occur which cause the beneficial effects. The effects of ultra-violet rays on the body may have a local reaction, or a more widespread effect, depending on the degree of the irradiation (output and general exposure to the rays).

Penetration of Rays into the Skin

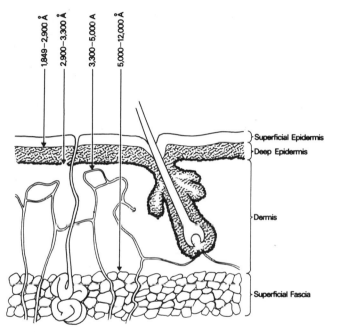

Local Effects

1 *Erythema Reaction*

A mild dose causes slight reddening of the skin, which is accompanied by no other symptoms, and soon fades. The reaction usually appears within 12 hours of the irradiation. There are four degrees of erythema; only the first reaction is a permissible application for the beauty therapist, but she should be aware of the consequences of overexposure and its effect on the skin.

A first degree erythema is a slight reddening of the skin, with no irritation or soreness, which fades within 24 hours.

A second degree erythema is a more marked reddening of the skin, with slight irritation. It fades within two to three days.

A third degree erythema is a marked reaction, which causes the skin to become red, sore, hot and swollen. The reaction lasts about a week and is very painful.

A fourth degree erythema is similar to the third degree reaction, with the addition of blister formation.

2 *Desquamation*
Ultra-violet exposure accelerates the skin's normal shedding process. The amount of peeling varies with the strength of the erythema reaction.

3 *Pigmentation*
Rays with wavelengths between 2800 and 3300 Å are absorbed in the deep epidermis, and initiate a chemical reaction which results in the conversion of the amino-acid tyrosine into the pigment melanin. The degree of pigmentation found depends on the client's natural colouring and the method of application. Constant duration treatments for germicidal purposes do not alter the skin's colour greatly, whilst progressive applications for cosmetic tanning and tonic purposes affect a considerable colour change over a period of time. The local applications appear to increase the skin's resistance to infection.

General Effects

Sufficient ultra-violet exposure:

(*i*) Increases the body's general resistance to infection.

(*ii*) Gives a general tonic effect.

(*iii*) Produces a Vitamin D formation, if of sufficient intensity and duration.

(*iv*) Produces pigmentation, and an improved skin condition.

INDICATIONS FOR TREATMENT

1 Sluggish complexion, with uneven texture and pH value.

2 Seborrhoea, for improvement of skin texture and to regulate secretions.

3 Acne vulgaris, to promote healing by its anti-bacterial and peeling effects.

4 To provide additional protection against natural sunlight and heat effects in the delicate or sensitive skin conditions, and permit a tan to form without discomfort.

5   For cosmetic tanning purposes, to produce or maintain a tanned complexion.

CONTRA-INDICATIONS FOR TREATMENT

1   A very sensitive skin or one that reacts to sunlight (photosensitive skin).

2   Ultra-violet should not be used in combination with certain other treatments, which alter the body temperature. Ultra-violet should not be applied until the temperature has returned to normal.

3   When a client is taking medically prescribed drugs classed as sensitive to ultra-violet: gold, the sulphonamides, insulin, thyroid extract and quinine.

4   Vitiligo.

5   Acute eczema or dermatitis or any unknown skin complaint.

6   An unnatural rise in temperature from any source.

APPLICATION OF ULTRA-VIOLET IRRADIATION

Assessment of Exposure Required

The most satisfactory method of assessing the dosage required is by observation of the erythema reaction created by a patch test or short primary exposure. The following factors determine the intensity of the reaction:

(*i*)   The output of the lamp.

(*ii*) The duration of the exposure.

(*iii*) The distance between the lamp and the client.

(*iv*) The sensitivity of the client to the treatment.

Equipment

Ultra-violet lamps vary in their output according to the type of lamp, its size and the source of the ultra-violet rays. The bulb type is most commonly used in facial applications for general skin effects and cosmetic tanning. It produces only longer ultra-violet wavelengths. Quartz tubes are also used, either in single or multiple form, to cover small or widespread areas. The hot quartz lamp produces a mixture of short and long rays and is suitable for tanning, tonic, cosmetic and germicidal purposes.

The glass bulb ultra-violet lamp has a hot quartz lamp inside it (high pressure mercury vapour), and the short wavelengths cannot pass through the glass of the bulb, so providing only the cosmetic tanning wavelengths.

The lamp chosen should be of sturdy construction, with a stable base, and sufficient reflector span to permit general exposure of larger areas, i.e. the back. The cross arm section should permit a free range of heights and angles, to accommodate the need for variation in the distance between the client and the bulb during the complete sequence of the treatment programme. The reflector must be free from dents, otherwise hot spots will result, which intensify the reaction and could cause burns.

Application

The effect of the ultra-violet rays on a client may be tested to determine sensitivity by giving an extremely short duration irradiation at a distance of 1 m (3 ft) and requesting the client to remember the effect (if any) apparent after 4—8 hours. The distance and duration of subsequent treatment may then be determined, using the principle of inverse squares, which all ray lamps obey.

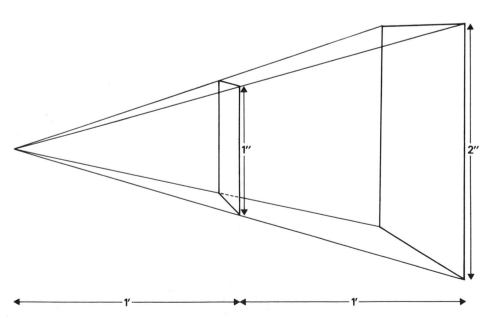

1″   2″

|←————— 1′ —————→|←————— 1′ —————→|

Inverse Square Law

The intensity of radiation varies inversely with the square of the distance from the lamp. Thus the intensity of the radiation at 30 cm (1 ft) is four times that at 60 cm (2 ft) and nine times that at 1 m (3 ft). This law applies to infra-red, visible and ultra-violet rays, so when a lamp obeys the law of inverse squares, four minutes at 60 cm (2 ft) and nine minutes at 1 m (3 ft) are required to produce the same effect as 1 minute at 30 cm (1 ft).

Both bulb and tube lamps require 1—2 minutes to reach maximum output or intensity, so they must be switched on in preparation for the treatment, and placed in such a way that the rays do not fall on unprepared individuals. A curtained area or individual cubicle is required for ultra-violet treatments. The high pressure lamp should be moved as little as possible prior to, or after, the irradiation until it has cooled, otherwise its life is reduced. There is also a risk of spontaneous implosion within the bulb if it is moved or knocked whilst hot.

Treatment Timing

For progressive tanning treatments the applications should be applied in rapid succession, as soon as the erythema reaction has faded, possibly every other day until a tan is established. The progression should be planned according to the client's general colouring and skin reaction. Fair skinned clients may take 8—12 treatments to progress from a total exposure of 1 minute to the full 10—15 minute exposure which is their maximum treatment time. The total treatment time is given which may be divided into two body sections (front and back) for multiple lamps, or four body sections (upper and lower body areas, front and back) for single reflector or bulb lamps. The treatment might progress in the form of treatment: *1.* 1 min, *2.* 2 mins, *3.* 3 mins, *4.* 4 mins, *5.* 6 mins, *6.* 8 mins, *7.* 10 mins, *8.* 12 mins, or it may pause at any stage and repeat the previous exposure time if irritation or sensitivity is evident.

Darker skinned, or previously tanned, clients may commence on a 4 minute exposure and progress rapidly to 20 minutes total, remembering again that these are total times and are divided around the body. The treatment could take the form of treatment: *1.* 4 mins, *2.* 6 mins, *3.* 8 mins, *4.* 10 mins, *5.* 12 mins, *6.* 16 mins, *7.* 20 mins, again with pauses if necessary. The tan may then be maintained by regular but spaced exposures.

If the skin appears irritated for any reason, treatment should be suspended, otherwise severe desquamation will result and the skin will peel and be sore.

Preparation of the Client

The client lies supine on the couch, puts on the protective goggles and is made comfortable by the therapist. If the whole body and face is involved, the hair should be covered if tinted, as ultra-violet affects the colour. No creams, oils, etc., should be applied to the skin.

The lamp may then be placed in position 60—75 cm (2—2½ ft) from the client, depending on the result desired. The distance is measured from the client's highest point, breasts or buttocks, etc. If a multiple lamp is used the whole front of the body can be treated at once, so half the total treatment time can be timed. The client then turns over, the height of the lamp checked and the other half of the time applied.

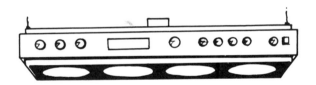

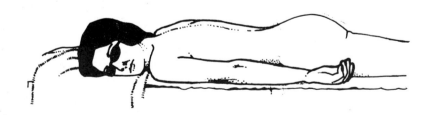

If a single lamp is used, the treatment is applied to just the upper half of the body, with the lower half covered, and then the lower half with the upper half covered. The exact position of the towelling protection should be marked to avoid a double exposure reaction in the central area. The client turns over and the process is repeated, with each section of the body receiving one quarter of the total exposure time.

If some areas of the client have become tanned naturally whilst others have not, such as breasts, the timing must always be worked out for the most sensitive less exposed patches, otherwise burning will result in the white areas. Cosmetic tanning can help to match up a tan to produce an all-over effect and avoid a patchwork result. Used carefully it can also prepare very sensitive skinned clients for overseas holidays and prevent them burning when exposed to strong sunlight. Even if a tan does not result from this course of special applications, it will have been very worthwhile for the client, saving her discomfort.

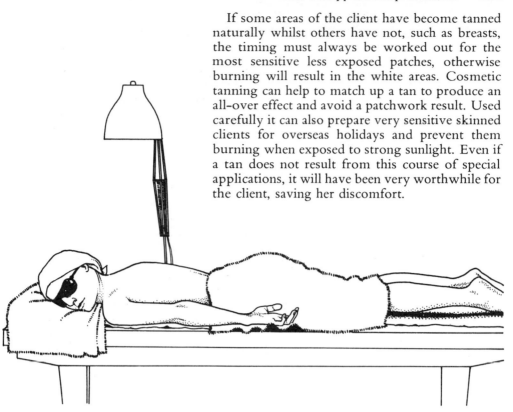

Records of Treatment

A record must be kept of the date, the lamp used, the area exposed and the time of exposure and distance from the lamp. The general effects, erythema reaction, and any related information should be noted.

Over-exposure

The skin becomes hot, red, extremely sore and there may be blister formation. In the event of over-exposure, the client must be advised to consult her own physician. The effect of over-treatment would not be evident immediately after the exposure, taking up to several hours to develop, so the possibility of its formation should not be ignored but discussed with the client to avoid anxiety. The precautions against an overdose lie in careful technique and to all the points mentioned previously. A strong reaction can occur if the client interferes with the exposure programme and undertakes excessive natural sun tanning at the same time. Wind exposure can also increase the skin's erythema reaction, and so verbal and visual investigation are necessary prior to treatment.

INFRA-RED AND RADIANT HEAT TREATMENTS

Infra-red rays are electro-magnetic waves with wavelengths of between 7000→10 000 000 Å. These rays are commonly known as heat radiation because the heating effect of the sun and of most heaters like electric fires in the home is almost entirely due to the infra-red radiation produced. When infra-red rays are absorbed by the tissues of the body, heat is produced at the place where they are absorbed. Various types of heat generators are available, which are usually referred to as either non-luminous or luminous generators. Treatment with the luminous generator is known as *Radiant* (visible heat), and *Infra-red* is used to describe the radiations from the non-luminous forms. Luminous generators produce red light and infra-red radiation while non-luminous generators produce no visible light of course, and produce less short wave radiation. Since both lamps produce infra-red radiation, the terms used to describe the lamps are rather misleading. The heat emitter is available in:

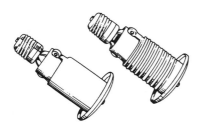

Infra-red and Radiant Heat Emitters

1   Non-luminous form, where the heating element is embedded in a fire clay material, and no visible rays are produced. Infra-red rays are produced with wavelengths between 150 000 and 7000 Å.

2   A luminous generator, where the element is apparent, and visible rays are produced in addition to the infra-red rays. The coiled filament surrounds a fire clay emitter and produces infra-red and visible rays of between 40 000 to 6000 Å when it reaches maximum output. Many of the R/H rays have wavelengths in the region of 10 000 Å.

3   A luminous form of bulb emitter, which produces radiant and infra-red, often called a duo ray is available. The bulb emits a warm glow and is ready for treatment within a few seconds of being switched on, making it a very convenient source of heat for treatment. The bulb type of emitters do not require a reflector to send the rays outwards to the client, because they have a built-in reflector system on the inner surface of the bulb.

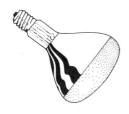

Bulb Emitter

Shorter infra-red rays penetrate to the deeper parts of the dermis, or to the subcutaneous tissues, while the longer rays are absorbed in the superficial epidermis (penetration of rays into the skin). Radiant (visible) heat is therefore more penetrating, but has greater irritant properties to the surface tissues, whilst infra-red, although less penetrating, is more readily absorbed by the tissues and is less irritating and is therefore more frequently chosen for beauty therapy applications.

An irradiation from either heat source produces heat in the superficial tissues, which is conducted to the deeper tissues by blood circulation.

Effects of Local Application of Infra-red Rays

Local irradiation by infra-red rays produces a rise in temperature, erythema (an increase in colour due to vasodilation), a calming effect on sensory nerve endings and increased activity of sweat glands. The sedative effect is enhanced by the general relaxation of the client, due to both the heat application and the relief of tension brought about by skilful client preparation and handling. All these effects correctly applied can be combined into a therapy routine to produce very satisfactory results.

Indications for Treatment

1 Any muscular tension present in the larger muscle groups.
2 Stiffness from over-exertion or unfamiliar work.
3 Any evidence of fibrous accumulations in the shoulder girdle muscles, i.e. trapezius.

The counter-irritation effect created by infra-red is especially effective for deep pain. The increased flow of blood from deeper structures to the surface capillaries washes away inflammatory products, and stiff muscles are eased.

The therapist must use her own professional judgement to decide whether conditions need medical approval prior to treatment. If actual pain is involved, or the client has a history of aches and pains, or back troubles, medical guidance should be sought by the client. Regular heat therapy may be advised for a wide range of muscular conditions and can act as a preventative measure to avoid tension or fibrositis developing.

Contra-indications

1   Any circulatory problems, such as fluid retention, swelling, varicose veins, etc.

2   Skin disorders, dermatitis, eczema, etc.

3   Diabetics, due to their less efficient skin circulation and lessened sensitivity to heat.

4   Clients suffering from respiratory illnesses, bronchitis.

5   Any clients who have metal used in fracture repairs in the area of treatment, i.e. plates or pins used in leg fractures.

6   Sprains would require medical approval prior to treatment.

Routine of Treatment

If using infra-red, the emitter should be switched on 10 minutes prior to treatment. If radiant heat, only a few seconds is required to bring the lamp to maximum emission or output.

The client is made comfortable on the plinth, with the area of treatment exposed and the skin free from oils, etc. The lamp is positioned so that the skin feels comfortably warm, 45—60 cm (18 in. to 2 ft) away and parallel to the client. The distance of the lamp is not so critical in heat treatments as the skin reaction can be seen and felt, and by keeping in close contact with the client an indication of how it feels can be obtained. The irradiation can last 10—20 minutes and can be followed by deep penetrating massage designed to relieve tension.

If the client's tolerance to the heat is poor, the lamp's distance from the client can be increased, using the inverse square principle, so that the client receives the same amount of radiation more gently and slowly. The simple rule of doubling the distance back from the client, requires four times the time necessary to produce the same effect, is a useful rule of thumb for therapists. So if 45 cm (18 in.) becomes 1 m (3 ft) the 10 minutes will have to become 40 minutes before the same benefit will be gained from the application.

The same principle can be used to keep the effect of the application as prolonged as possible after the initial application. After 10 minutes at the normal distance, the lamp can be placed further away from the client, and the heat continues its good work without causing skin mottling or a danger of scorching. Massage with oil can also be combined at this stage of the routine if indicated.

When the desired result is achieved, the lamp can be carefully moved away from the client, who can be left to rest warmly covered, to gain the most relief from the treatment.

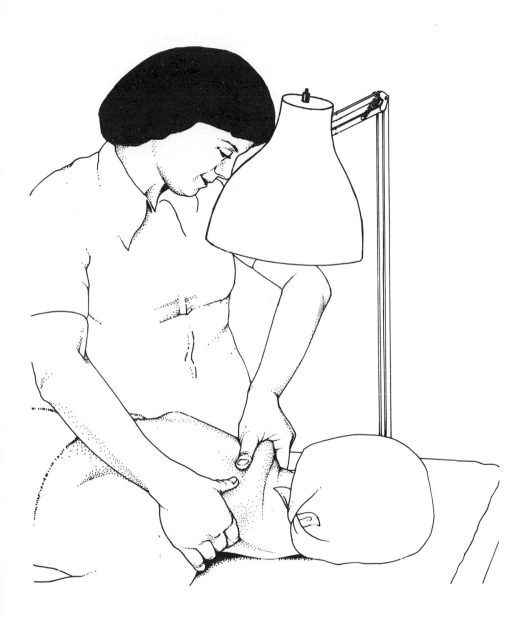

SAFETY PRECAUTIONS IN LAMP TREATMENTS

1   Check the apparatus carefully before use to ensure that reflective surfaces are clean and free from dents, otherwise hot spots will result.

2   If bulb fittings are used, check that they are securely in place. Many of the bulb type lamps have Eddison screw fittings and should be screwed in firmly, but not forced, otherwise the plastic lamp holder will fracture.

3   When handling lamps, ensure hands are free from oil to avoid accidents.

4   Check that the height and angle of the lamp is fixed securely, with screw fittings or wing nuts, to avoid it slipping and harming the client. Overhead solariums should be positioned carefully in the same manner.

5   Floor standing units should have their weight evenly distributed to avoid overbalancing. Standard single lamps are best positioned with the cross arm over one of the large feet rather than between them.

6   Indicate that the lamp is in use by a warning notice hung upon it, or in a prominent area.

7   Heat the lamp in a safe position, turned away from beds, trolleys, etc.

8   In ultra-violet treatments, goggles must be worn by the client, and the operator when in immediate contact with the client. Ultra-violet applications are best enclosed in a special cubicle or curtained area, to prevent the spread of the ulta-violet rays in general treatment areas.

9   Ultra-violet lamps should not be turned off during the course of the treatment, but only at its conclusion.

10 After use, the heat and ultra-violet lamps should be switched off and left in position until they cool down. This prolongs their life and is safer, as it reduces the risk of breakage or spontaneous implosion within the bulb.

Chapter 7

Electrical Body Treatments

Electrical treatments for the body are normally either for *general* application, providing stimulatory or relaxing effects, or are for *specific* application to one area of the body, producing localized stimulation or muscle contraction.

The more *general* treatments include: vibratory massage, indirect high frequency and galvanism.

The *specific* treatments include: muscle contraction and vacuum massage, which can help reshape the body.

The three most widely used systems are: vibrators, vacuum massage and muscle contraction, which between them can effectively complete the vast majority of salon treatments connected with figure reductions, reshaping or improvement.

GENERAL TREATMENTS

The general treatments may be applied in a wide variety of ways to achieve differing effects. *Vibratory* massage can create effects similar to manual massage, either relaxing or stimulating according to the application followed. *High frequency*, indirectly used, gives depth and power to the massage, creating a circulatory response and warmth deep in the tissues, to aid relaxation and dispel muscular and nervous tension. *Galvanism* is used to assist the dispersal of soft fat and 'cellulite' conditions.

All electrical treatment will, if chosen correctly, increase the effectiveness of an overall treatment programme. It can reinforce the reduction results produced by diet, and maintain client interest in general progress. It can ensure inches are lost from the correct areas, and hasten the reduction of established adipose deposits, ensuring that the diet is effective on these as well as subcutaneous fat.

No apparatus can produce a weight loss without a reduction in the client's food intake being achieved. The figure may be made to look trimmer through exercise or muscle contraction, through the toning, tightening effect on slack musculature, but a diet is necessary for actual weight loss. A temporary weight loss can be achieved through sauna and steam baths, but this small amount is simply fluid which is replaced by the body within 24 hours.

So nothing reduces body weight but reduced diet, or increased activity, and it is these elements, strongly reinforced by clinic treatments, that the therapist uses to reshape the client.

VIBRATORY
TREATMENTS

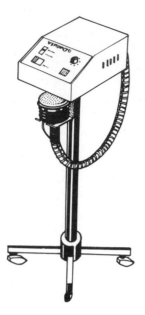

*Vibratory and Muscle
Toning Combined Unit*

There are three forms of vibratory treatment which may be applied to the body: the more generally used large gyratory vibrators, or for localized effects the smaller percussion or audio-sonic vibrators.

Gyratory vibrators for general body work are normally floor standing, with the weight of the motor supported by the main shaft or pedestal of the apparatus. This makes for greater safety as well as permitting long periods of use without undue fatigue. Hand held versions of these heavy duty machines are also available, which can produce similar effects for a lower outlay, but they are naturally more tiring to use. If the vibratory treatments are used simply to complement and reinforce the manual massage, rather than as treatments in their own right, a hand held gyratory unit may well prove adequate.

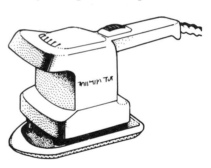

Hand Held Heavy Duty Vibrator

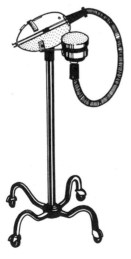

Gyratory Vibrator

Whatever form the vibrator may take it must be adequate for the task required, and should have an air cooled, heavy duty motor capable of running for long periods without overheating. The smaller vibrators normally used within facial therapy can be used on the body, but are suitable only for localized areas, such as the trapezius muscles of the shoulders, and the upper arm.

Gyratory vibrators operate on a vertical and horizontal plane, creating a circular movement whilst vibrating up and down, thus achieving effects similar in action to manual massage. By altering both the applicator heads and the method of use, effects similar to effleurage (sponge heads), petrissage (hard rubber heads) and tapotement (spiky and brush heads) can be obtained. This is useful guidance when deciding which applications are suitable and which contra-indicated.

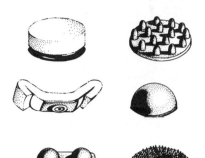

The sensation felt by the client during vibratory treatment, however, is totally different from the feeling of manual massage, and it can be rather impersonal and mechanical if not linked by some hand massage movements. In practice most vibratory treatments are applied in a combined form in this way gaining both the personal touch aspects of massage, and the power and depth of the vibratory unit.

Applicator Heads

Contra-indications to Vibratory Treatments

By adjusting the applicator heads and altering the pressure of the movements, most body conditions can be treated. Vibratory treatment has few contra-indications apart from the normal systemic physical conditions, skin disorders, etc., and is therefore a very useful salon treatment.

Contra-indications include:

1   Varicose veins which should be treated with care, using smooth surfaced applicators, or should be avoided, and the treatment linked manually.

2   A history of thrombosis or inflammation of the veins (phlebitis) would be contra-indicated.

3   Treatment of abdomen during menstruation or pregnancy, is contra-indicated. Treatment of the abdomen, when indicated, must at all times be light and controlled. The therapist should take care not to exert heavy pressure downwards into the abdominal cavity, due to the lack of bony support in this area, and the risk of disturbing the delicate structures present, the womb, fallopian tubes and digestive organs being very easily displaced or irritated.

4   Any identified lumps, hairy or pigmental moles, skin tags, epidermal warts, etc., should be avoided, as the less discriminating effects of vibration could cause abrasion of the skin and discomfort to the client.

5   Extremely hairy areas on men need careful treatment, and use of smooth surfaced applicators, if the treatment is not to cause discomfort. Spiky applicators where the hairs could catch and pull should not be used.

6 Very thin or elderly clients with a lack of subcutaneous tissue would be contra-indicated, or would require adapted applications.

7 A history of slipped disc would require the back area to be excluded from the routine.

8 Treatment of the colon can be undertaken in a similar manner to manual massage, but extra care must be exercised. As the therapist does not receive the normal responses felt through the hands, which guide her on pressure, speed and duration of treatment, a cautious approach is necessary. Vibratory treatment for constipation can be a very beneficial and effective solution to a common problem.

Method of Vibratory Treatments

The client is prepared for normal body treatment, and may have had some form of pre-heating to aid relaxation of muscle tissues. If the effect desired is relaxation only, then the application should concentrate on the soothing strokes and gentle vibratory effects of the treatment. If stimulation and figure reduction elements are needed, then a full range of applicators and a varied pattern of strokes are used. The concentration then is local rather than general, working on areas of established adipose tissue and heavy muscle groups. The manual aspects of a combined treatment are greater if relaxation is required, and reduced if simulation is the main aim. A general combined treatment may be 30—40 minutes, and may be increased or decreased according to the client's needs, and for reasons of convenience and cost. Vibratory treatments always show a time saving over manual methods.

A smooth surfaced applicator commences the treatment, being of sponge or soft rubber. This is used with a light application of a talc medium, applied via the therapist's hands with effleurage strokes. The treatment is applied with long sweeping strokes in an upward direction, towards the heart. The strokes follow the natural contours of the body, and can break contact gently or return with superficial strokes. The important point of technique is the smooth make and break of contact between the applicator head and the client's skin. Control of the heavy equipment comes only with practice and strength in the arms and wrists, and relies on working in the correct postural position.

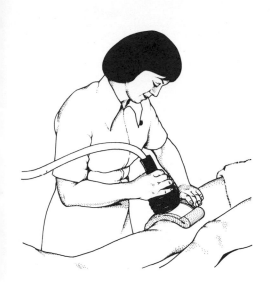

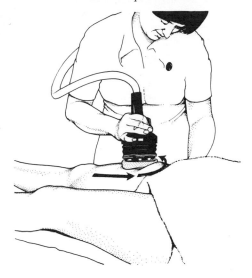

Different applicators may be used for variety, both simple round forms, and those pre-shaped to mould around an area, such as the leg. The size of the client will dictate the most suitable applicator head. Changing the heads unnecessarily should be avoided as it breaks the continuity of the treatment and can be irritating to the client.

Both legs may be treated superficially, interlinking vibratory and manual strokes, and then deeply using the ball studded applicator on the thighs. The deeper movements are performed in a kneading, compression manner, with the therapist's hand providing support and resistance to the strokes, and interlinking them with effleurage.

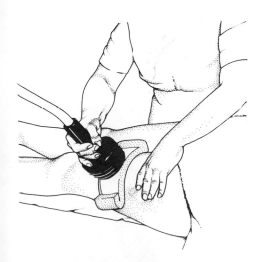

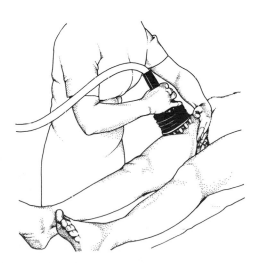

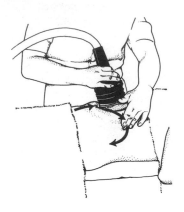

More superficial circular movements can then be performed using the brush type applicator to areas of adequate subcutaneous fat. Poorly textured skin and bad circulation will also benefit from the instant erythema produced by this method of treatment.

The legs may then be covered and the abdomen treated. The application commences with the sponge applicator, following the body contours, which is then followed by kneading along the ascending, transverse, and descending colon, using the ball shaped applicator. Manual movements interlink and re-establish relaxation, then the routine can proceed to stimulating movements on the sides of the waist if indicated. The studded or short brush type rubber applicator is used to produce erythema, and increase circulation in the area.

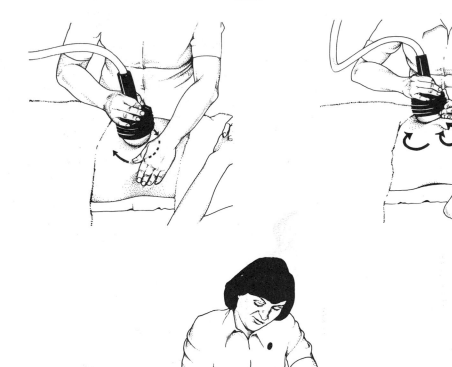

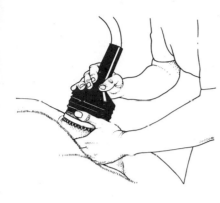

The abdominal area is then covered and the arms and chest treated. Commencing with stroking, and progressing to the short spiky applicator, on the upper arms, if indicated. Rough skin, heavy muscular or fat upper arms, and softening of skin over the biceps and triceps muscles, are all indications for the stimulating, slightly abrasive effects of this application. The skin should be bright pink and hot in the area after treatment if the full effects of vascular interchange and improved skin texture are to be realized. Just the arms may be treated, or the strokes can be extended to include the chest on either side. Choice will depend on the amount of subcutaneous tissue covering the sternum area. A very slim person would find vibration over this body area uncomfortable, and would feel the resonance up into the neck and head.

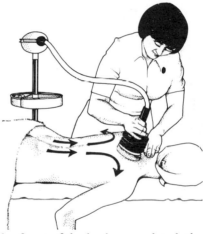

With the front of the body completed, the client turns over and the back is treated. Movements commence with sweeping strokes and progress through the range of suitable applicators for the bulk of tissues present. The ball shaped applicator may be used on the trapezius muscle, and the ball studded and the short brush type applicator used on the upper hip area of the gluteals. The ball studded applicator may also be used with its projections placed either side of the spine, lightly working down the back to the sacrum. The applicator must be kept under control to avoid irritation or damage to the spinous processes of the vertebrae.

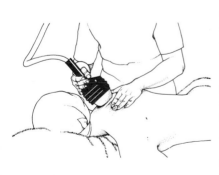

Manual effleurage is used to link and reinforce the movements, and to maintain client contact, and gives an indication of the client's response to the treatment. Verbal contact is also kept throughout, to guard against discomfort or irritation from the treatment.

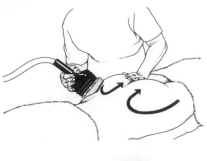

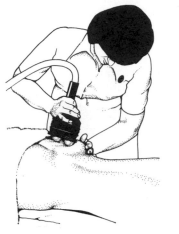

The back is then covered and the buttocks and back of the thighs treated to complete the sequence. A very short period of stroking movements may be given, quickly followed by more active movements, with deep and controlled pressure. The heavily studded and brush applicators may be used to create stimulation, and help to prevent or disperse adipose accumulations in the area. The treatment should endeavour to create its effects without separating the gluteal fold, or causing irritation to the sciatic nerve of the body, placed deeply under the indented area of the buttocks. Irritation or damage to this important large nerve of the lower body could result in sciatica (inflammation of the nerve) causing intense pain and temporary loss of muscular co-ordination in the lower body.

Use of supporting hand contact, and relaxing manual effleurage between differing applicators should prevent any discomfort occurring. On the larger, more resilient areas of the hips and thighs, deep effective vibratory treatment can be applied, using compression and stimulatory techniques. The supporting hand can act to produce a wringing effect, pulling out the muscle as it is worked upon, or act as a bolster, pushing the muscles towards the applicator. The client feels that a more active, vigorous, effective routine is being applied, which will help her weight accumulations. Like any concentration of effort on one area of the body, from exercise, massage or electrical therapy, this will have an effect if sustained, and forms part of an overall reduction programme.

Effects and Benefits of Vibratory Treatments

1   Vibratory treatments act as tremendous encouragement to the clients in their figure improvement plans, helping them to achieve results more swiftly, and maintaining interest in their reduction programmes.

2   As the effects of vibration are general stimulation of the circulatory system, the pattern of application can be varied to meet personal needs. The method of application follows body contours, and works with the venous return towards the heart. Its effects are on the subcutaneous tissues of the body, bringing about an increase in circulation, without any chemical change or muscular contraction.

3 The muscular system is improved by the fresh interchange of blood through the tissues, but vibrations do not excite the muscle fibres to bring about a contraction.

4 It produces a skin toning effect, both by the improved nutrition to the skin's dermal layer, and by increasing desquamation (skin shedding).

5 Tense muscle fibres are relaxed, and muscular pain relieved.

6 Established fatty deposits are made more available to the general circulation and lymphatic systems, to be used up by the body when on a reduced food intake.

7 Vibratory treatment can be extremely relaxing if combined with heat therapy and the more active stimulatory elements are excluded.

8 Gyratory vibrators penetrate into the subcutaneous and cutaneous layers of the tissues, having their greatest effect on the skin's surface. Bony areas should be avoided to prevent resonance.

Advantages of Vibratory Treatments

1 Adds variety to the treatment routines.

2 Saves time and prevents fatigue.

3 Is less personal, so it is useful in treating male clients.

4 A deeply effective result can be achieved with less energy expended by the therapist, so helping her to conserve energy for other work.

5 The time saving can help vibratory body work to be more profitable.

6 Clients enjoy vibratory massage, and feel it is helping them in their fight against figure problems. The feeling is gained of getting value for money, and a sense that something active is being achieved.

Care of Vibratory Equipment

In a busy clinic situation, the vibrator will be worked very hard, and must be chosen for its durability and ability to cope with this heavy and constant usage. Used correctly and serviced regularly, the vibratory unit will work for years without problems. Dust from the talc medium used does tend to clog the rotating rubber supports of the hand held units, and they should be gently tapped after use to dislodge any adhering talc particles.

The floor standing units, with their motors isolated, do not suffer this problem, but still suffer wear on the applicator heads. If in constant use, several sets of applicator heads are necessary to allow for cleaning, sterilizing and drying of the heads between treatments. Being of sponge or soft rubber consistency, the applicators should only be used with talc or on a clean skin, never with oil or cream. If vibrations are used following on from oil massage, it must be thoroughly towelled from the skin before commencing treatment. If in prolonged contact with oil or cream the rubber will soften, perish and eventually disintegrate, scattering particles of perished or hard rubber on the client during treatment. The pads and applicator heads are also more likely to split, tear away from the base of the applicators or become loose, failing to make good contact on the base.

To stay in good order, and to have a long working life, the applicators need to be washed after use, in a mild detergent solution, dried thoroughly on disposable paper to remove surplus moisture, and sterilized in an ultra-violet or vapour type (formaldehyde) cabinet. If dry and clean when placed inside, they need only 20—30 minutes for sterilization. With the most important point being the overall cleanliness, applicators may alternately be placed in a mild antiseptic solution for 10 minutes after washing and then be placed in a closed cupboard until required. Removal of body oils, skin particles, talc, etc., with the initial washing, is very necessary as no sterilizing cabinet can work effectively if the items placed within it are soiled.

A light dusting of talc on the dry sterilized sponge applicators before storage helps to keep them in good order and delays perishing.

A breaking away of the top surface sponge or rubber from the base may respond to instant repair using an adhesive to bond the two surfaces. If caught in time this can delay costly replacements. It may also point to incorrect use of the applicators if it is a recurring fault. The sponge applicators particularly tend to be used in a grinding, rather than the correct sweeping, fashion which places a great strain on the layers of the surface of the applicator, which then part. Not being designed for such use, the soft heads break down under the strain. When firm kneading movements are needed, they should be produced with the correct flat, ball studded or spiky headed rubber applicators which are designed from tougher material, able to take the strain. So a constant need for repairs or replacements may point to operator inefficiency or carelessness in use.

AUDIO-SONIC VIBRATORY TREATMENTS

Within the field of vibratory treatments which may be applied to the body is audio-sonic, or sound wave vibrations, which are applied where specific effects are needed, such as relief on tense contracted muscle fibres, particularly on the back. Audio-sonic may also be used where ordinary percussion or gyratory vibrations would be contra-indicated, as on hyper-sensitive or very tense areas.

The audio-sonic unit comes in a hand held form, so it is really suitable only for localized areas of the body, or for facial therapy. The audio-sonic vibrator works on a different principle from the mechanical vibrators, using sound waves to create its effects. It puts the air filled cavities of the body and soft tissues through a process of sounding vibrations which bring about gentle stimulation, and relieve tension in the muscles. The tissues on which audio-sonic vibrations will be most effective are those which offer least resistance, such as soft tissue. The vibrations can travel along a muscle path and appear effective in relieving tension and discomfort caused by fibrositis nodules in the upper back, particularly in the trapezius muscle. The surface sensation of audio-sonic is very slight, appearing to slightly impair sensation, but its depth of vibratory effect can penetrate down to 5 cm (2 in.) on certain sound frequencies. This level of sound vibration is sustained through the entire depth of the vibration, and does not rapidly dwindle as it leaves the skin's surface.

These special effects allow the audio-sonic unit to be used on conditions of hyper-sensitivity or extreme tension, where even manual massage could not be tolerated to relieve discomfort. So it is very effective in unknotting the fibrositis lumps found frequently during massage of the back. Its action appears to unravel the tension in the nodules by gently shaking or vibrating them out, like knots out of a ball of string. Its deep effects also make it useful for treatment of soft fat deposits when found in conjunction with sensitive

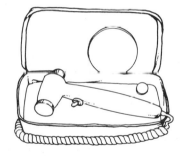

Audio-sonic Vibrator

or vascular skin conditions which would contra-indicate normal vibratory treatment. These conditions are very common, particularly in older clients, and seen in evidence on the legs, upper arms and abdominal areas. It can also be used for longer periods than the gyratory vibrator, on conditions such as adipose deposits on the buttocks or inside thighs, where discomfort, excessive skin irritation or erythema often cause a premature halt to be called to the treatment before really effective results are obtained.

The depth of audio-sonic frequencies makes it uncomfortable over bony areas, as it resounds unpleasantly along the bones. The frequencies may be altered, changing the sound pitch and reducing or increasing the power of the vibration. The smoothness of the vibration felt by the client is due mainly to the lack of surface 'banging' experienced with most other forms of vibration. If the wave path is compared with percussion vibrations, it can be seen how the action of the sound waves is sustained to the deeper tissues. For this reason care should be taken in its use, and it is not advisable over the abdominal area.

Audio-sonic used on the trapezius muscle, along the length of its upper fibres to the occipital cavity of the skull, seems very effective in relieving migraine attacks in some clients. It can be used for short duration periods on clients to assess its effects, gradually building up the period of use as the client becomes accustomed to its effects. Audio-sonic may be applied in addition to manual massage, or combined with heat treatments such as infra-red rays, for a localized treatment of the back.

Comparison of Audio-sonic and Percussion Vibrations

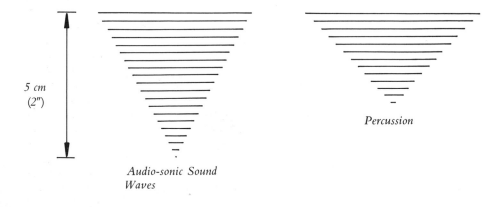

5 cm
(2")

Audio-sonic Sound Waves

Percussion

Because of its reduced surface effects, but deep stimulating actions, audio-sonic has a special role to play in body therapy, and although only available as a small hand held unit, can still be very effective when indicated.

Indications for Use

1 Fibrositis nodules in the trapezius muscle.
2 Soft fat conditions, 'cellulite', etc.
3 Hypersensitive or vascular skin conditions.
4 Where deep relaxation is required on contracted muscle tissues.
5 Localized adipose deposits in sensitive areas, i.e. inside thigh.

Contra-indications

1 Inflammation of the skin, sepsis, etc.
2 Extremely bony areas, or very slim clients.
3 History of slipped disc.
4 Must not be used heavily over the abdomen, or during menstruation or pregnancy.

Method of Application

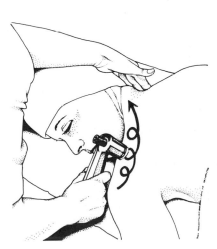

Audio-sonic vibrations are applied to the body in a similar manner to gyratory vibrations, following the path of the muscle where tension is present, or contouring with the shape of the body. The strokes are applied in a smooth, stroking manner, or with circular movements tracing the same path. The smooth plastic applicator head is used for general work, and the hard, rounded ball shaped applicator for concentrated effects such as around joints. The level of intensity is altered by increasing or decreasing the level of sound frequencies, by the control knob on the head of the vibrator. The vibration can be felt to alter in consistency as the frequency is altered, and with practice the correct depth of vibration is reached.

Talc or oil may be used as a medium for audio-sonic vibrators, or more normally simply a clean skin. The hard plastic used in the applicator discs is impervious to oil, etc., and is simply washed clean after treatment.

HIGH FREQUENCY TREATMENTS

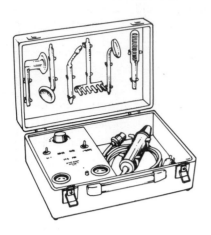

The high frequency current may be applied indirectly and directly (for germicidal effect). The high frequency current alternates so rapidly that it does not stimulate motor or sensory nerves. It has a frequency of more than 500 000 Hz (cycles per second), and is termed an oscillating current. Indirect high frequency passes through the surface of the body and produces a stimulating, anti-congestive effect, with no chemical formation on the skin's surface. Direct high frequency is an external application which dries, refines and heals the skin. It produces a germicidal effect, through ozone formation at the skin's surface, above which the glass electrode is held. High frequency has an irritating noise, produced during the application, and so every attempt should be made to put the client at ease prior to the application so that she can gain maximum benefit.

General Characteristics

1 *Stimulation of Surface Tissue*
   High frequency has great penetration power and generates heat within the tissues, which increases the interchange of blood and tissue fluids. Improved nutrition and elimination produce an improved skin texture and oil and moisture balance.

2 *Relaxation*
   The generated warmth within the tissues produces a sedative effect, increasing relaxation and relief from tension. The current flows through the surface of the body (indirect method), but due to the speed of the oscillations it does not excite muscle fibres.

3 *Germicidal, Drying Effect (Direct Method only)*
   Directly applied the high frequency current produces a germicidal, antibacterial effect, limiting the sebaceous secretion and drying and healing pustular infection.

4 *Destructive (Fulguration, Direct Method only)*
   Incorrectly applied, direct high frequency could have a destructive effect on skin tissue and sebaceous glands, so adhering to the correct sequence of application for therapy purposes is essential.

Though more commonly thought of as a facial treatment, high frequency is also very valuable in body therapy, for inducing relaxation and improving the overall skin texture. Combined with manual massage, the indirect method generates warmth deep in the tissues, bringing about relaxation which has a very sedative effect on tense, nervous clients. The increased interchange of tissue fluids occurring at the skin's surface improves its biological activity and helps it to function more efficiently. The improved nutrition to the skin, and increased removal of waste products through the lymphatic system, improve the skin texture and clear small imperfections. Rough, dry or blemished skin conditions can be greatly improved. Oily skin conditions, acne, etc., can be controlled by the use of high frequency directly given to the area, to produce a drying, germicidal, slightly destructive effect on the overproductive sebaceous glands in the area.

As part of the overall treatment of the body, high frequency has a special place, relieving physical tension, bringing suppleness to taut, constricted areas, and acting as a cosmetic treatment to the skin. Applied correctly high frequency indirectly used gives depth and power to the therapist's massage, and its sedative effects make it a popular client treatment.

Indications for Use

1 Tense, highly strung individuals needing relaxation.
2 Muscular tension in the back.
3 Poor skin texture, rough or extremely dry and flaking.
4 For clients who suffer from poor circulation, chilblains, cold hands or feet.
5 Oily or blemished skin conditions, i.e. acne, requiring medical approval (direct high frequency).

Contra-indications

1 Epilepsy.
2 Asthma.
3 Metal plates or pins in the body (fracture repairs or replacement surgery).
4 High blood pressure, or defective circulation, oedema, etc.
5 Pregnancy.

Indirect High Frequency

The client is prepared for general body massage, and oil or talc applied to permit free movement of the hands over the body. Oil massage is preferable if the skin is dry, talc if it is more oily. The deeper and firmer the massage with high frequency, the more relaxing, and the lighter in contact the hands are, the more stimulating will be the effect.

All jewellery should be removed from both the client and the therapist to prevent induced electricity from building up and being discharged, causing discomfort and possible loss of contact. The apparatus should be prepared, placed conveniently, and the glass saturator electrode attached to the holder to form a firm connection. Plugs, switches and leads should be checked, with the intensity dial at zero and the machine switched off for safety. As the therapist has to remain in contact throughout the treatment, the routine has to be planned to allow her to return to the machine to switch off when the front of the body is completed. The routine is then repeated for the back and buttocks area.

Application, Indirect

The client is given the saturator to hold, and advised to maintain contact throughout the treatment in order to complete the circuit and facilitate an even flow of high frequency current through the superficial tissues. A brief explanation of the sensation to be experienced will dispel nervousness and increase the client's enjoyment and benefit from the application. The therapist places one hand in contact with the client's thigh and commences the massage, whilst the second hand turns on the machine, and gradually increases the intensity until the client's immediate tolerance level is reached. Verbal contact gives guidance as to general effect, and may indicate a possible increase in intensity level when the client has relaxed and become accustomed to the high frequency current. The second hand (nearest to the high frequency machine) is then placed in contact, and both hands perform rhythmical massage movements over the area. The movements may be superficial (stimulating) or deep (relaxing) to achieve the desired effect. Contact must be retained by at least one hand throughout the routine to prevent a break in the current flow and subsequent prickling and discomfort to both client

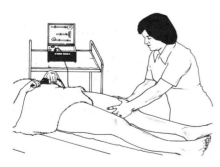

Indirect High Frequency

and therapist. This discomfort is due to high frequency transient current, caused by sudden changes in the electrical circuit when hand contact is lost.

Areas of increased subcutaneous tissue may have the intensity increased, according to the client's tolerance, to achieve a more stimulating, regenerating action. With both hands in contact the current is evenly spread, but if one hand is removed the effect is intensified, and care should be taken to avoid creating a feeling of pressure and discomfort.

When the necessary reaction is achieved, the skin will appear stimulated, with increased local warmth and colour and an improvement in texture. The underlying muscles should feel relaxed and warm, soft and free from tension.

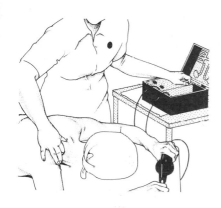

The body may be completed by working on the right leg, right arm, chest, left arm, abdomen and left leg, returning to the high frequency unit at the foot of the bed. The treatment may be concluded by releasing one hand from the leg, reducing the current intensity to zero, and switching off the machine. The second hand may then be released, and the saturator removed from the client, prior to further treatment. The client turns over, the saturator is then returned and the high frequency unit moved to the head of the bed, so that the back and buttocks can be completed freely. This then permits closer control and variation of the intensity level when treating the back, this being the area most likely to suffer from muscular strain, tension, etc. All deep kneading, effleurage and friction movements may be used as long as contact is maintained.

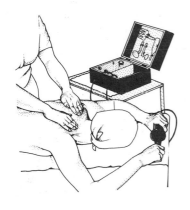

The treatment of the back is concluded as before, and the high frequency machine placed safely out of the way whilst the client has the oil or talc removed, and is helped on with the gown. The glass saturator should be cleansed and sterilized after use, and retained in a sterile container until required.

Any area of the body can be treated with high frequency applied locally, in the same manner as described. The intensity needed should be gradually worked up to, whilst building the client's tolerance and acceptance of the treatment. Once a competent application has been achieved by the therapist, it may be effectively given to any area of the body, with slight adaptation.

If the client experiences unpleasant tingling in the hand whilst holding the saturator electrode, an application of talc on the palm will help the problem. The sensation is sometimes caused by perspiration on the skin, or may be due to stiffness in the joints of the hand. The indirect high frequency current tends to concentrate on weak areas, and whilst it may be beneficial to circulation improvement, may be uncomfortable to the client.

DIRECT HIGH FREQUENCY TREATMENTS

(Germicidal and Drying Effect)

Directly applied high frequency has an extremely stimulating effect on the surface blood circulation and, due to the production of ozone as a by-product, its action is also germicidal, anti-bacterial and drying to the skin. Its main application is within the treatment of seborrhoea and acne conditions, which may be present on the back and centre chest areas in younger clients.

Preparation

The area is prepared with talcum powder to permit a smooth passage of the electrode over the contours, to absorb the natural secretions formed during treatment. A glass bulb-shaped electrode replaces the saturator, and the client is not connected into the high frequency circuit as in indirect high frequency, but receives the treatment *directly*. The current is obtained with the bulb electrode held in contact with the skin.

Application

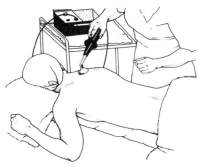

Direct High Frequency

The application commences at the centre back, the apparatus is switched on, and the intensity increased slowly to the client's maximum tolerance. Circular movements cover the area with the current intensity and pressure regulated to the skin's sensitivity and degree of subcutaneous tissue. The more superficial movements create the greatest stimulation, as the high frequency current ionizes the air when a slight gap exists between the electrode and the skin. The ionization appears as a small spark, which activates the sensory nerve endings.

The high frequency output terminates in the low pressure gas-filled glass electrode, which offers complete protection to the client and operator from the risks of electric shock. In normal use the gas becomes ionized and gives a blue/violet glow in the tube of the chosen electrode. Ozone is produced as a by-product in the air between the skin and the electrode and causes a chemical reaction on the skin's surface. The spark created by providing an air gap should not exceed 6 mm ($\frac{1}{4}$ in.) in general therapy practice, as its effect becomes destructive to skin tissue beyond this length. This technique of 'sparking' can be used to advantage on scar tissue, or to activate a sluggish complexion, by improving lymphatic circulation and achieving an anti-congestive effect. Sparking must be applied with care by an experienced therapist to prevent client discomfort and subsequent skin irritation and flaking.

Erythema, increased warmth, and a generally stimulated appearance will indicate when the desired effect has been achieved. The treatment may then be concluded by reducing the current to zero, switching off the machine, and releasing the electrode from contact. The talcum should be removed with damp tissues, and the skin left free from tonic preparations in order to maintain the refining, drying germicidal effects of the high frequency.

Application time varies according to the purpose of the treatment, with rough textured skins requiring a low intensity given for 8—10 minutes, and oily or blemished skins needing 10—15 minutes at a higher intensity. Longer treatments, regularly applied, are needed for acne conditions if they are to benefit from the controlling elements of the high frequency on sebaceous secretion and bacterial growth. The direct high frequency application to the back often forms part of a 'back pore' treatment, which includes deep cleansing, steaming, massage with medicated cream, mask, direct high frequency, and concludes with acne lotion.

Long term benefits of direct high frequency include refined skin texture, increased cellular activity of the skin's basal layer, and an improvement in the skin's defence against bacteria.

GALVANIC TREATMENTS

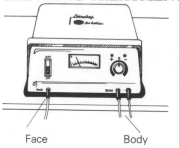

Face   Body

Galvanic Face/Body Unit

Galvanic treatments for the body are becoming increasingly popular as a means of treating areas of soft fat, fluid retention etc., collectively known as 'cellulite' by the client. Treatment concentrates on releasing trapped adipose and fluid deposits in the surface tissue – which give it its soft dimpled appearance – by use of galvanic current penetrating active anti-cellulite substances into the subcutaneous tissues (iontophoresis). The galvanic process, or penetration, concludes a treatment routine of skin peeling, massage/heat, and muscle contraction, to form a cellulite sequence that provides excellent results for the client.

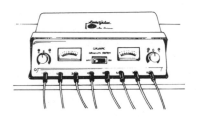

Multi-pad Galvanic Body Cellulite Unit

Galvanic treatments have many uses in therapy, in facial treatment they are used for desincrustation, and for iontophoresis (penetration of active substances through the intact skin). In body cellulite conditions, iontophoresis is again used, with special anti-cellulite lotions, to disperse stubborn fat deposits or areas of fluid retention on the thighs, buttocks, abdomen and inside arm areas – in fact anywhere the soft, cellulite condition is seen to be present. The process of iontophoresis improves the functioning of tissues in the body, and, in conjunction with skillfully applied massage and an elimination type of diet, can help to disperse unsightly bulges and dimpling of the skin.

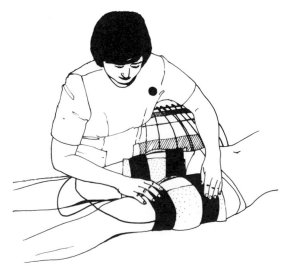

Cellulite Treatment is Popular with Clients

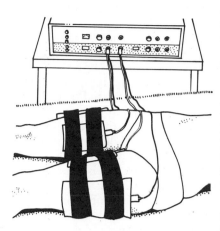

Combined Galvanic and Interferential Unit

The galvanic current for completing cellulite treatments may come from a small galvanic face and body machine, which provides for 2 paired sets of electrodes (4 pads). This allows small areas of the body to be treated, and is a good introduction to cellulite routines. However when a full body service is offered, a large multi-pad galvanic cellulite body system is needed, with 8 sets of paired electrodes (16 pads). This allows several areas of the body to be treated simultaneously and penetration of the active substances to be completed within a half hour treatment application, or concluding the one hour cellulite routine of peeling, massage heat, muscle contraction/vacuum and galvanic iontophoresis for cellulite.

There are many combined galvanic units available, which give the therapist a choice of treatments to offer. Some units combine galvanic current, with a high frequency facility, whilst on others, the galvanic current is available on an interferential treatment system. If the galvanic unit is intended for full body treatment it should have a multi-pad capacity, otherwise the body areas would have to be treated in rotation, which would be time consuming, and satisfactory results would be difficult to achieve. Whatever the source of galvanism, its use for iontophoresis is similar in effect, though the method of achieving the action may differ from one machine to another. The therapist should ensure that she has a full knowledge of the particular system before use on clients, either by practising on herself, or other staff, until the effects and sensations of the treatment are known. Full instruction should be given

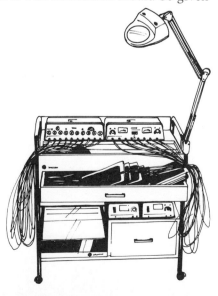

Faradic Muscle Contraction and Body Galvanic Cellulite Systems

by the manufacturer as to the equipment's method of use and its effectiveness, either from instruction notes, training guide, etc., or by attending training sessions.

Galvanism works by penetrating active substances into the subcutaneous tissues, where they act on the ineffective circulation to bring about an improvement in the vascular and lymphatic interchange in the area. This is completed in a natural and harmless way, and is aided by the actual effect of the galvanic current on the tissues. This improves the function of the cellular membrane, and allows the trapped fluid and fat to be dispersed and eliminated, or used up by the body as fuel – when a reduction diet is being followed.

The substances used in cellulite treatments are based on natural diuretics (elements which help the body naturally release retained fluids). These include citric oils, herbal and marine elements, ivy extracts etc., and will vary according to manufacturer.

The diuretic or fluid loss effect caused by the penetration of the active lotions under the active pads, causes the client to pass more fluid as urine, and stubborn areas of cellulite disperse over a period of time. The client must have medical advice as to the suitability of the treatment if she has a medical history of kidney infections, infections of the bladder or urinary tract, as the treatment can cause irritation on rare occasions due to the active substances the body is passing through the urine. The client should be warned about the additional water she will pass, so she does not become anxious. This effect will be accelerated if the client uses an anti-cellulite product on the problem area at home, and is also drinking herbal teas to speed her elimination process.

Application

The actual application of galvanic iontophoresis is undertaken on a warm, clear skin, whether it is concluding the one hour cellulite routine, or being applied independently within a half hour galvanic application. The more preparation the skin has received, the less galvanic current will be needed to overcome skin resistance, which is a factor in galvanic treatments. So combining galvanism into the longer cellulite routine, improves both client comfort and the results obtained. The cellulite lotion is applied evenly all over the affected area, with gentle effleurage strokes, prior to applying the pads.

Galvanism works by using paired sets of electrodes (conductive rubber pads), which allow the ion active (electrically active) cellulite lotions to be drawn into the skin, towards the attraction of the opposite electrode or pole. The client and her skin offer resistance to this flow of constant direct current (DC); in a form which is measured on the equipment as units of milliamps (thousandths of an amp). When the pads are in place, their damp sponge envelopes and the client's body complete the circuit, its resistance giving a reading on the meter on the equipment.

The polarity of the pads is fixed so that it's possible to know which pad will commence as the negative pole and which as the positive pole. This is always with a black lead connected to the negative pole and a red lead connected to the positive pole. As cellulite treatments are completed mainly on the negative polarity, this being the most penetrating polarity, this means the black lead will go

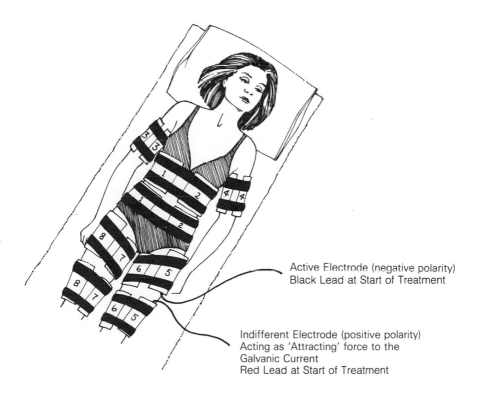

Active Electrode (negative polarity)
Black Lead at Start of Treatment

Indifferent Electrode (positive polarity)
Acting as 'Attracting' force to the
Galvanic Current
Red Lead at Start of Treatment

Body Galvanic System—Body Padding

to the active pad over the cellulite affected area, and the red lead will be attached to the indifferent pad acting as the attracting 'magnet' pad to draw the substance into the skin from underneath the active working pad. The large covered pads must be firmly strapped in place, and checked for moisture and skin contact. They are paired to allow the galvanic current to flow comfortably from the working pad to the indifferent pad, carrying the ion active substance into the surface skin under the working pad where it has to do its work.

Preparation complete, the galvanic current is applied on a negative charge, and increased in intensity slowly until the client is just aware of a sensation in the skin. No discomfort should be experienced, just a feeling of warmth. As galvanism works by attraction of opposite poles, there is no need for a high current intensity, as the cellulite lotion is attracted into the skin, not pushed in. It will seldom be necessary to use a skin resistance reading of more than four on the milliamp meter, often less, and client sensation should be used as the best guide to a safe and effective treatment.

After 5—6 minutes on the negative polarity, the intensity control is smoothly returned to the zero point, and a few minutes of the positive polarity is applied at even less intensity. This completes the tissue interchange, and gives effective results, but should not be overdone, as this more active pole can cause skin irritation, red wheals, etc. Initially use caution, or use only negative polarity until skin reaction is known. At the conclusion of the positive polarity, the intensity control should be returned smoothly to zero.

The cellulite lotion remains in the skin, it is not washed away, but continues to do its work. After releasing the client from the straps, and covered pads, the area can be lightly dried and talced if necessary for client comfort. The sponge envelopes should be washed and placed in the sterilizer until needed again.

Cellulite treatments are completed 2—3 times a week if the galvanic routine is completed independently, or once a week if applied within the one hour cellulite routine. Cellulite products are designed for clinic and home use, as it is obvious that if the client does not become involved in her improvement, results will be poor. With a home diet and exercise plan, plus correctly advised cellulite products, results will be excellent, and indeed cellulite treatments are some of the most popular the therapist has to offer.

**Contra-indications to
Galvanic Iontophoresis**

1　Over open abrasions, inflammation or stings.
2　When sunburnt, or on hypersensitive areas such as the inside thighs, if extreme discomfort is felt.
3　During the first few days of menstruation.
4　Any condition of defective circulation or impaired sensitivity to heat, such as in diabetic conditions.
5　Oedema from unknown source, due to lessened sensitivity in the area.
6　History of nervous disorders, or damage to the nervous system, pinched nerves, paralysis of a nerve, dermatitis etc., should be considered contra-indicated, or medical approval would be needed prior to treatment.

There is no international convention of colour coding leads on galvanic equipment. If using equipment other than the kind described in this book, then therapists must consult the equipment manufacturer to determine which lead acts as positive at the start of treatment.

Readers requiring additional information on the full range of galvanic treatments now available are advised to read my book: *Beauty Guide 3 – Galvanic Treatment*, also published by Stanley Thornes (Publishers) Ltd.

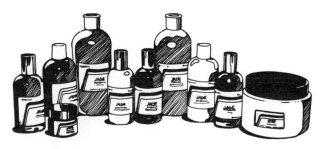

Anti-cellulite products for clinic and home use

Chapter 8

Specific Reduction Treatments

These treatments are capable of reshaping the body, either within a diet programme or, if the client is simply out of proportion, by toning the muscles or hastening the removal of adipose deposits or fluid in the area. It has been seen how specific exercise can reshape a figure, toning the muscles and changing the body's contours. Muscle contraction treatments act in the same way and can be extremely effective. Vacuum massage does not contract muscles but works to improve the body's circulation and removal of waste products through the lymphatic system.

In combination muscle contraction and vacuum massage can be extremely effective in regaining an attractive, healthy figure, and they are both highly successful salon treatments. They do, however, require special skill in application and demand a thorough understanding of the body's muscular, nervous and circulatory systems. Ineffective treatments, or client discomfort, can nearly always be traced back to lack of proficiency and knowledge on the part of the operator.

VACUUM MASSAGE

The vacuum, or suction, treatment is based on the principle of creating reduced pressure within clear plastic cups applied to the body in patterns which relate directly to the lymphatic system of the body. The cups are attached to the vacuum machine by plastic tubing, and the suction effect produced by the combined pump and motor of the equipment. The inverse pressure effect causes the skin and subcutaneous tissues to arch upwards to fill the cavity, thus creating considerable erythema, stimulation and vascular interchange in the area.

The treatment is effective by moving in flowing strokes towards the nearest lymphatic node to hasten the removal of waste products in the area. Both gliding and static pulsing is used within beauty therapy, but to be really effective, the areas of treatment need not only to be activated, but also to have the circulation in the area hastened. This is accomplished by general patterns of vacuum strokes for an area, which can be repeated until the desired effect is produced. If static pulsing is included within the treatment, it is preceded by and followed by the more commonly used gliding method.

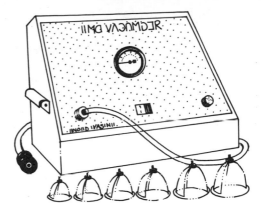

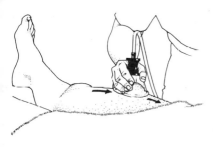

The degree of lift into the cup can be monitored visually, and the amount of reduced pressure created is shown in inches or centimetres of mercury on the meter of the machine. The softness or resilience of the tissues to which the vacuum is applied alters the lift into the cup, and care should be taken to avoid excessive arching of the skin. To avoid bruising, discomfort, or dilation of surface blood vessels, the tissues should not be allowed to fill more than 20% of the cup, regardless of its size. The speed at which the vacuum is applied also alters the lift, with faster movements being far more comfortable to the client, as this prevents the full amount of arching being achieved.

Effects and Benefits of Vacuum Treatment

1 Increased vascular and lymphatic flow.

2 It favours regeneration of the tissues, and absorption of intra-muscular and subcutaneous infiltrations by improving the blood supply in the area.

3 Stimulates the metabolism if used generally.

4 Produces erythema and increases desquamation.

5 In conjunction with a reduction diet, it can hasten the removal of fatty deposits from established weight accumulations.

6 Reduces swelling (oedema) if due to poor circulation or tired legs.

7 Helps prevent chilblains.

Indications for Use

Any condition which would benefit from the effects mentioned may have vacuum massage applied to good effect if not contra-indicated. Conditions in which it is commonly used in clinic practice include:

1 Heavy hips and thighs, particularly if out of proportion to the rest of the figure.
2 Abdominal and midriff weight accumulations, particularly after pregnancy.
3 Heavy lower legs, with thickness or swelling of the ankles.
4 Heavy upper arms, particularly where the adipose tissue is interspaced between and over strong muscular tissue.
5 Subcutaneous fat on the back and over the shoulder area, particularly if a 'dowager's hump' is present.
6 Large buttocks, or low slung buttocks, particularly if out of proportion to the rest of the figure.

Vacuum massage, often in conjunction with muscle toning, is most effective if the client is out of proportion or slightly overweight rather than generally overweight or obese, where diet would be the main solution.

Preparation

Many of the problems experienced when applying vacuum can be minimized by careful preparation and attention to technique. The client should be carefully checked for contra-indications and, if not suitable, should be advised on alternative measures. Younger clients are the most likely candidates for vacuum treatments, having fewer contra-indications, so permitting fast results to be achieved.

The client may be prepared for vacuum by some form of pre-heating, either general, such as sauna, or locally with lamps or a few minutes' massage. The muscles and subcutaneous tissues need to be warm and relaxed if the treatment is to be achieved comfortably, and if it is to be effective.

The cups used within the application should contour closely to the area of treatment, and be the correct size in respect to the bulk of tissues present.

The lubricant used to permit the gliding effect should be warm in temperature, and thin in consistency. A fine massage oil is ideal for the purpose, being normally of vegetable origin. A constant check should be kept to see adquate oil is present so that the cup does not drag, particularly on dry skin where the oil is absorbed into the epidermis.

Method of Application

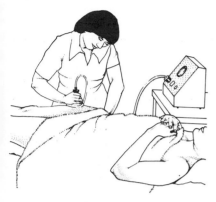

The client is prepared for general body treatment, and the warm oil applied to the area to be treated. If combined with manual massage, vacuum treatment could be applied to those areas of the body needing extra help, after massage of the section has been completed. More normally vacuum massage is given as a half hour treatment to one or more areas of the body, such as hips and thighs, or midriff and abdomen. Areas such as lower legs, or heavy upper arms, or backs, are all treated in the same independent way. Vacuum may also be applied as general all over body treatment, though this is more unusual.

The client is kept as warm as possible throughout the application, exposing only those areas under immediate treatment. The equipment is checked for pressure by blocking the air inlet inside the cup with a finger or thumb, and the reading adjusted on the equipment. The gauge should be regarded as a guide to the reduced pressure being used, rather than purely as an intensity control. After assessing the softness or firmness of the area to be treated, allowance can then be made for the resistance, or lack of resistance, that the skin and underlying tissues are likely to present. A low percentage of lift should be used initially to build up the client's tolerance and accustom her to the treatment. This can then be increased when suitable, to reach an effective level. Erythema, evident skin reddening, warmth and increased circulation in the area should all be present at the conclusion of the treatment. To avoid discomfort, the pattern of strokes should overlap slightly, and care should be taken to avoid passing over any one area repeatedly, or a bruise will result. Adjacent areas should be treated alternately, keeping the cups moving in a rhythmical way, backwards and forwards, to prevent sensitivity building up.

The method of application is to work methodically, in the pattern for the area, lifting the skin into the cup and arcing smoothly towards the nearest lymphatic node. The position of the lymphatic nodes acts as guidance when treating any area of the body, as strokes will always move in a straight line towards them. With this in mind, no confusion need arise as to the pattern of treatment.

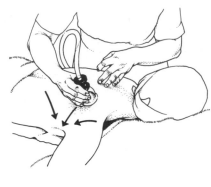

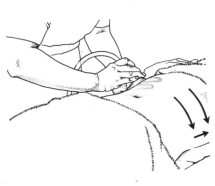

The methods of application suggested are, however, useful guidance for treatment planning, giving client position, likely treatment durations, and the cup sizes for the area.

The therapist works with even rhythm, adopting a pattern of work that can be described as lift, move and release, forming flowing strokes towards the regional lymph node. Where the nodes are placed so that the strokes will converge like the pivot point of a fan, alternate strokes should be shortened, otherwise soreness and bruising will result. The armpit, groin and lower abdomen are all areas where this technique should be used.

The application works up and down, or from side to side with the strokes being away from or towards the therapist, depending on area. The cup is released at the end of the stroke by a fast flicking movement of the wrist, or the vacuum may be broken by slipping a finger under the edge of the cup. If the cup becomes too firmly attached due to unexpected softness of skin, the vacuum should be broken in this way, and not by pulling. Otherwise blood vessels will be ruptured and the skin will bruise.

Practise should be limited initially to work on firm musculature until confidence and skill grows with this difficult treatment. Progression to soft areas like the inside thigh, abdomen, etc., should be delayed until full handling abilities are established. Vacuum massage is a treatment which improves by diligent practise, as skill is developed by dealing with all types of body conditions, skin textures and physical reactions.

At the conclusion of the specific reduction treatment, the client should ideally be warmly wrapped and left for half an hour, to maintain the heat produced for as long as possible for maximum effect. If this is not possible, the client should be advised to dress warmly, and to maintain the heat as much as possible. Without pre-heating, and maintenance of the created warmth after treatment, results will not be so effective and more treatment will be needed to obtain the same results.

The short treatments need to be applied at least twice a week, ideally 3—4 times or even daily, as in the hydro situation. Then the treatment has a build up effect, which is particularly useful if the client is trying to reduce her body weight, rather than simply reshape her contours. The skin toning effects are then very beneficial, especially to the mature client whose skin is less elastic and inclined to become crepey.

Measurements of the treated area should be taken at regular intervals within a course of treatment, whether the client is on a reduction plan or is simply reshaping the figure. The measurement should be taken on the fullest areas, and recorded on the client's card to show results achieved. Occasionally full body measurements should be taken to check overall body proportions, and assess progress.

Contra-indications to Vacuum

1   High or low blood pressure, or history of thrombosis.

2   Over varicose veins, or history of phlebitis.

3   Immediately after childbirth, or during pregnancy. (Medical permission is required after childbirth before applying vacuum, and 2–3 months would normally have elapsed before it would be given.)

4   Never treat the breasts, due to sensitivity.

5   Do not apply over scars, unless very old. Scar tissue does not stretch in the same way as normal skin, and discomfort can result. Recent scars are naturally contra-indicated.

6   Oedema from a systemic cause, kidney malfunction, etc., may not be treated by vacuum massage. Fluid retention may be assisted greatly by vacuum massage, but medical permission is needed, to confirm the nature of the problem.

7   Very bony areas should be avoided during treatment, if they come within the general application area, as bruising and discomfort will result.

8   During menstruation, the abdominal area should not be treated.

9   Skin abrasions, sunburn, bruises should be avoided.

10   Skin diseases are contra-indicated to vacuum.

11   Hypersensitive skin, or fine skin prone to thread veins.

THE LYMPHATIC SYSTEM
AND REGIONAL
LYMPH NODES

Vacuum massage is concerned mainly with the lymphatic circulation, and treatment follows the regional lymph nodes in any area.

The lymphatic system is closely interlinked with the vascular circulation, and many lymphatic vessels lie in close proximity to the larger veins. The system is responsible for the interchange of tissue fluids and primarily concerned with the removal of waste products through the lymph. This lymphatic fluid is carried along vessels interspaced with lymphatic nodes, these consisting of small solid masses of lymphoid tissues, which act as a filtering system to the lymph.

The lymphatic nodes are also concentrated in certain areas of the body, being superficially placed and forming a clustered or bead-like appearance. When inflamed, these nodes can be felt beneath the skin, like almond shaped elevations. These regional nodes include the *submandibular*, beneath the mandible, the *occipital*, at the base of the skull, the *axillary*, in the armpit, the *supratrochlea*, in the elbow, the *inguinals*, in the groin and the *popliteal*, behind the knee.

It is these superficial nodes with which therapy treatments are concerned, these having little direct contact with deeper lymphatic structures. For, although all lymph eventually returns to the vascular system through the thoracic duct and right lymphatic duct, into the left and right brachiocephalic veins respectively, therapy treatments can have no direct effect at such a deep level. Vacuum massage indirectly and safely hastens the local removal of lymphatic fluid, whilst increasing the circulation generally in the area.

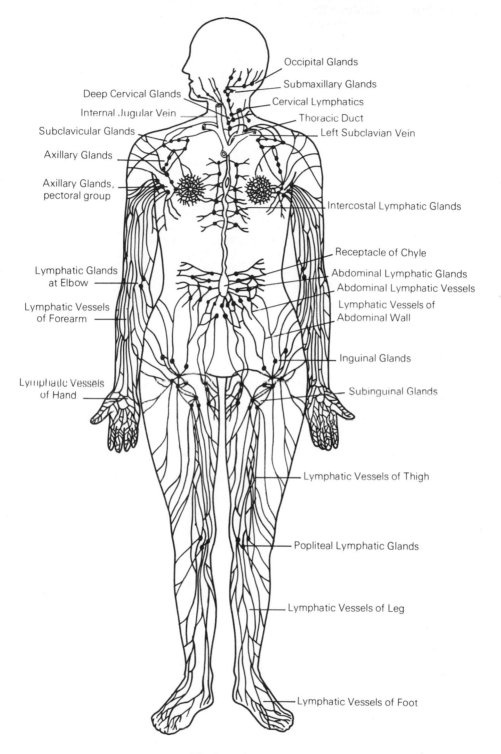

Occipital Glands
Submaxillary Glands
Deep Cervical Glands
Cervical Lymphatics
Internal Jugular Vein
Thoracic Duct
Subclavicular Glands
Left Subclavian Vein
Axillary Glands
Axillary Glands, pectoral group
Intercostal Lymphatic Glands
Receptacle of Chyle
Lymphatic Glands at Elbow
Abdominal Lymphatic Glands
Abdominal Lymphatic Vessels
Lymphatic Vessels of Forearm
Lymphatic Vessels of Abdominal Wall
Inguinal Glands
Lymphatic Vessels of Hand
Subinguinal Glands
Lymphatic Vessels of Thigh
Popliteal Lymphatic Glands
Lymphatic Vessels of Leg
Lymphatic Vessels of Foot

The Lymphatic System
Regional Lymph Nodes

Application: Gliding Cup Method

Areas or Zones of Treatment (half hour duration)

The Abdomen and Midriff

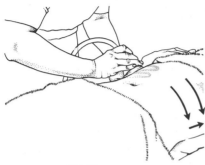

Vacuum on Midriff

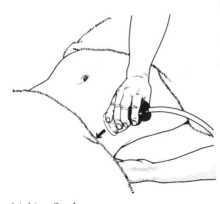

Linking Stroke

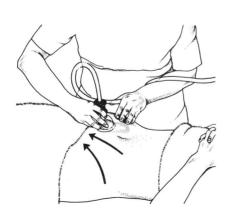

The client lies with the abdominal area comfortable, either flat or with a towel support under the knees. With a knee support the abdominal skin is less taut, and in the case of relaxed abdominal muscles of poor tone, harder to treat. The midriff and abdomen are often treated together, but if this is not necessary, more concentration can be given to one section. If the abdominal area is very sensitive, the treatment time can be divided between the abdominal and buttocks areas. The treatment is applied moving round from one side of the midriff to the other, then progressing across and back over the abdomen several times, then the whole routine is repeated. The shape of the bony rib cage is followed to permit the vacuum cups to form a complete contact, then a stroke links the strokes upwards into the armpit area (axilla node). This linking stroke may be a little slower, to avoid discomfort from the folds of skin normally present in this area in the overweight client. A small or medium size cup is used in the area, and the cups may be released at the end of the stroke by the therapist's other hand if the skin is very soft. This avoids trauma to the area.

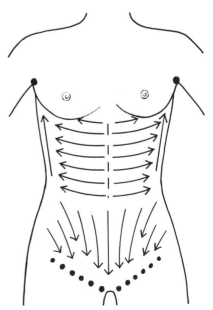

Treatment Plan for Midriff and Abdomen

Hips and Upper Thigh

If weight has accumulated on the outer part of the thighs, and on the buttocks, a convenient method of treatment is to place the client on her side, with the hip and thigh slightly flexed, and her body weight comfortably supported. Areas not concerned in treatment can be covered, for warmth and modesty. First one side of the body may be treated, then the other, moving up and down with overlapping strokes. If required the inside thighs can be treated, using small cups and lower pressure, with the client in a supine position.

The outer thigh and buttocks area require a medium to large cup for treatment, with the largest cup having the greatest effect. On areas of established adipose tissue, the maximum effect will be created by using the correct amount of lift, vigorous fast strokes and the largest cup size possible for the area. Twice the established rate of massage strokes is permissible in vacuum massage, and keeps down discomfort for the client whilst permitting the treatment to be effective.

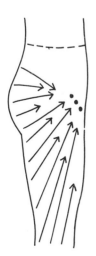

Treatment Plan for Hips and Upper Thighs

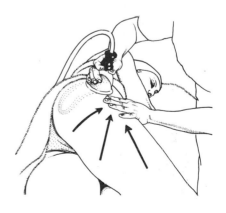

Front and Back of the Legs

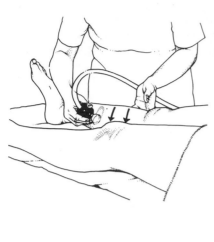

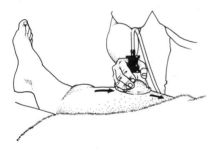

The application is normally divided between the front and back areas of the legs, with concentration on the areas of greatest need. Either the lower or upper parts of the legs may be deleted and all attention centred on one section. The thighs are the most common problem area for women, and these may be treated working from leg to leg on the fronts until the desired result is achieved, then the application is completed on the backs in the same manner. Medium or large cups may be used.

If the whole leg is to be treated, first small cups are used, with moderate vacuum pressure to complete the front of the lower legs. These are then wrapped and the thighs treated. On turning over, the calves are treated in just the same way, and then the back of the thigh. Firm effleurage movements upwards towards the knee may be applied manually between the strokes on the lower leg, to help the venous and lymphatic return to the heart from this area. This helps the dispersal of fluid caused by tiredness around the ankles, and helps prevent the formation of varicose veins or chilblains.

The inside thigh area may be very sensitive in some clients and, in this instance, both outside thigh areas should be completed, then the cup size decreased and pressure lowered to treat the inside thigh area.

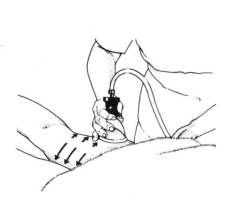

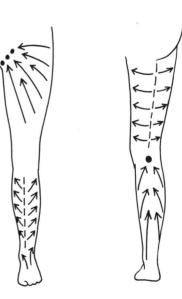

Treatment Plan for the Legs

Back and Nape of Neck

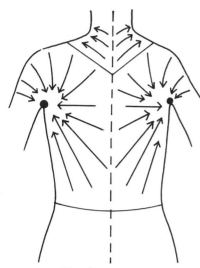

Treatment Plan for the Back

The client lies prone on the couch, with only a small towel as head support. The shoulder blades should not protrude and the client may need to have her arms repositioned until as flat a surface area as possible is achieved. The application lifts carefully over the bony areas of the back, attempting to keep the application as smooth as possible. Protruding bones which break the vacuum and release the cup may be avoided in the strokes, or slightly more lift used when passing over these areas. Alternate converging strokes may be shortened to avoid over-treatment near the armpit. Small or medium cups may be used on the back, depending on the subcutaneous fat present. If the neck is included, a very small cup is needed.

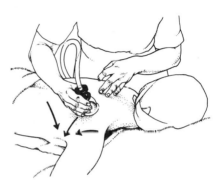

Arms and Shoulders

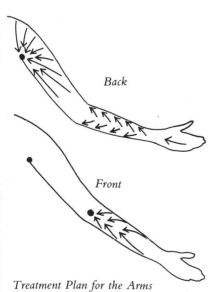

Back

Front

Treatment Plan for the Arms

If the arms are heavy in proportion to the rest of the figure, they may be treated independently, or the treatment of the back can be extended to include them. If clients have lost a lot of weight, they may be left with over-heavy upper arms, which spoil the overall effect. Vacuum can be used to good effect in this instance, as normally the problem is not one of poor muscle tone, or slackness, but of muscular, solid arms, with well established adipose deposits. So vacuum rather than muscle toning is indicated.

Very small cups are used on the lower arm, and small to medium on the upper arm, depending on the bulk present. The armpit bruises very easily and care should be taken not to over-treat the area.

Lower Back and Buttocks

The buttocks area is normally well covered with adipose tissue and can take extensive vacuum treatment, applied with the largest cup that will contour to the area. The cups should be lifted well during the application, to bring about the maximum vascular response in the area. The treatment alternates from one side of the buttocks to the other, working up and downwards, covering the area three to four times on each side before moving on. In this way the client can tolerate a far more vigorous treatment without discomfort. The gluteal fold should not be pulled apart during the treatment, and if the correct lift and control is used in the strokes in this area, separation should not occur. The strokes should be taken well down to the sides of the body, to move towards the regional lymph nodes of the groin (the inguinals). Also due to the effects of gravity, much of the body's bulk will rest close to the plinth, rather than on the upper surface of the buttocks.

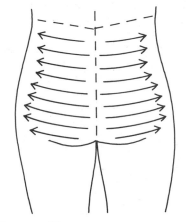

*Treatment Plan
for the Buttocks*

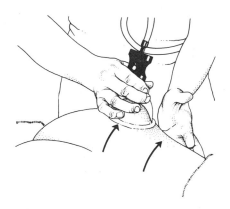

STATIC OR PULSATING VACUUM TREATMENT

A more recent form of vacuum treatment, the static or pulsing method, combines both elements of vacuum within modern treatment units. The gliding method is provided to commence the treatment, using the normal system of reduced pressure within a cup connected to the pump and motor of the machine by plastic tubing.

The units also provide for multi-cup application, where localized areas of the body can be treated by pulsing static cups, which remain in contact throughout the application. The cups retained by a constant low level of vacuum which can be altered to provide differing periods of increased arcing within the cups to bring about stimulation of the area. Clear perspex cups of differing sizes, graduated in pairs, are used attached to the machine by individual tubes. The level of the vacuum can be adjusted, also the period in which the skin is more firmly drawn up into the cups. The low vacuum periods linking the pulse and resting the tissues can be prolonged or of short duration.

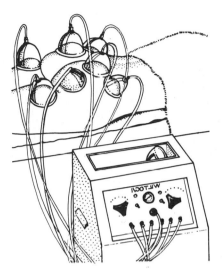

Pulsing Suction Equipment

Initially treatment should have longer holding periods (low vacuum), and short periods of increased arcing. When the client's tolerance is developed, and the effects of the first few treatments is known, then the periods of greater lift into the cups can be increased, both in intensity and duration.

Until the client's sensitivity is known, and the possibility of bruising or capillary dilation is assessed, vigorous treatments of high intensity and high skin arcing should not be applied. Only clients with large adipose deposits, or who are really overweight, should be treated by this static method. Contra-indications for vacuum must also be carefully checked. Without adequate bulk being present, the treatment cannot be applied, as the cups must be applied to the upper surfaces of the client, and will not hold in contact on the sides of the body, with the client prone or supine. This is due to the weight of the leads connected to the machine, which tend to pull the cups off if insufficient bulk is present or too low a pressure is used. The client, can, however, be turned on to her side to treat the outer surface of the thigh, thus presenting an upper surface on which the static method can be applied.

Application

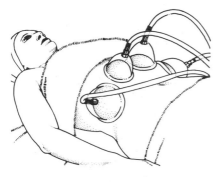

The area is first treated by gliding method vacuum following the normal method of treatment, with the air inlet of the piping closed at the machine connection terminal.

The treatment progresses to application of the multi-cup method, by adjusting the intensity to a low level of vacuum, and quickly applying the necessary cups of varied sizes to the area. As the cups are applied, their air inlet holes are closed one at a time, and the cup makes contact, holding on to the tissues and drawing them up gently. The cups need to be applied swiftly so that the chosen level of pressure is spread evenly between the 4 or 6 cups applied, rather than concentrated on to one cup, giving a strong reaction. The inside surface of the cup may be spread with a little massage cream to help the adhesion, and prevent cups losing contact when using low pressures. Otherwise the

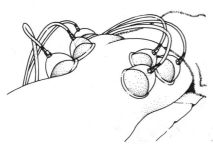

oil previously applied will suffice. When the cups are all in position, holding on a constant pressure, and the skin reaction is assessed, then the pulsing effect can be added into the sequence. If this is attempted whilst the cups are being applied, they will fall off. The lift into the cup can then be increased, and the length and degree of arcing during the pulse altered. The machine may have its controls divided into intensity, pulsing, and it will also incorporate a vacuum gauge. On a larger person even a very low reading on the gauge may result in a very fierce lift into the cups, due to the skin softness and lack of resistance, so visual judgement is the best guide to a safe and satisfactory treatment.

The cups can be placed in unison on both sides of the body, as when treating the midriff or buttocks, or may need to be graded down an area such as the thigh.

The cups should be chosen for their suitability for the area and must be able to contour closely. The cups for static pulsing vary in size, being in pairs, but are, naturally, much larger than gliding cups being designed for the larger client, or one with large local fatty deposits.

CARE AND MAINTENANCE OF VACUUM EQUIPMENT

Vacuum units are normally of a very robust construction, having few external working parts in which faults can develop. The pump and motor, which are often combined, are enclosed and seldom need attention.

The machine simply needs to be kept clean, but the connecting leads and cups need rather more careful attention to ensure a long life. The perspex cups should be washed out in warm soapy water, or can be wiped out with a cloth soaked in cleansing solution, containing anti-bacterial elements. The cups should be stored safely so that they do not become chipped or grazed by other implements. The outer edges must be smooth, free from cracks, etc., to form a good vacuum with the skin. The cups may be cleansed by the fluid method, in sterilizing baths, or within a vapour or ultra-violet cabinet. Due to their size, simple cleansing and disinfection is usually acceptable for normal clinic use.

Oily matter which becomes lodged within the connection tubes should be removed by immersing the tubes in a hot detergent solution and leaving them to soak. If done regularly, this prevents a discoloured oily build up which looks unpleasant. For stubborn deposits a cotton tipped orange stick can be used to clear the tube or, as a last resort, a small section can be cut off the end of the tube. In time tubes do become a little slack and do not form a good connection at the cup, so a small piece removed also remedies this problem, though eventually, of course, it reduces the tube to an unworkable length.

Care of the applicators is an essential part of the therapist's duties with any treatment, but in specific reduction, if it is not consistently followed, the routines will be inefficient and the therapist hampered, not aided, by her equipment. The routine of cleaning the equipment, quickly washing the cups, unravelling the leads (multi-cup method) and replacing the unit for further use, is a system which the therapist would be wise to adopt.

Cleaning and preparing as one works is a sure sign of a professional therapist, and it is essential when dealing with specialized routines, involving a range of applicators and connections.

MUSCLE CONTRACTION
TREATMENTS
(FARADISM)

Muscle toning treatments are perhaps the most popular and successful of all the figure improving routines available within the clinic. Closely resembling natural exercise in effect, yet requiring little effort on the part of the client, apart from regular attendance for treatment. Faradism can effect a reduction of inches, but does not alter body weight unless combined with diet.

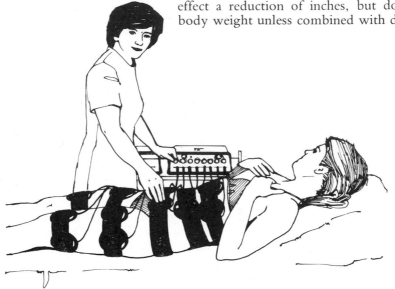

PHYSIOLOGICAL
EFFECTS OF FARADIC
TYPE CURRENTS

The name 'faradism' was originally applied to the current obtained from a faradic cell. This was an uneven alternating current which produced spasmodic fierce contractions, controlled by the physiotherapist for treatment of damaged or denervated muscle tissues. Modern equipment used for beauty therapy purposes combines various types of currents, which produce similar physiological effects, without discomfort, and these are termed 'faradic type' currents. The current is surged or interrupted so that the contraction produced closely resembles natural exercise and is acceptable to the client.

The primary sensation is stimulation of sensory nerves, prickling, slight irritation and resulting erythema in the area. When the electrode is placed accurately over a motor point, and sufficient intensity of current is applied muscle contraction takes place. The surging or interruption of the current produces relaxation and prevents muscle fatigue or discomfort. The working muscles exert a pumping effect on blood and lymphatic vessels in the immediate area, improving cellular function and removal of waste products.

Indications for Faradic Treatment

1   Where figure reshaping or a reduction in inches is required. For greatest success, clients should ideally be within 7—8 kg (1 stone) of their correct weight, and if they are very overweight the treatment will not be so successful, with slower results being obtained.

2   For rehabilitation of the waistline after pregnancy (post-natal permission is needed if treatment is within 3 months of the birth).

3   For toning and firming the contours whilst body weight is being lost through diet.

4   To reshape or tone thighs or buttocks which are out of proportion to the figure or inclined to adipose deposits.

5   To re-educate muscle tissue which has become poor in tone as a result of prolonged disuse or incorrect use: the abdominal muscles on women being an example, where overweight and poor muscle tone causes the abdominal contents to press outwards against the muscular abdominal wall causing protrusion.

6   To firm and tone the pectoral muscles underlying the breasts, particularly after childbirth and lactation.

7   To maintain an attractive firm figure and prevent weight accumulating.

Application of Faradic Treatment

Muscles can be exercised *individually* or in *groups*. Where the individual muscle is treated by the *motor points* method, the contraction is very clear, and the muscle works by contracting towards its origin. The insertion and origin coming closer together, the muscle shortening on its long axis, and movement occurring at connecting joints. Accuracy is needed to trace the motor point of the muscle so that the current may flow easily along the nerve path, otherwise the primary reaction of prickling and erythema will cause client discomfort.

MOTOR POINTS

Due to the time consuming problems of picking out individual muscles, the points method is seldom used in the clinic situation, but there are some distinct advantages to its use in certain cases. First in training, 'pointing' the muscles establishes the location of the best nerve connections of each superficial muscle, and this knowledge produces more accurate group pad placings. Then in treatment there are individuals who need help to obtain a specific muscle contraction, and the points method has the advantage that each muscle performs its own individual action, and does not simply form part of a more general contraction as in the group system.

When shortening of the rectus abdominis muscle after pregnancy is necessary, it can be made to work independently rather than forming part of a general abdominal contraction, where it could be carried by other stronger muscles. By contracting the muscle specifically with points, it shortens and gains strength and gradually flattens the abdominal bulge. The pectoralis muscle of the chest and the adductors of the inside thigh are other examples of muscles which can be carried by surrounding or adjacent muscle groups, with little improvement being gained to weak muscles.

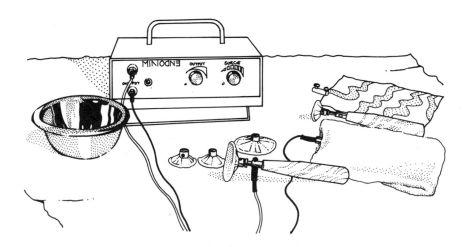

Motor Points Equipment

The motor point system is applied by connection to a one-outlet faradic unit, or by using only one outlet on a multi-outlet clinic machine. The connection will be to a linked set of leads which attach to a terminal, or two leads to two connections on the smaller units. One of the leads is connected to a thin sheet of tin 10 cm (6 in.) square (the 'indifferent'), covered in lint or sponge previously soaked in warm saline solution (salt), so that no metal is exposed. The second lead is attached to a handle with a mushroom or button type electrode head, which acts as the point. The connections must all be tight, clean and protected from the client. The lint covered electrode heads come in a wide range of sizes for differing muscle sizes and shapes, being from 13 mm ($\frac{1}{2}$ in.) diameter up to 5 cm (2 in.). The motor point connection may also be a small sheet of tin instead of a mushroom handle, and would also need sponge or lint covering.

The 'indifferent' plate is then placed on the origin of the muscle, or on a good connection point such as the lower spine. Any indifferent connection that allows a good response without discomfort, such as a nerve trunk, is satisfactory. This is then firmly strapped to the area so that it is fully in contact. If under the client's back, the body weight may need the additional support of a small towel in the centre back to hold the pad firmly against the spine. If the indifferent plate is loose, current seepage will occur and cause skin prickling and unwanted contractions around the plate. It also causes a loss of power on the active, working point.

The faradic unit may then be turned on, the surge rate adjusted if not automatically pulsed, and the moist button or point electrode applied to the motor point of the chosen muscle. A pinch of salt in a small bowl of water improves the conduction of the current, and this saline solution should be used for soaking the lint coverings on indifferent and active electrodes.

The surge rate should be 50—60 pulses a minute if not automatic, and this gives a fairly fast comfortable contraction, close to natural movements and nervous stimuli. The sensation that will be experienced should be explained to the client to allay anxiety and gain co-operation. The intensity of the current can then be gradually increased to overcome the primary reaction, and if the button is in the correct position, when sufficient intensity is applied visible contractions will commence. If the intensity used seems adequate and no contrac-

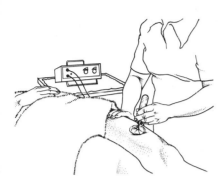

Muscle Contraction on the Thigh

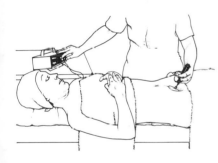

Muscle Contraction on the Abdomen

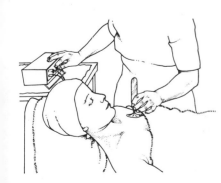

Muscle Contraction on the Breast

tion occurs, the intensity should be reduced and a new position tried. From experience it is learnt where the motor points are likely to be in relation to the shape and size of muscle, and it is beneficial to plot the position of each superficial muscle of the body before progressing to group work. Although each body will be slightly different, filling in or 'plotting' all the points personally found during practice on a full figure diagram of superficial muscles will build knowledge and confidence when applying faradism to all types of figures.

The intensity or size of the current used gives only guidance as to the degree of contraction that can be expected from a muscle, as several other factors alter the contraction achieved. The size and tone of the muscle, and the amount of fatty tissue overlying the area through which the current has to pass all alter the possible contraction. As muscles grow stronger, they require less and less intensity to achieve active contractions, and this gives guidance as to the improving strength of the muscular tissue.

When treating an area by the points method, only a few contractions on each muscle should be applied to avoid muscular fatigue being produced. Weak muscles fatigue very quickly, and this is shown by tremor and an unwillingness to contract. The muscles appear to struggle to perform the contraction. Although not desirable in general treatment, it is useful to note at what point this occurs, so that overtreatment can be avoided when later using the less specific method of group pad placings, where individual contractions are less visible.

Each muscle may be exercised by contracting actively 6—10 times, or less if considered sufficient, until the whole area is completed. The intensity is slowly reduced and the machine turned off, or contact quickly broken during a rest phase of the circuit. The client may then be dried thoroughly and the back plate removed.

With the indifferent plate in the centre back position, the whole of the front of the body can be treated, from the ankles to the chest. With the client prone, the indifferent plate can be placed on the upper spine area, as it cannot be placed under the abdomen. A side hip position may be used, or even the centre back placing, as long as the points are not used in close proximity to the plate, otherwise contractions would commence around the indifferent plate as well as under the active button holder.

If two covered plates of metal are used, one large and one small, as the indifferent and active electrodes, both have to be strapped to the body firmly. The indifferent plate is placed at the origin and the active plate at the motor point or insertion of the muscle.

No current is lost by this method, the current having only to travel through the length of the muscle fibres to obtain a clear contraction. Its laborious application makes this a system little used in points faradism, but the principle of working muscles along their length is seen in use in general padding layouts and it does produce some of the best and clearest contractions.

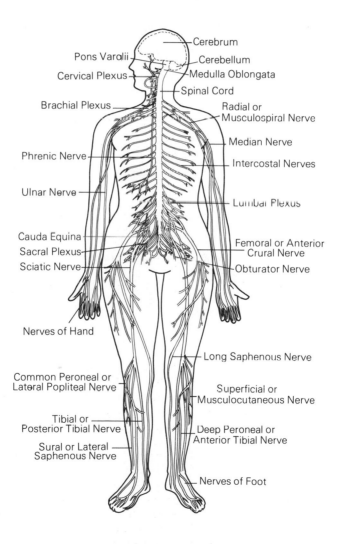

Cerebrum
Pons Varolii
Cerebellum
Cervical Plexus
Medulla Oblongata
Spinal Cord
Brachial Plexus
Radial or Musculospiral Nerve
Median Nerve
Phrenic Nerve
Intercostal Nerves
Ulnar Nerve
Lumbar Plexus
Cauda Equina
Femoral or Anterior Crural Nerve
Sacral Plexus
Sciatic Nerve
Obturator Nerve
Nerves of Hand
Long Saphenous Nerve
Common Peroneal or Lateral Popliteal Nerve
Superficial or Musculocutaneous Nerve
Tibial or Posterior Tibial Nerve
Deep Peroneal or Anterior Tibial Nerve
Sural or Lateral Saphenous Nerve
Nerves of Foot

The Nerve Supplies to the Body

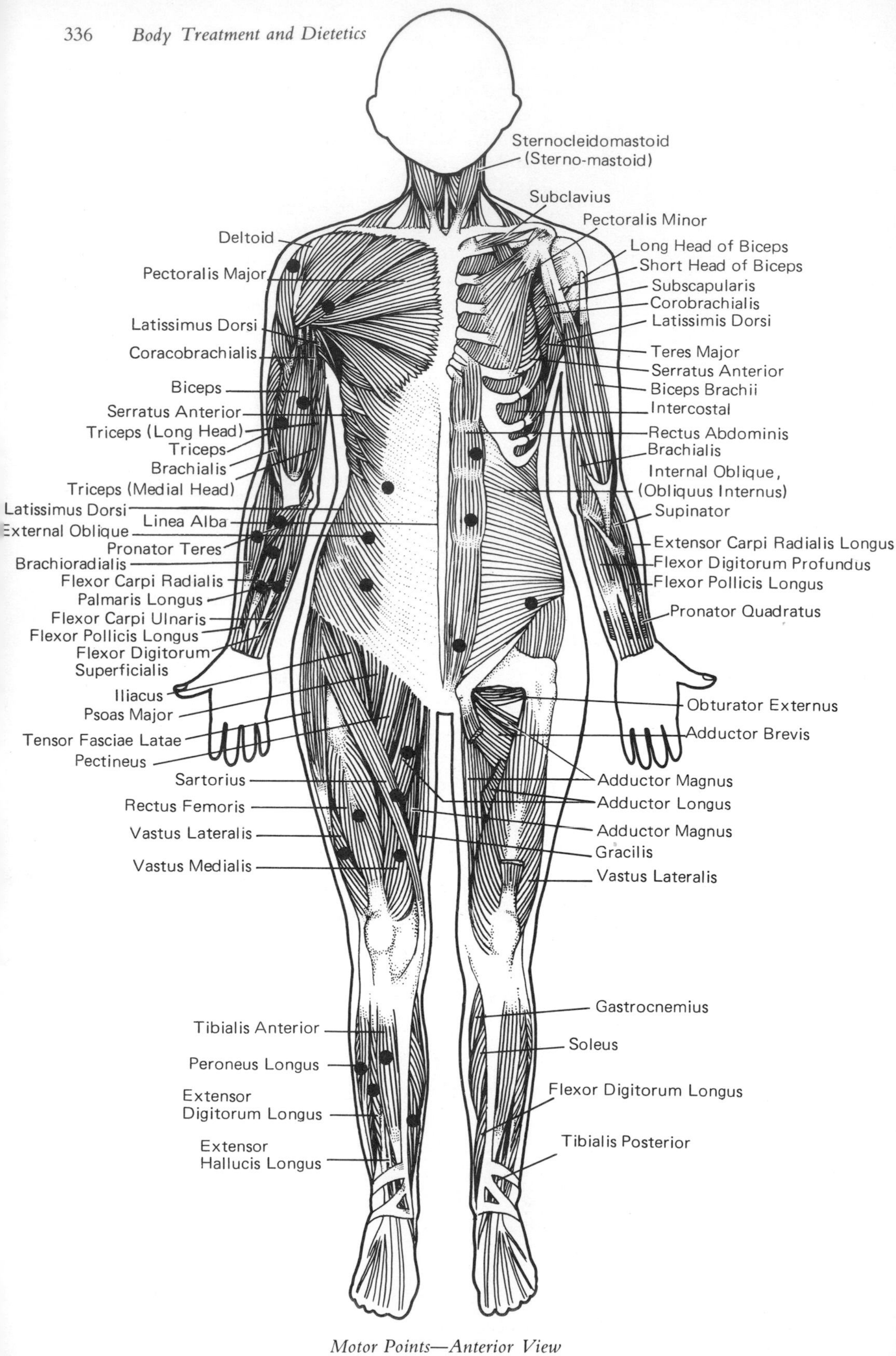

Sternocleidomastoid
(Sterno-mastoid)

Subclavius

Pectoralis Minor

Deltoid

Long Head of Biceps

Short Head of Biceps

Pectoralis Major

Subscapularis

Corobrachialis

Latissimis Dorsi

Latissimus Dorsi

Coracobrachialis

Teres Major

Serratus Anterior

Biceps Brachii

Biceps

Intercostal

Serratus Anterior

Rectus Abdominis

Triceps (Long Head)

Brachialis

Triceps

Internal Oblique,
(Obliquus Internus)

Brachialis

Triceps (Medial Head)

Supinator

Latissimus Dorsi

Linea Alba

External Oblique

Extensor Carpi Radialis Longus

Pronator Teres

Flexor Digitorum Profundus

Brachioradialis

Flexor Pollicis Longus

Flexor Carpi Radialis

Pronator Quadratus

Palmaris Longus

Flexor Carpi Ulnaris

Flexor Pollicis Longus

Flexor Digitorum
Superficialis

Iliacus

Obturator Externus

Psoas Major

Adductor Brevis

Tensor Fasciae Latae

Pectineus

Sartorius

Adductor Magnus

Rectus Femoris

Adductor Longus

Vastus Lateralis

Adductor Magnus

Gracilis

Vastus Medialis

Vastus Lateralis

Gastrocnemius

Tibialis Anterior

Soleus

Peroneus Longus

Extensor
Digitorum Longus

Flexor Digitorum Longus

Extensor
Hallucis Longus

Tibialis Posterior

Motor Points—Anterior View

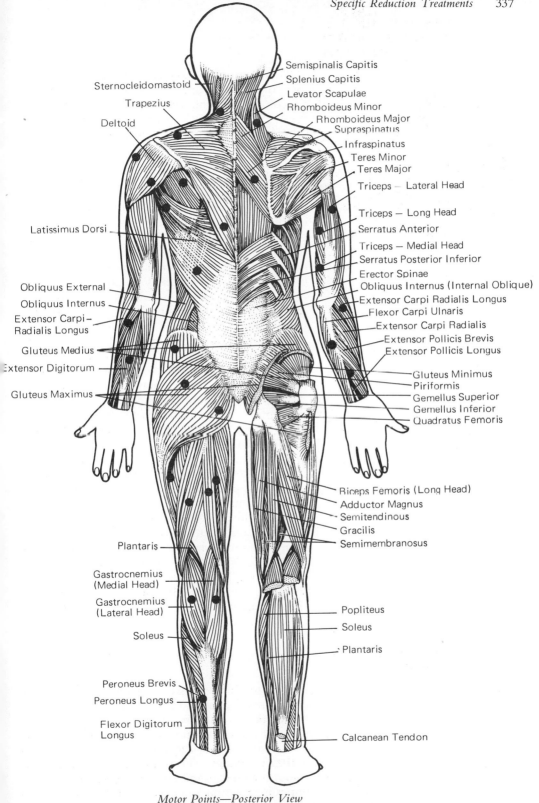

Semispinalis Capitis
Splenius Capitis
Levator Scapulae
Rhomboideus Minor
Rhomboideus Major
Supraspinatus
Infraspinatus
Teres Minor
Teres Major
Triceps — Lateral Head
Triceps — Long Head
Serratus Anterior
Triceps — Medial Head
Serratus Posterior Inferior
Erector Spinae
Obliquus Internus (Internal Oblique)
Extensor Carpi Radialis Longus
Flexor Carpi Ulnaris
Extensor Carpi Radialis
Extensor Pollicis Brevis
Extensor Pollicis Longus
Gluteus Minimus
Piriformis
Gemellus Superior
Gemellus Inferior
Quadratus Femoris

Sternocleidomastoid
Trapezius
Deltoid
Latissimus Dorsi
Obliquus External
Obliquus Internus
Extensor Carpi–
Radialis Longus
Gluteus Medius
Extensor Digitorum
Gluteus Maximus

Biceps Femoris (Long Head)
Adductor Magnus
Semitendinous
Gracilis
Semimembranosus

Plantaris
Gastrocnemius
(Medial Head)
Gastrocnemius
(Lateral Head)
Soleus

Popliteus
Soleus
Plantaris

Peroneus Brevis
Peroneus Longus
Flexor Digitorum
Longus

Calcanean Tendon

Motor Points—Posterior View

PASSIVE MUSCLE EXERCISE, GROUP METHOD

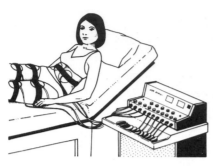

Passive muscle exercise operates on general areas of the body, or groups of muscles, so making for convenient application. Large areas of the body can be treated with multi-outlet faradic units, these having 6—8 outlets which allow 12—16 pads to be applied. The therapist uses her knowledge of muscle groups and their function, plus expertise with the equipment, to create effective layouts which bring results. For with muscle contraction the therapist must also be a technician able to control the equipment and adjust its actions on the client in response to physical effects noted. By monitoring the treatments throughout the client can be helped towards a much more active level of contraction without anxiety or discomfort.

The principle of group padding is to exercise the muscles in a similar manner to that of movements performed naturally. So reference to muscular movement employed in exercise (Chapter 4) will be a guide to all layouts. The motor points of the muscles are also essential to consider, so that the pads are placed where they can obtain the best contraction, with the lowest intensity, so avoiding discomfort. It has been seen that muscles seldom work independently, but rather in groups, with this movement being reflected in the cerebral cortex of the nervous system; so to exercise muscles as a group is close to the natural manner. For this reason padding layouts come in many different variations, many of which are successful. If choice can be based on how muscles work together, and naturally form movements, rather than on standard layout charts, treatments will be more successful. The routines can also be adapted for differing body types and devised to personally fit clients' needs and differing levels of tolerance to the treatment.

EQUIPMENT (CLINIC FARADIC UNITS)

Modern clinic units incorporate a wide variety of different controls to alter the form the treatment takes: *regulators* for the variable surge or pulse of the contraction (duration and relaxation of current), and *intensity controls* for the number of outlets provided. The terminals may have leads colour matched to indicator lights which show the outlet is in action and save confusion. This *colour coding* is really essential when up to eight outlets are in use, that is with 16 pads attached to the client; otherwise the therapist may find herself turning up the wrong set of muscles.

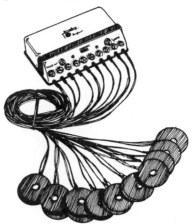

Clinic Faradic Unit

The really large clinic units also have facilities for altering the rhythm of treatment and adjusting the muscles' rest period between contractions, which is useful for a small percentage of clients.

Many units have a fixed surge rate, set at a fairly normal rate of surge (50—60 a minute), and in most salon applications this is really no disadvantage as the variable surge controls tend to stay turned to a standard rate of surge ($8\frac{1}{2}$—9 on many dials). In some cases a fixed surge may ensure safety and prevent accidents occurring.

Whatever controls the equipment incorporates, the therapist should become familiar in its use before applying treatment to clients. The sensation experienced by the client is unusual enough to cause anxiety, without the additional worry of an operator unsure of the application.

The semi-conductor pads are made of rubber impregnated with graphite, which makes for more comfortable treatment and makes protection unnecessary. They do still, however, require moistening before application. Their construction means that the current enters the skin over an area rather than being concentrated on one small part of the body, and the resistance of the pads keeps the current down to a suitable size. Thus, removing the pain or shock element and making the treatment more acceptable to clients. The connection leads are either permanently attached, or more commonly push into connection points on the back of the pads. To save wear and tear on the leads, the pads may be left in their working situation, and cleansed with disinfectant and detergent in situ.

Each outlet is like a separate contraction point and can be controlled individually, although the surge rate is common to all outlets in use. In some cases two smaller units can be used together to complete a group layout by placing them side by side and matching their surge rates. Portable faradic units are available which can operate from a mains supply or battery: useful for home visiting treatments.

There is nothing magical about the larger, more impressive clinic units, for they are only as good as the operator controlling their use and application. Although initially faradic muscle contraction appears complicated to use, the treatments will all be successful if muscular anatomy is known and the client's condition accurately assessed.

BASIC PADDING LAYOUTS

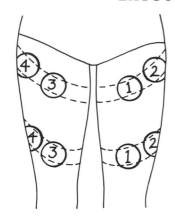

Longitudinal Placing

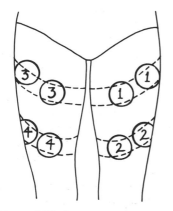

Diagonal Placing

The method of padding in most common use is what is termed a 'split body' layout, where each side of the body is dealt with separately. This method works on the principle of exercising groups of muscles as they might contract voluntarily to cause a movement. With this method differences in muscle bulk, tone of muscles, etc., can be accommodated by balancing the variable output controls to obtain equality of movement on both sides: development of one side of the body often being greater through sports activities, right handedness, etc.

Pairs of pads are placed each side of the body, to make the muscles of the group work together. The pads may therefore be placed in a similar fashion on both sides, but may be using different levels of intensity to achieve visible contractions. The pads may be placed diagonally in pairs, such as on the quadriceps group on the thigh, or some of the pads may be placed either end of the muscles to make use of the longitudinal reaction used effectively in point work. Working muscles in this way causes the greatest degree of muscle shortening, and allows it to contract as fully as possible. This is not as essential on the thighs where general toning and tightening is needed, but would be essential on the abdominal area.

If the pads are not placed in close proximity to the motor points of the muscles in the area, much of the current is ineffective, missing the motor points. The insulating, buffering capacity of fatty tissue in the area compounds the problem and contractions will be poor. A slim person with reasonable muscle tone will form contractions even with slightly inaccurate placings, but an overweight, out of condition person will not, so accuracy is then vital.

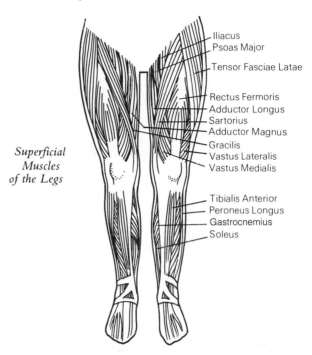

Superficial Muscles of the Legs

Iliacus
Psoas Major
Tensor Fasciae Latae
Rectus Fermoris
Adductor Longus
Sartorius
Adductor Magnus
Gracilis
Vastus Lateralis
Vastus Medialis
Tibialis Anterior
Peroneus Longus
Gastrocnemius
Soleus

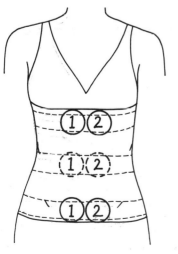

When pads are placed around an area to be exercised, a transference of current occurs, with some of the current being lost or seeping away to affect connecting muscles. This then reduces the need for strong intensity on surrounding muscles, when pads are subsequently placed to reinforce the effect of general contraction in the area. An example of this effect is on the rectus abdominis muscle, where the pads are normally placed close to the symphysis pubis and sternum attachments. An amount of transference occurs between the internal and external obliques and the transversalis muscles, and the specific effect on the rectus abdominis decreases. If padding is then completed, the sides of the trunk are found to need less intensity to form movements. So the purpose of the routine has to be decided, whether a general toning of the area is needed, or specific shortening of the rectus abdominis.

The natural movements that are being copied are therefore abdominal retraction as in isometric contractions, which a general padding of the area can achieve, or sit-ups which pads placed longitudinally can accomplish.

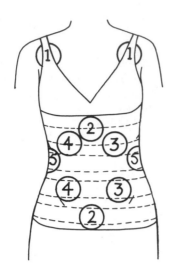

General Retraction Placing

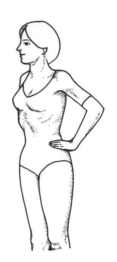

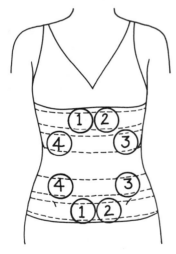

*Longitudinal Placing
for Shortening
Rectus Abdominis*

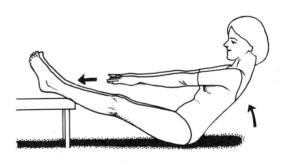

As the abdominal muscles are worked locally, without involving the rest of the body in activity, a very concentrated effect can be created, equal to vigorous active exercise of the area, without physical effort. Of course there is less expenditure of energy, so less weight-reducing elements than active exercise, but the specific effect is very successful in reshaping in this area. Both men and women suffer greatly from weak abdominal muscles, women mainly from childbirth and men from overindulgence.

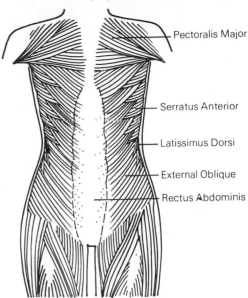

- Pectoralis Major
- Serratus Anterior
- Latissimus Dorsi
- External Oblique
- Rectus Abdominis

Superficial Muscles of the Abdomen

Treatment of the back is difficult with group faradism, as maintaining the pads in good contact requires elaborate strapping or use of small weighted bags. Not a very common area of treatment, its placings would normally be planned with consideration for the shape of the latissimus dorsi and trapezius, being large muscles with multiple bone attachments. The layout should be applied to avoid excessive movement of the arms, or rotation of the trunk caused by the insertion of these large muscles into the arm and pelvic girdle bones.

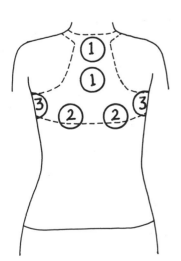

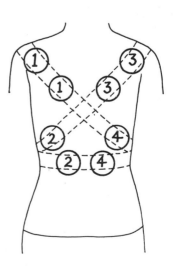

Hips and thighs are often treated together, and as long as the antagonistic effects of muscle movements in the area are considered, a wide area can be treated simultaneously. Being well covered with subcutaneous fat, the buttocks may need additional padding to achieve effective contractions, and this can be achieved by reinforcing the standard padding layout with extra pads.

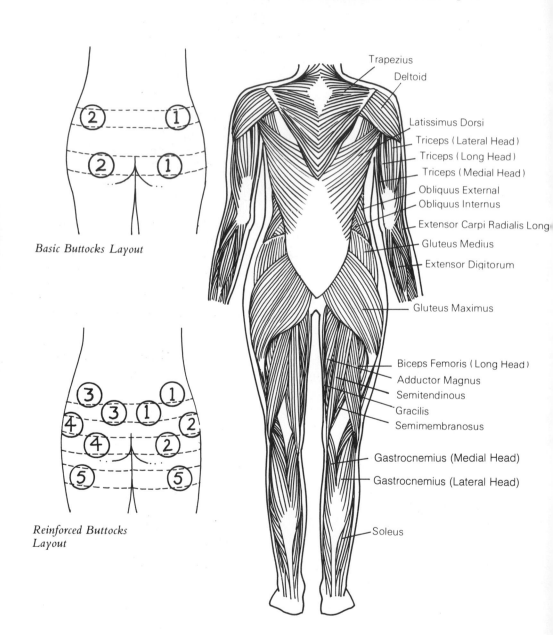

Basic Buttocks Layout

Reinforced Buttocks Layout

Trapezius
Deltoid
Latissimus Dorsi
Triceps (Lateral Head)
Triceps (Long Head)
Triceps (Medial Head)
Obliquus External
Obliquus Internus
Extensor Carpi Radialis Long
Gluteus Medius
Extensor Digitorum
Gluteus Maximus
Biceps Femoris (Long Head)
Adductor Magnus
Semitendinous
Gracilis
Semimembranosus
Gastrocnemius (Medial Head)
Gastrocnemius (Lateral Head)
Soleus

Superficial Muscles of the Back

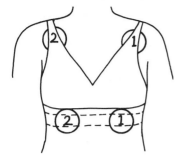

Split Body Padding
(Post-natal and Lifting)

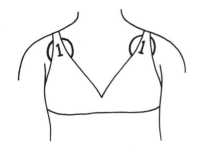

Upper Pectoral Padding
(Maintenance)

The position of the breasts can be improved with muscle contraction work on the pectoralis major. The positioning can be either with the body split, with two pads placed either side of the body, above and below the breast (four pads in use), or one outlet can be divided to simply exercise the upper pectoral area (two pads in use). The 'split body' method is preferable as breasts often differ in size, occasionally considerably, and differing levels of intensity are needed either side. For toning, lifting and post-natal work this method is necessary. With an outlet divided between the upper breast areas, the contraction is weaker and the intensity split between the pectoralis major muscles. For a slim person who is simply maintaining her figure, this method is adequate, particularly if combined with a more general padding layout. When only a small number of outlets are available, it also allows this area of the body to be included, rather than neglected.

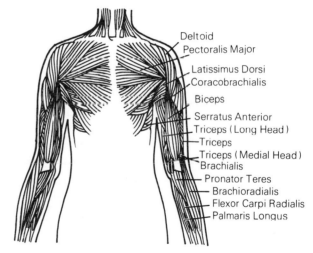

Deltoid
Pectoralis Major
Latissimus Dorsi
Coracobrachialis
Biceps
Serratus Anterior
Triceps (Long Head)
Triceps
Triceps (Medial Head)
Brachialis
Pronator Teres
Brachioradialis
Flexor Carpi Radialis
Palmaris Longus

Superficial Muscles of the Breasts and Arms

Arms can be prevented from becoming slack in the triceps area by regular application of faradism to reinforce the work of natural exercise, particularly isometrics, in the area. A natural contraction should be aimed for, without excessive involvement of the forearm or elbow joint.

In some cases outlets can be divided between the two sides of the body, as seen in treatment of the pectoralis major. The rectus femoris is commonly seen treated in this manner in error, with a pad placed on either thigh from the one outlet. The load which the contraction has to lift is excessive

Upper Arms Padding

and a high intensity is needed to initiate a contraction. To judge whether a padding placing is going to be effective, certain points can be considered.

1 The placing should never make muscles work against each other. As natural antagonists, certain areas of the body should not be treated at the same time. The back and the front of the trunk and the back and front of the legs are two examples, where muscles would be trying to work eccentrically and concentrically simultaneously. As this would be impossible naturally, it should not be applied artificially, and would lead to discomfort, irregular contractions, excessive movement in the area and, worst of all, ineffective results.

2 The load the contraction has to lift should be considered. A slim person offers little resistance to muscular stimulation; a large person offers a great deal more, due to poor tone, large adipose deposits and sheer bulk.

3 The job the placing has to do should be considered: to tone or maintain a figure, or completely reshape or flatten an area, such as after childbirth, or connected with a severe weight loss. The pads can then be placed along a muscle working it specifically, or within a group, or placed generally to exercise a whole area, with extra pads for reinforcement if needed.

4 The way the muscles work naturally should be followed as closely as possible when planning padding layouts. If in doubt, the muscles' action can be tested manually, by asking the client to perform exercises chosen to work the area. Tests for muscle strength (see Chapter 2 Figure Diagnosis) form the basis of many muscle contraction treatments, and offer valuable guidance as to the client's general and specific muscle tone.

REASONS FOR POOR OR UNEVEN MUSCLE CONTRACTIONS

1 Dividing pads between either side of the body.
2 Greater skin resistance under one of the pads.
3 Pads not placed on identical areas of muscle bulk either side of the body. Repositioning is then needed in relation to the medial line of the body, and *inferior* and *superior* aspects of the body.

4 Pads becoming dried out, or dirty, where a faradic 'burn' might result.

5 Incorrectly positioned pads, i.e. too close to joints or tendons, or affecting connecting or adjacent muscles.

6 Poor contact of pads with the skin's surface, due to the straps being too loose or the indifferent plate not being firmly held against the body (points method).

7 Loose or faulty connections, giving intermittent performance.

8 A stronger contraction being obtained from one pole (electrode).

Careful consideration of all these factors, allied to padding layouts based on muscle groups, will ensure a good, comfortable even treatment. When a difference is experienced in contractions from the negative and positive poles, it will usually diminish after 10 minutes.

POLARITY

A simple explanation of the relationship of polarity to modern therapy faradism may help to dispel the confusion which exists. Modern apparatus uses various types of current which, while differing considerably in wave form, produce the same physiological effects as the original faradic current. These are termed 'faradic type' currents, which have the advantages of providing more comfortable smooth contractions, acceptable to clients who have a choice of whether or not they undertake treatment.

When the motor point system of faradism is used, the larger plate, termed the 'indifferent', is the *positive* electrode (the anode), and this is placed so that it will not cause contractions of muscles other than those being treated, and particularly not the antagonists. The *active* electrode (the mushroom handle or small plate) is then termed the 'negative' electrode (the cathode), and this is placed over the motor point to produce clear contractions.

Terms in Use

Positive electrode
Anode
Indifferent electrode
Less effective in initiating an impulse

Negative electrode
Cathode
Active electrode
Greater stimulation produced

When the group system is used for 'slimming' through firming slack musculature, several pairs of electrodes are needed, and all muscles of a group are made to work together, to re-educate their action. With this system it is difficult to discern any difference in strength of the muscle contraction from either pole. The electrodes (semi-conductor pads) are of equal size so that current intensity is similar and the muscles are contracting as a group. The polarity is considered to be constantly alternated between each pair of pads, and for most purposes in group work the polarity is not of importance. More emphasis is placed on making sure that the pads are correctly postioned on nerve trunks and motor points, to obtain a good all round contraction.

Contra-indications

1   Open cuts or stings under the area of treatment.
2   Not directly over varicose veins.
3   Defective circulation from systemic causes.
4   Not during the first 2—3 days of menstruation, on the abdomen.
5   A history of thrombosis or phlebitis.
6   Not after operations or childbirth until medical permission is given.

Method of Application – Group Faradism

The client diagnosed as benefiting from muscle contraction is measured carefully, and these measurements are recorded on the client's clinic card. The largest measurement for each area is recorded, taken around the fullest part to be treated. Several measurements may be necessary if specific figure shaping is desired, e.g. when the shape of the legs needs improvement, rather than their overall size.

The client is helped on to the bed, which is prepared with overlying straps, placed in readiness for securing the pads on to the client. The straps are firmly placed round the client, leaving just sufficient slackness to slip the pads underneath. Pads are applied systematically, working from one end of the machine's outlets to the other, to avoid the leads becoming tangled. The pairs of pads are placed according to the needs of the area, following suggested patterns of padding. Muscles are padded up in sequence, first one side of the body then the other, to keep the layouts co-ordinated and even. The abdominal placing, for example, would be applied rectus abdominis, first one side then the other, then the external obliques and underlying internal obliques, in sets of pads.

When correctly in place, the padding is checked for comfort and the client reassured about the sensation to be experienced. The surge rate is set, and the intensity of the current gradually increased until visible contractions are produced. The intensity may be increased one muscle at a time, or a group of pads worked together. Or the intensity gradually increased on all the pads simultaneously to produce a general movement, rather than producing movement in each muscle area separately.

The method of 'bringing up' contractions and producing comfortable movements will depend on the area of treatment. The thigh, for example, contains one large muscle, the quadriceps, which is divided into four sections, three superficial, one deep, and requires a general increase of intensity on all the pads placed to work the muscles. The muscle would naturally work in a co-ordinated manner, not in individual sections as when treated by the points method. So, although knowing the individual motor points of the muscle sections helps the placing of pads, it is also important to know the muscle's normal movement, which in this case is a combined one, with the muscle becoming as one unit for most movements.

With an initial treatment, visible contractions may not always be possible if the client has poor muscle tone or local fat deposits. The area of treatment can be palpated, and the client questioned on the physical reactions experienced. If activity is present deep in the muscles, this will act to re-establish tone and strength, and will help to build towards stronger contractions. Clear contractions are what are needed for results, but if the client can be guided towards this goal, rather than bullied towards it, then a less traumatic routine will result.

After a few minutes of adjustment to the current, it may be gradually increased and then left at a comfortable level for 15—20 minutes initially. Treatment durations can increase over the course of 10—12 treatments, and total times are normally 30 minutes per session. Treatment may be applied daily, and needs to be given at least 2—3 times a week to achieve a build up effect.

If accurately placed, contractions are very concentrated in effect and excessive periods of application only lead to muscle fatigue. It is important to obtain sustained levels of contraction by adjusting the current intensity during treatment, rather than applying prolonged treatment which can lead to aching and tired muscles.

The therapist should stay in close proximity to the client during treatment and can apply a minor treatment, such as manicure, eyebrow shaping, etc., if the client is quite comfortable. Several clients can be supervised at once, in individual cubicles, within a clinic specializing in muscle toning treatments. With the client comfortably settled, warmly covered, the treatment can progress with periodic checking and adjustment from the therapist. This makes the treatment more profitable, and makes better use of the therapist's time. New, anxious or difficult clients will always require the therapist's undivided attention, however, if the full potential of the treatment is to be realized.

At the conclusion of the treatment, the intensity levels are reduced individually on each variable control, gradually bringing all the controls to zero, then switching off the unit. The pads are removed in reverse order to the application, to avoid tangling of leads, and the pads replaced neatly on the trolley in working sequence ready for cleansing. The straps are then released, the client is helped into a sitting position and the area of treatment thoroughly dried and talced if necessary. A few minutes may be spent in the sitting position to recover balance and overcome any feelings of dizziness caused by the changes in circulation produced by the treatment.

Measurements are normally taken only prior to the treatment, but occasionally they may be taken again after the treatment, to encourage the clients in their home efforts. Care should be taken to measure in the same position exactly in this case, and this can be achieved by marking the level with ballpoint pen. Then the toning effect of the treatment can be judged.

Muscle contraction treatment achieves the best results if applied regularly and when reinforced by natural exercise. If a weight as well as an inches reduction is required, then a diet must be involved. No electrical treatment, however well applied, can reshape a client who is overweight; however, it can help considerably to hasten results when a diet plan is being followed.

There is the temptation for clients to rely heavily on the salon treatments available, without considering it necessary to co-operate with diet and exercise plan. Without reducing the client's belief in the treatment, it is important that they should realize the importance of supporting home routines and diet.

INTERFERENTIAL CURRENT

(Muscle Contraction and Cellulite Treatment)

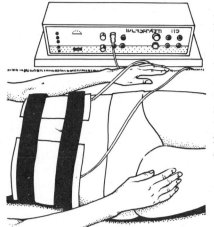

Muscle contraction and improvement of vascular and lymphatic circulation can also be achieved by application of *interferential* currents to the body. The interferential units offer a great number of variable applications, from muscle toning, treatment of cellulite conditions, through to general circulation stimulation. Being very diverse in their applications, the treatments will only be fully understood in practical application. The most important points of treatment may provide guidance initially.

Four Field Electrodes

The Interferential Current

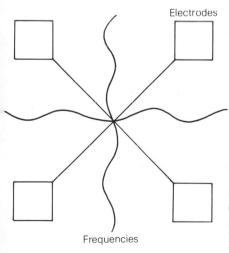

Electrodes

Frequencies

Superimposition Field

Interferential current is the result of crossing two medium frequency stimulating currents, both of which are independently generated within the machine, and introduced separately into the area to be treated. One of the circuits has a frequency of 3900–4000 cycles per second, the other has a frequency of 4000 cycles per second. The two electrode plates of the currents are in diagonally opposed positions, and only the field in which the two currents cross causes an effect on the tissues (this area or field is termed the 'superimposition field'). It is therefore considered as an endogenously generated alternating current (produced within the tissue itself) rather than an exogenously generated current (produced outside the body).

The crossing of the two currents generates low frequency waves with a frequency spectrum of 0—100 cycles per second. This frequency range is closely similar to the body's own oscillations or body frequencies and is therefore considered more biologically sympathetic in treatment. The treatment naturally tunes itself to the client's physical condition, and a more comfortable treatment can be accomplished. Interferential treatment produces less surface reaction on the skin and, well applied, provides a very natural and smooth method of toning the body systems.

Application and Effect

The difference between the currents generated by the machine provides a working frequency of 0–100 cycles per second which allows muscle contraction at the low frequency level, and circulation stimulation at the medium to high frequencies. Most machines have controls which provide a range of 0—10 cycles per second for body treatments, muscle toning and slimming effects, including 'cellulite', and a range of 0—100 cycles per second for facial work and vascular and lymphatic stimulation.

So the interferential system can be said to combine strong active elements and gentle soothing elements which, when used together in treatment, produce a wide range of effects on the client. Most units also produce facilities for galvanic iontophoresis, to create a treatment for cellulite from within the body itself, as well as by means of active substances.

So the equipment provides several different systems of treatment within the one unit, all of which can be used separately. The price for this convenience and wide variety of treatment is naturally rather high and will only be justified if the therapist becomes fully conversant with all aspects of treatment, and can promote them skilfully.

The interferential unit is considered a sophisticated and advanced piece of equipment, but one that is coming into increasing use as clients become more discriminating in their treatment demands.

Application and General Body Application

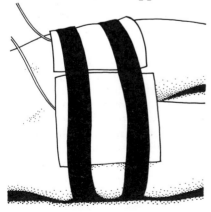

Four Field Electrodes

The pads are applied so that the area of treatment falls under the area where the path of the two frequencies cross. The further apart the pads are placed the deeper will be the effect; the closer together the more superficial will be the effect. The 'four field' principle is either built into the applicators, or applied via four connections to individual covered plates which are placed around the area of treatment. For convenience of use, many of the applicators have the activating electrodes built in within the manufacture, and the fibrous rubber pads are connected by one attachment lead to the machine. This saves time in treatment and makes for greater client safety.

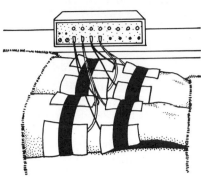

Individual Plate Electrodes
(Total Thigh Application)

When individual plates are used, they must be covered by moist sponge envelopes and be placed so that the leads are positioned alternately red and white. This then forms the 'four field' system between the plates. The main action being in the area where the currents actually cross, with the effect diminishing away from this point.

The action can be best understood by considering the different applications available for the body. Depending on the action required, the varying levels of frequency can be applied in a progressive fashion, both for intensity and duration.

The treatment commences on the body using a constant frequency of 100 cycles per second, with minimum intensity applied, for a few minutes to prepare the client for further treatment. This has a relaxing effect and increases the vascular and lymphatic circulation. The client finds the sensation comfortable, visibly relaxes and is then more prepared to have more active treatment.

The intensity is then increased on this frequency but given rhythmically, to a comfortable level until the body becomes tuned into the treatment, and strong vascular and lymphatic circulation is achieved. Although nothing can be seen at this stage, the tissues are being activated strongly which prepares the way for following muscle contraction if needed. This frequency is used to improve vascular circulation and remove toxic infiltrations, so may be used for 'cellulite' conditions and to help prevent varicose veins or tired aching legs and joints. It is preferable, occasionally, to stay on the higher frequency levels until general circulation is improved before progressing to the lower frequencies where muscle contraction takes place. For older clients this is found to be particularly beneficial, for it is often general functioning of tissues that are at fault rather than simply poor muscle tone. Diagnosis, once again, is vital to determine the client's condition.

The frequency is then changed to 0–10 cycles per second rythmically applied to obtain deep muscle action, which acts like a massage from within the body. The intensity can be gradually increased until it reaches an effective level, where it is left for 10—20 minutes, depending on area.

So the different proportions of treatment time given to the high, medium or low levels of frequency will depend on the nature of the problem.

Clients who are overweight, but whose muscles are firm, will benefit from a percentage of treatment given to high frequencies, to improve metabolism in the area, reduce pressure on the vascular network and reduce swelling or 'cellulite' conditions present. The muscle contraction being of secondary importance.

Older clients who have poor muscle tone, slack skin tissue, aching joints and dilated or varicosed veins will benefit from an equal allocation of 1—100 and 1—10 cycles per second frequencies, as their problems are both muscular and circulatory. The interferential current may be used over varicosed veins, as the action is produced from within the body rather than externally.

TREATMENT APPLICATION

Legs. Slimming Effects

The applicators are applied, either preformed pads or individual pads in the 'four field' position, centring the area of treatment in the superimposition field. The frequency is then applied for general reduction effects in the routine of 100 cycles per second constant for 2—3 minutes, then changing to rhythmical frequencies, increasing on the 0—100 level for 5 minutes, and then switching to 0—10 cycles per second for a further 5—10 minutes. As tolerance builds these times can be increased on the 0—100 and 0—10 scales until 8—10 minutes is spent on the high frequency (0—100) and 15—20 minutes on the low frequency (0—10). This half hour treatment can then be applied 2—3 times a week, gradually increasing the intensity used, but not prolonging the duration of the application.

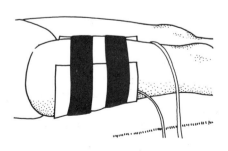

Four Field Electrodes
(Outer Thighs)

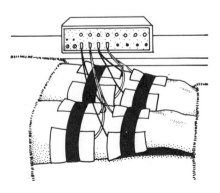

Individual Plate Electrodes
(Total Thigh Application)

'Cellulite' Conditions

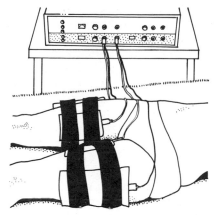

'Cellulite' conditions can be treated successfully with interferential currents, combined within the one machine, or can have special apparatus of a similar construction used, which is specifically planned for the treatment of 'cellulite'. The improvement in 'cellulite' experienced with interferential treatment can be seen almost as a bonus, as the main object of the treatment is muscular activity.

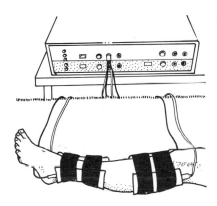

On the combined machine, the padding for 'cellulite' problems is similar to that of muscle contraction, but the frequencies are slightly different in emphasis. The application commences on the outside thigh with five minutes at 100 constant, 10 minutes at 0—100 increasing, and 10 minutes at 0—10. The treatments are applied in quick succession, ideally daily, and after the sixth treatment the 0—100 increasing and 0—10 levels are increased in duration to 20 minutes each. The intensity level is kept low to hasten the absorption of subcutaneous infiltrations and removal of toxic substances, and to mobilize fatty particles and improve metabolism.

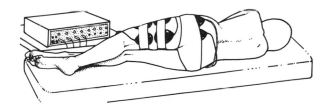

Upper Inside Thigh Treatment

Being a sensitive area, the inside thigh is often difficult to treat by traditional methods, but can be successfully improved by interferential current. As the body is able to moderate the current by its own biological frequencies, a more active treatment can be tolerated by this method than any other. The treatment is applied with two 'four field' pads, or four separate plates, and the worst

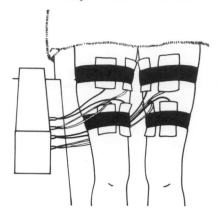

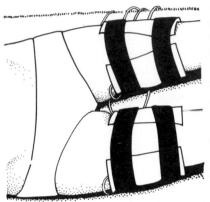

points placed under the central area. If the condition is superficial fat, then pads with the electrodes placed close together will be ideal, giving a superficial action. If the problem is muscular weakness, plus slack skin, then the separate plates or pads should be used placed further apart, to give a deeper effect within the muscles. The treatment is given on 100 constant for five minutes, 0—100 increasing rhythmically into a comfortable beat sensation at low intensity for five minutes, and then switching to 0—10 for a further five minutes, again at low intensity.

If the skin is slack and crepey, the current can be held at the lowest level of 1 or 2 on the 0—10 scale for five minutes, to provide extreme skin stimulation in the area. Client's tolerance should be built up to this special treatment addition, as not all clients find it comfortable. All areas of slack skin, upper arm, abdomen etc., can have this technique used upon them, to good effect.

After several treatments the 0—100 and 0—10 frequencies can be gradually increased in intensity and duration to 10 minutes each. The preparation frequency and skin toning aspects should remain of constant duration, although the intensity of the 0—10 scale will by then have increased, so vigilance is required when holding steadily on the 1 or 2 level to ensure treatment is still comfortable.

Inside Knee or Ankle Treatment

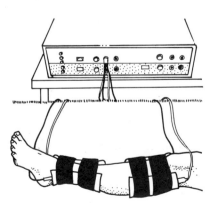

If oedema (swelling) and 'cellulite' conditions are present in these areas, they should be treated first before progressing to more general improvement, such as muscle contraction. The swelling must be medically checked and assessed as being due to poor circulation rather than from physical illnesses. It may then be treated by applying the frequency 100 cycles per second for five minutes constant, and then increasing on this level for five minutes, gradually building up the intensity on the rhythmical frequency. The treatment will be most successful if applied frequently at a low intensity. Once the oedema is improved, the 1—10 frequency can then be added if still needed to deeply activate the muscular tissue. If applied prematurely, however, it will slow the good results obtainable on the 'cellulite' or circulation defects.

If both legs and arms are to be treated simultaneously, they may be attached to further outlets on the larger units. This can mean that both sides receive identical levels of intensity, which may not be desirable, but it is time saving. If a considerable difference is noticed in the strength of either arms or legs, then the treatment should be applied independently, one limb after another. If a large amount of body therapy is undertaken large, multi-outlet machines, with independently controlled outlets are desirable.

Abdominal Area

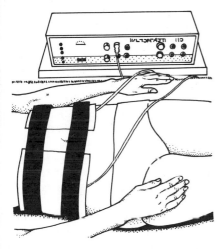

Due to the deep acting power of the interferential current, the active electrodes must be carefully placed when treating this area. The superimposition field must not be allowed to be centred over delicate internal organs, so the superficial muscles and subcutaneous tissue only must be treated.

This is accomplished by using pads with built-in 'four field' electrodes, placed directly over the abdomen, so that the action is on superficial tissues only. Or by placing similar pads, one on each side of the waist, both having separate attachments to the machine so that they work as independent 'four field' positions. The main point being that the frequencies *must not* cross in the middle of the abdominal cavity, whatever the padding. So the pads must be placed anterior to the body so the frequencies cross superficially or posterior. again so the currents flow through surface subcutaneous tissue.

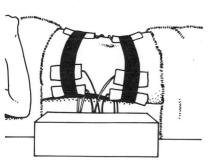

For weak muscles in the abdominal area, the application would be 5 minutes on 100 cycles per second constant, then increasing 0—100 for 5 minutes, taking the intensity increase very slowly, then switching 0—10 for 5 minutes, at the same level as the higher frequency. The tolerance to the treatment being decided on the higher level, and simply maintained on the lower muscle contracting frequencies. The treatment for slack skin can also be very successfully applied in this area (1 or 2 constant for 5 minutes on the 0—10 scale).

The intensity and duration can be increased gradually over the course of treatments on both the 0—100 and 0—10 scales, until an active half hour treatment is achieved in the area.

Breasts

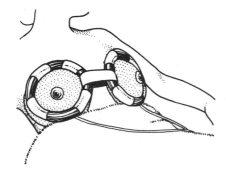

Breast Electrodes

Special attachments are available for treatment of the breasts which provide a deep and effective activation of the whole pectoral muscle area, and the breasts themselves. The ringed applicators are placed over protective sponge coverings and the nipples placed through the apertures to ensure the breasts are correctly positioned. The 'four field' electrodes are built into the rings and should be placed diagonally around the breast for greatest effect. The rings may then be strapped around the body, adjusting for the client's size. A semi-reclining position is most satisfactory for treatment, but whilst attaching the ring electrode and sponges, the client can adopt a forward leaning position. This then brings the fullness of the breast naturally into the cup, rather like putting on a bra, and makes positioning more easily accomplished. During treatment the whole area becomes warm through increased circulation to the area, and muscular tissue, skin tone and texture are improved. Results can be quite dramatic with post-natal conditions, or where an extreme weight loss has produced a dropped bust condition.

Extremely dropped bustlines, with 100% sag, cannot be lifted with this or any other method of therapy, and clients can only be advised on the possibility of plastic surgery. Prevention of loss of muscle tone, and maintenance of an attractive figure throughout life being the main indications for its use.

The application should be applied 100 constant for 2—3 minutes, 0—100 rhythmically increasing for five minutes, and 0—10 for five minutes initially. The medium and low frequencies can be increased to 10 minutes and increased in intensity as the course of treatment is progressed. Treatment needs to be applied regularly, ideally daily for best results, and needs to be reinforced with natural exercises.

Chapter 9

Business Organization

METHODS OF WORK

Qualification in body treatments may form part of a *total* training in beauty therapy or may be *independently* undertaken. A large percentage of therapists have both facial and body treatment skills, which enable them to work in a wide variety of work situations. More interest in body therapy may lead them to concentrate on this aspect of the work, in clinics specializing in figure treatments. Some therapists may train purely in body aspects but, like facial specialists, will find their employment prospects a little more restricted.

GENERAL SALON WORK, HEALTH AND BEAUTY CLINIC

In a clinic offering facial and body aspects of treatment, it is often possible for a therapist to concentrate mainly on figure improvement work. Body therapy tends to be fairly strenuous if a large proportion of the work is manual, so the daily routine may include pre-heating, massage, exercise instruction and client guidance, divided by periods of electrical treatment. The advantage of holding facial and body qualifications is obvious in salon practice, as it provides quieter periods in the daily work schedule, to avoid fatigue spoiling the quality of the work applied.

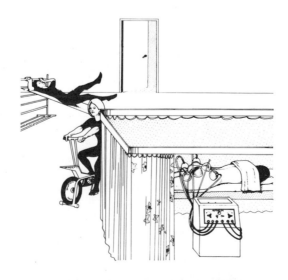

Fatigue can be avoided with careful treatment planning, even if no facial work is offered in the clinic, and it concentrates exclusively on figure improvement. Alternating active work, such as massage or exercise, with periods of muscle contraction, or pulsating vacuum treatment, allows the therapist to conserve energy to help through a strenuous day.

A wide range of treatment possibilities based on personal assessment and choice makes the work varied, interesting and very satisfying as results are achieved. Helping clients to maintain or regain their figure and improve their health is a very worthwhile and rewarding aspect of therapy.

EXERCISE AND HEALTH CLUBS

Here the emphasis will be on exercise work, backed up by heat therapy, massage and electrical treatments. The clients are encouraged to help themselves towards personal fitness, through use of exercise equipment, saunas, showers, pools and occasionally sports facilities. The treatment side of the club reinforces the client's efforts and acts to help them achieve personal figure improvement and improved fitness and stamina.

Clients may be regular visitors who hold club membership, or they may be clients who come to obtain a particular result, such as post-natal problems in women, or a medically advised weight loss in men. So the therapist will have to be capable of encouraging the client's own efforts in diet and exercise areas, as well as being skilled in treatment aspects.

The health club idea grows in popularity and can be found within larger hotels, country clubs and exclusive blocks of flats in city centres, or may be run independently as a therapy concern. The sports and self-help emphasis makes exercise and health clubs very popular with men and women, and provides another very exciting area of work for the therapist.

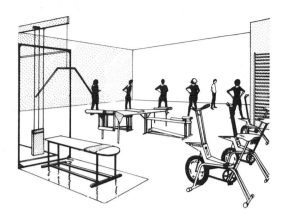

THE HEALTH HYDRO

The health hydro work situation is normally divided into facial therapy and body work aspects, and therapists have to decide to concentrate on one aspect of their training. This practice is changing as the standard of general therapy training is improving, and the therapists are better able to work in close liaison with nutritional, health and homeopathic experts, and can fulfil their wishes regarding the therapy treatment, under their general guidance.

Due to the total supervision and controlled and restricted diets of the hydro guests, a more remedial programme of health, face and figure improvement is normally attempted. This sort of total approach will appeal to therapists interested in body treatments, based on diet, exercise, manual massage and electrical muscle-toning applications.

Therapists will find their work divided between exercise instruction, in groups, and treatment aspects. A very concentrated approach to treatment can be applied, with daily massage, electrical therapy, foam baths, wax baths, sauna and steam treatments, all forming part of the overall treatment plan. A wide range of large scale apparatus and luxurious facilities makes the therapist's work within a hydro very varied and congenial.

Residence is normally required whilst working within the hydro situation, due to the slightly varied work hours, compared to a salon and, in some cases, the isolated position of the hydro. These points are compensated by longer periods of time off, and personal use of some of the hydro's facilities during free time.

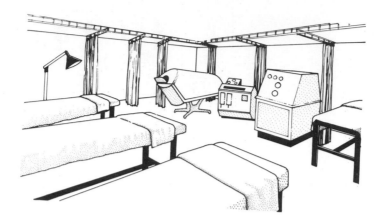

Treatment Area

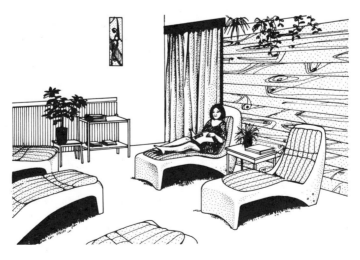

Resting Area

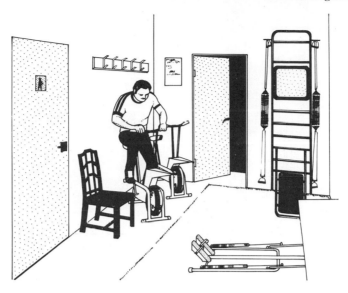

Exercise Room

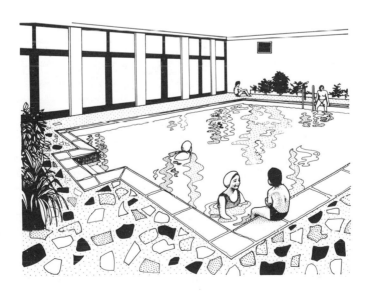

Pool and Activity Area

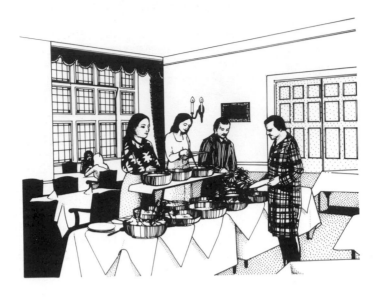

Light Diet Room

PRIVATE PRACTICE

Due to the large scale nature of the equipment required in body therapy, it does not readily lend itself to a mobile or home visiting practice. Certain treatments, such as massage, or muscle contraction, can be added to the mobile therapist's list of treatments, as long as sufficient care is taken in the choice of clients. The intimacy of body treatment places the therapist in a very vulnerable position when working within a private dwelling, rather than in a business establishment. Male clients should never be treated by female therapists unless in a supervized clinic or health club, and never on a home visiting basis.

Private practice *can* be successful, however, normally limited to female clients, within a private house, or business premises, perhaps in association with other professional services, opticians, dentists, etc. The therapist will normally work alone, or in partnership, to provide a full body service on a personal rather than a large scale level. Space will normally restrict the active exercise that can be accomplished, so this is applied on an individual basis through client instruction during consultation. Sauna, steam bath and waxing therapy may all be offered, with the smaller or individual units being installed. The private practice will normally have all the component parts of a larger clinic, applied on a more individual basis.

Closer contact with the client is possible, and this can provide excellent treatment results as the applications can be altered or modified on a very individual basis. All aspects of electrical therapy can be offered, according to demand, and a very successful business practice built up.

The responsibilities and also the rewards of a private practice are greater than working as an employee. Financial backing or personal capital is required to set up a figure practice, being initially a fairly heavy investment. Planning permission is necessary before setting up, whether in a private house or business premises, to ascertain that the facilities are suitable for the planned venture. In residential areas this approval may not be easily acquired, due to parking restrictions, and objections from neighbours. Houses and office premises situated close to city centres may not prove such a problem, and may only require a change-of-use ruling.

In many areas a licence to practise is necessary, issued by the Department of Health or through the Environmental Health Offices. Details will be available from civic offices in the area of proposed trade. The licence to trade will be issued on the basis of the suitability of the therapist to perform safe and competent treatments, and will be limited to aspects of work in which actual qualification is held. Main areas that will be considered are saunas, and body treatments, facial work, and epilation, with ultra-violet and lamp work being considered as separate areas from main therapy. Premises and staff are inspected, very often before the licence is granted.

A licence to practise can be revoked for misconduct, poor hygiene or running immoral premises; complaints by individual clients being investigated by public health or consumer protection officers. All this maintenance of standards helps the qualified and competent therapist. Differences exist between counties and countries as to which treatments may be applied, and which restricted, and it is wise to investigate this point before planning a clinic layout.

A business may also need to be registered if it is not trading under the owner's name, and personal and business insurance must be obtained before commencing work. It is necessary to be vigilant about keeping accounts for tax purposes, with all expenses recorded, so that they can later be set against profits when yearly turnover is submitted.

Business taxation is complicated and requires

the help of an accountant to prepare the figure for submission to the tax authorities, so that tax liability can be assessed. The therapist has to be able to keep a record of all outgoings and income over the yearly period. Standard expenses, such as rent, light, heating, laundry, cleaning and telephone costs have to be listed, plus incidentals like flowers, magazines, repair costs, etc.

Working independently does require more business acumen, but the minor problems of keeping accounts, stock control, VAT and PAYE are more than offset for many therapists by the rewards of greater job satisfaction and higher financial rewards.

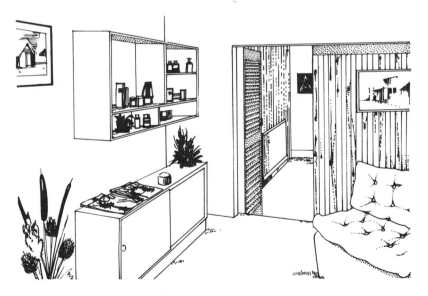

Private Therapy Clinic

TREATMENT, PLANNING AND PROMOTING

Figure treatments differ according to their location, but are similar in principle. The circumstances of the client, whether residential as in a hydro, or coming for periodic treatment, make a difference to the manner in which the treatment is applied. An exclusive health club, with entry open to members only, requires a different approach from a city centre figure shaping clinic, catering mainly for younger men and women.

The average age of the clientele will give guidance as to which treatments will prove profitable. Older clients enjoy relaxation treatments and appreciate the personal attention, so do not begrudge the cost involved. Younger clients like fast results, so effective equipment and good facilities to encourage self help is needed.

Weight reduction forms the basis of most figure improvement programmes, so this element should be strongly featured in the clinic treatments and promotion. Any apparatus that helps to keep the client interested in a diet programme indirectly helps that client to reduce.

Most therapy practices have a mixture of elements, and it is wise when setting up the business initially to allow a fair measure of flexibility until a clear pattern of client needs emerges. Skilful promotion can sell almost any beneficial treatment to a client, if a good measure of confidence in knowledge and techniques has been achieved, and a sense of trust established. Advertising promotions linked with the time of year, or any new apparatus the salon has acquired, are normally very successful, if all resulting enquiries are dealt with sympathetically by a knowledgeable receptionist who is capable of converting them into treatment bookings. Because the beauty therapy business appears fairly complicated to the average person, advertising, stressing the qualified status of the staff, is a sensible step.

Staff membership of professional organizations, including those which operate in conjunction with the major examination boards, denotes a high standard of skill and illustrates to the potential client the value placed on her receiving a safe and successful treatment.

FACTORS WHICH
INFLUENCE CHARGES
FOR THERAPY
TREATMENT

The location of the salon and the overall cost of its overheads, business loans, rent, rates, equipment and staff costs, must be considered when deciding the scale of charges that will operate. The highest cost is usually that of the skilled staff involved, and where personal attention is required throughout the duration of the treatment, this fact must be reflected in a high cost per hour. Treatments requiring more general supervision, or not demanding such a high level of skill, i.e. sauna applications, etc., can be costed on a lower basis, due to the reduced staff costs involved. Remedial figure therapy, where skill and experience are of paramount importance, in the choice of electrical and cosmetic applications, will be the most expensive aspect of the clinic's treatments, due both to staff costs and the additional equipment expenditure involved.

Many salons with the main bulk of the treatment carried out by the therapist, operate a charge per hour basis, formulated at a figure which returns a certain percentage of profit, related to the overall costs and capital investment involved. The level of this price per hour must be set according to the location of the salon, its competitors' prices and the type of clientele it attracts. This method demands good facilities, a wide equipment choice and skilled staff, experienced in treatment promotion, to achieve success. Bookings of treatment courses have benefits for the client and the business as the forward planning enables the appointments to be placed at convenient times in the week, and forms a solid base for other bookings. The arrangement also permits a discount to be given to the client, usually a bonus treatment, on advance course payment of the 8 or 12 treatment booking.

Specialized treatments such as wax baths, massage with infra-red heat, galvanic iontophoresis, will naturally be costed at a higher rate, due to the additional equipment costs, greater preparation time and additional skill involved in the application.

Specialist qualification, training and experience are required in order to promote these treatments, and these factors may be reflected in advertising in order to build this aspect of work. The clients for the specialist services will be drawn from a wider area, particularly if similar facilities are not available within a reasonable proximity, and this enlarges the reputation and status of the business.

STARTING A FIGURE TREATMENT SERVICE

When initially planning a figure treatment unit, attention must be given to the client's flow of movement through the clinic, to make the best use of the space available. Areas must be set aside for changing, resting and treatment, and a small figure unit providing all aspects can be installed in a relatively small area, if ventilation and lighting are adequate.

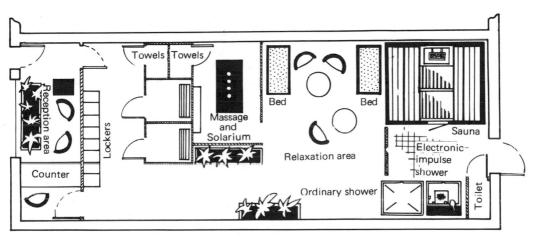

Commercial Sauna Unit

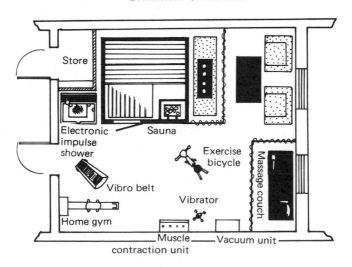

Small Sauna Unit (Private Practice)

If the sauna, steam and wet areas are placed separately but adjacent to the treatment cubicles, the therapist is able periodically to check the clients using these facilities whilst fulfilling her treatment schedules. Or if supervisory staff are caring for the sauna, shower and rest areas, a qualified member of staff is close at hand in case of client difficulties.

The treatment unit may be set up initially to provide heating treatments, massage and exercise instruction, plus basic heavy duty apparatus. The better equipped the figure clinic is, however, the greater will be the range of possible treatments and potential income from the service. It is important primarily to ensure that all basic forms of treatment are offered, rather than concentrating investment into one elaborate piece of equipment or fashionable system of treatment that may go out of favour. It may also get inadequate usage to justify its expenditure. The clinic should have the three main systems – muscle contraction equipment, vibratory and vacuum massage – before looking for more sophisticated apparatus.

A FIGURE TREATMENT UNIT

(Basic Equipment)

In addition to sauna/steam baths and showers, a basically equipped treatment unit should include:

1   A strong massage plinth, with a wipe clean surface, well stressed legs, and back rest that can lift up into a tilted position. The plinth should be of a suitable height, 10 cm (28 in.), to avoid stooping to perform the massage.

2   A mobile trolley, large enough to take a vacuum unit or muscle contraction machine, plus commodities, towels, etc.

3   A sterilizer for equipment heads, applicators, etc.

4   Sink or vanity unit providing storage for spare leads, pads, and general equipment used in body therapy, as well as washing facilities.

5   Vacuum suction unit, with a selection of suitable cups.

6   Clinic model muscle contraction unit (8–12 outlets), plus pads and leads, and body straps.

7   Floor standing or hand held heavy duty vibrator.

8   Talc, oil, salt, small bowls, towels and towelling gowns.

9   Blankets, pillows (large and small).

10   Disposal materials, wall mounted in dispensers for rough and smooth tissues.

11   Scales (floor or balanced type).

This body treatment unit could then provide a range of applications, including manual massage, combined manual and electrical massage for general body treatment, muscle toning treatments, specific reduction treatments, relaxation therapy, back massage and diet and exercise instruction. The combination of treatments that these basic and standard pieces of equipment can accomplish can be seen in Chapter 1. Purpose and Organization of Treatment. All the main elements of figure treatment are represented, manual skills, inches reduction and stimulatory treatments to aid weight reduction, as part of a diet controlled programme.

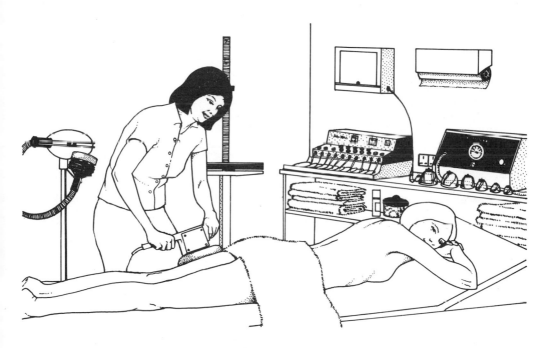

ADDITIONAL EQUIPMENT TO EXTEND THE TREATMENT RANGE

1   Lamp treatment: ultra-violet, radiant heat and infra-red rays, to provide for sun tanning effects, deep heat treatments, combined heat and massage routines for tension in the back. (Single or multiple lamps (solariums).)

2   Paraffin waxing equipment, baths or single wax heating units, to permit localized waxing applications or general body applications.

3   Pulsating vacuum unit, to treat conditions of obesity, or established adipose deposits, which may also be combined with faradism.

4   Interferential and galvanic equipment, either combined or in separate apparatus, to provide for iontophoresis (galvanic) and a wide range of advanced muscle toning effects on all areas of the face and body (interferential muscle contraction).

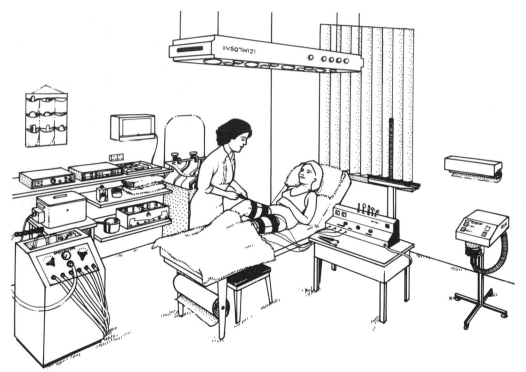

It can be seen that a figure treatment unit has to be well equipped from the start, with a large proportion of costs going to installation of sauna and steam baths, showers and purchase of heavy duty equipment. The exercise facilities can be added to with the provision of more wall bars, cycling machines, etc., if demand is sufficient. The important thing is to keep the treatment facilities in constant use by promoting treatments to clients using associated services. Often a figure service will be added to an existing beauty clinic or hairdressing salon, and special introductory schemes can be introduced to permit clients to discover the pleasures and benefits of body treatment.

QUALIFICATIONS AND METHODS OF TRAINING AVAILABLE

Beauty therapy qualifications may be obtained in a variety of ways, either within an educational situation (Further Education College or Technical College) or by commercial means through a training school. Nationally recognized qualifications offered by the National Health and Beauty Council, International Therapy Examination Centre, C.I.D.E.S.C.O., Confederation of Beauty Therapy and Cosmetology Ltd. and by the City and Guilds of London Institute denote both a competent level of practical skill and a sound background knowledge of anatomy, physical science, nutrition and cosmetic chemistry, related to the practical therapy. The qualifications are obtained by examination only, after a specified period of training, laid down by the examination board, according to the level of course undertaken.

City and Guilds Beauty Therapist's Certificate 761 (2-year full time Further Education Course)

This certificate covers all aspects of facial and body treatments, and is provided on a two year basis at selected colleges throughout the British Isles. Students must be at least 18 years old, and have a minimum academic qualification of three 'O' level G.C.E. subjects. Due to the competition for places, colleges can be very selective in their choice of applicant, and may demand a higher level of G.C.E. passes than the minimum requirement. Tuition is divided between theoretical and practical aspects of therapy, permitting confidence to develop in client handling and practical techniques. The longer period of training makes this an ideal course for the younger woman, and allows skills to become established under the guidance of an experienced lecturer.

International Health and Beauty Council International Health and Beauty Therapy Diploma

This course is more widely available, on a one or two year basis, at Further Education Colleges, private schools and training establishments. The course covers all aspects of salon work, facial and body treatments, figure improvement and cosmetic applications, plus background theory related to the practical subjects. Certain colleges combine the two courses, over a two year period, and in this way benefit from the wide range of subjects covered, whilst establishing practical skills through salon sessions and client handling. More frequently the course is run over a one year period, and attracts a proportion of more mature applicants, who may have previous experience in nursing, commerce or cosmetic work.

International Therapy Examination Council

Courses concentrating purely on body therapy are available through this organization, which also acts as an examining body. Available through private schools and some educational training establishments, the qualifications offered permit employment in health clinics, figure treatment salons and private practice.

C.I.D.E.S.C.O. Le Comité Internationale D'Asthetiques et de Cosmetology

Represented in the British Isles by the British Association of Beauty Therapy and Cosmetology, training is provided in private schools and some educational establishments. Different levels of qualification are available, according to the length of tuition.

Beauty Education International 'Beauty Club'

An international organization whose aim is to raise the standards of beauty therapy by means of training, education, equipment information and supply, and management consultancy. The aim is to motivate, communicate within the beauty industry through membership, news letters, instructional material (books, tapes, etc.), and supply information about basic and post-graduate training.

Beauty Education International acts as a reference point for all those involved in beauty therapy and, through their own club, keeps them informed of the latest developments in the industry around the world. Membership is open to all those who work within the Beauty Industry or related fields—all are welcome to join and learn.

BENEFITS OF PROFESSIONAL MEMBERSHIP

Professional membership of therapy organizations provides a means of keeping up to date with new techniques, equipment and information, through periodic meetings, news bulletins and social gatherings of members. It maintains a professional status for the members, and serves to promote a high standard of practical and theoretical knowledge. It builds a good relationship with the medical profession and other well-known organizations, which creates a good working atmosphere based on mutual trust and respect.

Insurance for professional work is available either linked with annual membership, or is offered at preferential rates related to the level of skill acknowledged by the insurance companies.

Most beauty therapy organizations have a membership list or a national register of qualified operators, listing their qualifications and range of treatments. These lists are available to the general public, either from private or press enquiries, or through public libraries, etc. This practice of joining the larger organizations is growing as younger operators see the advantages of gaining a professional status, which it is hoped will eventually lead to government recognition of the need for full registration to safeguard the public from untrained therapists.

CONVERSION CHARTS

Height Conversion

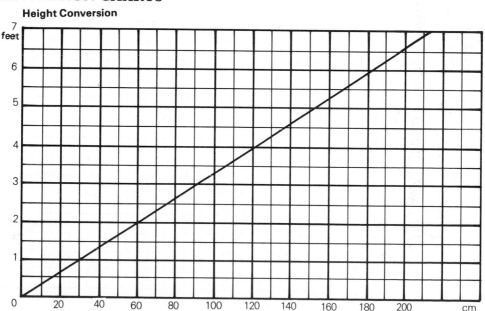

Measurements Conversion (inches/cm)

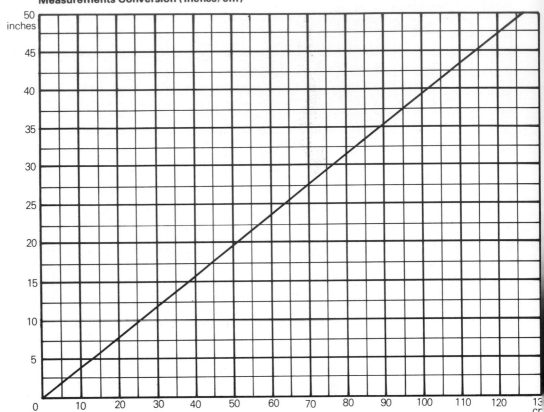

Volume Conversion

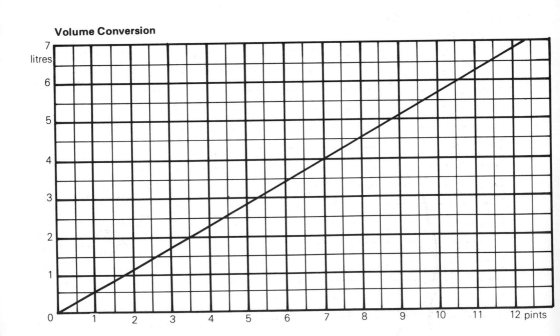

Weight Conversion

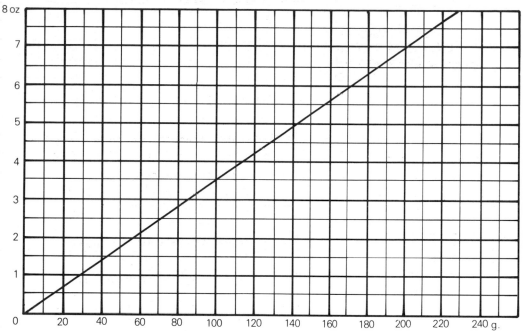

Temperature Conversion

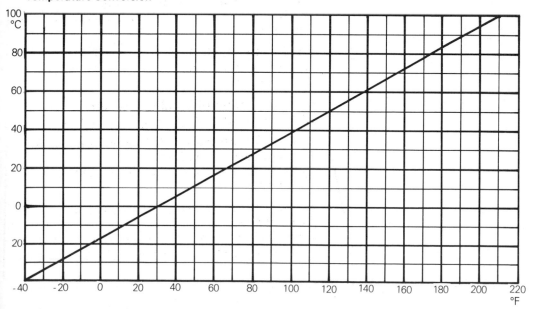

Useful Addresses

Further information on courses is available from the following examination boards and professional organizations:

Aestheticians' International Association Inc,
5206 McKinney, Dallas, Texas, USA

American Electrolysis Association,
Corresponding Secretary Sandi Strum, 211 Jonnet Building, 4099 William Penn Highway, Monroeville, PA 15146, USA

Association of Suntanning Operators
32 Grayshott Road, London SW11, UK

Beauty Education International—Beauty Club
E. A. Ellison & Co Ltd, Brindley Road South, Exhall, Coventry CV7 9EP, UK
Esthetic and Beauty Supply,
180 Bentley Street, Markham, Ontario, Canada, L3R 3L2 (Tel. 479 2929)
There is also a Californian office, USA

British Association of Beauty Therapy and Cosmetology,
Secretary Mrs D. Parkes, Suite 5, Wolesley House, Oriel Road, Cheltenham GL50 1TH, UK

British Association of Electrolysis,
16 Quakers Mede, Haddenham, Bucks HP17 8EB, UK

British Biosthetic Society,
2 Birkdale Drive, Bury, Greater Manchester BL8 2SG, UK

City and Guilds of London Institute,
46 Britannia Street, London WC1 9RG, UK

Le Comité Internationale D'Esthétiques et de Cosmetologie, (CIDESCO),
CIDESCO International Secretariat, PO Box 9, A1095 Vienna, Austria

Confederation of Beauty Therapy and Cosmetology,
Education Secretary Mrs B. Longhurst, 3 The Retreat, Lidwells Lane, Goudhurst, Kent, UK

Institute of Electrolysis,
251 Seymour Grove, Manchester M16 0DS, UK

National Federation of Health and Beauty Therapists,
PO Box 36, Arundel, West Sussex BN18 0SW, UK

International Therapy Examination Council
3 The Planes, Bridge Road, Chertsey, Surrey KT16 8LE, UK

The Northern Institute of Massage,
100 Waterloo Road, Blackpool FY4 1AW, UK

Skin Care Association of America,
16 West 57th Street, New York, NY, USA

South African Institute of Health and Beauty Therapists,
PO Box 56318, Pinegowrie 2123, South Africa

EQUIPMENT DESIGN AND DEVELOPMENT

Beauty Education International
Design and development of equipment/clinic planning/market research in the industry through:
Ellison, Brindley Road South, Exhall, Coventry CV7 9EP, UK
Esthetic and Beauty Supply, 180 Bentley Street, Markham, Ontario, Canada, L3R 3L2
There is also a Californian office, USA

EQUIPMENT MANUFACTURERS

Ann Gallant Beauty Therapy Equipment
From Esthetic and Beauty Supply, 180 Bentley Street, Markham, Ontario, Canada, L3R 3L2
(Tel. 479 2929)
There is also a Californian office, USA

Beauty Gallery Equipment by Ann Gallant,
E. A. Ellison & Co Ltd, Brindley Road South, Exhall, Coventry CV7 9EP, UK

Cristal (Equipment),
86 Rue Pixérécourt, 75020 Paris, France

Depilex Ltd and Slimaster Beauty Equipment Ltd,
Regent House, Dock Road, Birkenhead, Merseyside L41 1DG, UK

Electro-Medical Services,
Bermuda Road, Nuneaton, Warks, UK

George Solly Organization Ltd,
50a Queen Street, Henley-on-Thames, Oxon
RG9 2DF, UK

Soltron Solarium and Sun Beds
Josef Kratz, Vertriebsgesellschaft mbH,
Rottbizer Straße 69-5340, Bad Honnef 6,
W. Germany (Tel. 02224/818-0)
(Telex jk 8861194)

Nemectron Belmont Inc,
17 West 56th Street, New York, NY10019, USA

Silhouette International Beauty Equipment,
Kenwood Road, Reddish, Stockport, Cheshire
SK5 6PH, UK

Slendertone Ltd,
12–14 Baker Street, London W1M 2HA, UK

Taylor Reeson Ltd,
96–98 Dominion Road, Worthing, Sussex, UK

TREATMENT PRODUCT SUPPLIERS

Ann Gallant Beauty Therapy Products
From Esthetic and Beauty Supply, 180 Bentley
Street, Markham, Ontario, Canada, L3R 3L2
(Tel. 479 2929)

Elizabeth of Schwarzenberg,
13 Windsor Street, Chertsey, Surrey
KT16 8AY, UK

Clarins (UK) Ltd,
(Oils and body products)
150 High Street, Stratford, London E15 2NE, UK

**Gallery Line by Ann Gallant—Skin Care and
Body Products,**
From E. A. Ellison & Co Ltd, Brindley Road
South, Exhall, Coventry CV7 9EP, UK
(Tel. 0203 362505)

**Germaine de Capuccini, Professional
Cosmetics**
Mallorca, 81-08029 Barcelona, Spain

Pier Augé Cosmetics,
Harbourne Marketing Associates, Oak House,
271 Kingston Road, Leatherhead, Surrey, UK

Thalgo Cosmetic/Importex,
(Marine based products)
5 Tristan Square, Blackheath, London SE3 9UB,
UK

MAGAZINES AND TRADE PUBLICATIONS

Beauty Therapy Club by Ann Gallant
(International club for all those involved in the
beauty industry–publications/fact
sheets/guides/books, etc.)

Details from:
Ellison, Brindley Road South, Exhall, Coventry
CV7 9EP, UK

Esthetic and Beauty Supply,
180 Bentley Street, Markham, Ontario,
Canada, L3R 3L2 (Tel. 479 2929)
There is also a Californian office, USA

Health and Beauty Salon Magazine

Hair and Beauty Magazine

Hairdressers' Journal

Trade publications for the hair and beauty
industries, details from International Beauty
Press, Quadrant House, The Quadrant, Sutton,
Surrey, UK
(Health and Beauty Salon Magazine Editor—Ms
Marion Mathews, Tel. 01 661 3500)

A Note on Beauty Education International—Beauty Therapy Club

Beauty Club offers a unique service to the beauty industry; through COMMUNICATION, MOTIVATION and EDUCATION the Club can provide all the necessary information for success in this exciting and profitable field; through its own Newsletter it keeps its members informed of all the latest developments in the industry around the world.

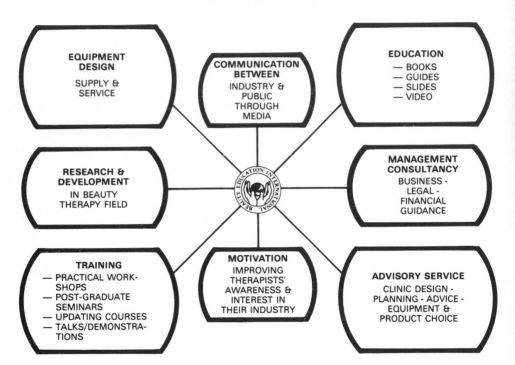

EQUIPMENT DESIGN

SUPPLY & SERVICE

COMMUNICATION BETWEEN INDUSTRY & PUBLIC THROUGH MEDIA

EDUCATION
— BOOKS
— GUIDES
— SLIDES
— VIDEO

RESEARCH & DEVELOPMENT

IN BEAUTY THERAPY FIELD

MANAGEMENT CONSULTANCY
BUSINESS -
LEGAL -
FINANCIAL
GUIDANCE

TRAINING
— PRACTICAL WORK-SHOPS
— POST-GRADUATE SEMINARS
— UPDATING COURSES
— TALKS/DEMONSTRA-TIONS

MOTIVATION
IMPROVING THERAPISTS' AWARENESS & INTEREST IN THEIR INDUSTRY

ADVISORY SERVICE
CLINIC DESIGN -
PLANNING - ADVICE -
EQUIPMENT &
PRODUCT CHOICE

What Membership of Beauty Club can Offer

- A feeling of belonging to a truly international club.
- Regular Beauty Club Newsletters to support this linked-in club feeling.
- The right to wear the Beauty Club Badge which shows your interest in the beauty world.
- Beauty Club Member's Card for preferential buying terms and discounts on a selected range of salon equipment and products.
- Information and expertise from leading experts in the field.
- News of latest advances in the industry.
- Technical fact sheets for easy reference on products, equipment and treatment systems, etc.
- Guidance and practical support on retailing products for home use.
- A link into Beauty Education International for: Books, Beauty Guides, Technical Information, Research and Development Programmes, Clinic Planning Guidance, Stock Management.
- Training—practical workshops, post graduate seminars, up-dating courses, talks/demonstrations.
- Motivation—improving therapists' awareness and interest in their industry.

Anyone who is interested in the beauty industry, and wants to keep up to date and in touch with the latest knowledge and tehniques available to help them in their work is eligible to join.

ANN GALLANT

Int. B. Th. Dip. D.R.E.

Index